Lisa Needham
Pharmacy Practice

Handbook of Pharmacy Health Education

Handbook of Pharmacy Health Education

SECOND EDITION

Edited by

Robin J Harman

PhD, MRPharmS
Independent Pharmaceutical
and Regulatory Consultant
Farnham, Surrey

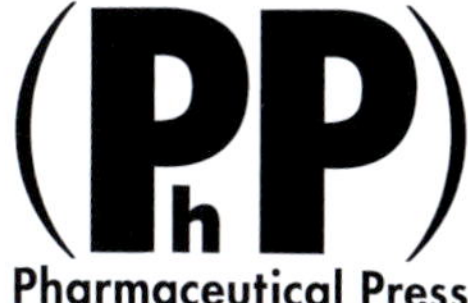

Published by the Pharmaceutical Press
1 Lambeth High Street, London SE1 7JN, UK

First edition published 1991
Second edition published 2001
Reprinted 2002

Text design by Barker/Hilsdon, Lyme Regis, Dorset
Typeset by Type Study, Scarborough, North Yorkshire
Printed in great Britain by Cambridge University Press, Cambridge

ISBN 0 85369 471 0

A catalogue record for this book is available from the british Library

Contents

Preface

THE INSTINCTIVE HOPE of all parents of newborn babies is that their offspring will be perfectly healthy in every respect. Great concern and distress arise if there are immediately apparent visible defects in the neonate: these could include limb or other developmental physical defects or the well-recognised facial appearance of trisomy-21 (Down's syndrome). Other problems present at birth will only become apparent with time: problems with hearing and genetic malfunctions (e.g. lactose intolerance) appear in the initial months of life.

The human body is an entity of such immense complexity that it defies belief, and has so far defied complete understanding. It is a considerable miracle that minor or major defects are nearly always completely absent at birth. One has only to consider the intricacy of the physical appearance of the brain to be astounded that such a high proportion of births are untainted. Similarly, the absence of a single chemical enzyme can cause devastating diseases: phenylketonuria is due to the absence of phenylalanine hydroxylase; coeliac disease is caused by an intolerance to gluten in the diet. In spite of this, almost all babies are born with every component of structural, chemical, electrical and psychological functioning intact!

This desire for the presence and continuance of good health is commonly maintained throughout life: it begins with parents' concern for their offspring, and is then transferred, with developing personal awareness, to the individual. With further development and increased age, individuals develop a concern, not only for themselves, but for others. The aspiration for good health for themselves progresses to concern for their parents, their siblings, their friends and their partners. It comes full cycle with their instinctive hope of good health for their own children and then grandchildren.

There is an, as yet unresolved, debate as to the degree of influence upon health of genetic and environmental factors. Some choose to put the determination of health solely on genetic factors. This produces a somewhat negative view that it doesn't matter what the individual does, it is decided by their genetic make-up. Others believe that environmental influences are paramount: that the guidance provided by parents and the physical circumstances in which individuals are brought up determine the health of the individual. A greater proportion incline to a composite view: some aspects are determined genetically, others are influenced by environment. Such a view is essential if one is to believe in the virtues of health education as a positive influence on the health of the individual.

The promotion of health is an activity carried out consciously or unconsciously by almost everyone during the course of their lives. It is not the exclusive preserve of any one group of individuals, be they healthcare workers or otherwise. However, different groups of healthcare personnel have varying opportunities to convey messages about the promotion of health. The two groups that the majority of people have the greatest contact with regarding health matters are general practitioners and pharmacists. (Certain groups of people will have greater contact with others (e.g. social workers and nursing staff), but these are a minority.) Most general practitioners will take every opportunity they can during a consultation to reinforce healthy practices in their patients. However, time is limited, and it is not unusual for many people subsequently to be unable to recall accurately details of the conversation with their general practitioner.

There is, consequently, an immense opportunity for pharmacists to be one of the prime educators in healthy behaviour. Visits to pharmacy premises are undertaken for a number of reasons:

- to have a prescription dispensed
- to purchase non-prescription medicines
- to seek advice for the treatment of a condition which is felt does not require the advice of a general practitioner, or
- to purchase items that are sold through most pharmacy outlets.

Each of these reasons can provide opportunities for pharmacists to consider other issues that can benefit an individual's health. However, one should be circumspect about choosing to try to advise people. It can be of tremendous help to some members of the public to feel that there is someone to whom they can talk about health issues over which they may be confused. Equally, it can be a highly negative encounter if pharmacists try to force a conversation with someone who is not receptive to hearing such advice. Some people may be in a hurry to get to an appointment, they may be concerned about a close relative and not want to delay leaving the pharmacy, or they may feel that they know enough already about a particular health topic and do not welcome additional advice.

As in all matters of counselling, experience in dealing with people will guide pharmacists to the most appropriate opportunities for giving information about health matters.

This book provides an overview of the most important issues on which pharmacists can provide advice on health matters. Such advice can only be given confidently in the presence of a clear understanding of the issues: of what happens if a particular course of action is undertaken or not carried out. Detailed information is, therefore, given on all aspects of the topic.

Chapter 1 – Health, disease and health education explains how disease can arise and the factors which affect health, including 'fixed' factors, social and economic factors and lifestyle. The effects of the access of individuals to specific health and social services are also discussed. Measurements of health are described, and the occurrence of 'modern' epidemics considered. General issues in the promotion of health and the role of pharmacists are explained in detail.

The occurrence of diet-related diseases is described in **Chapter 2 – Dietary management**. This chapter explains the body's energy requirements and how dietary reference values and food tables can be used to assess an individual's dietary requirements. In order to understand how diet can influence health, it is essential to appreciate the different ways in which dietary constituents are utilised in the body. The role and source of all components of the diet are detailed, from carbohydrates, fats and cholesterol to the trace elements (e.g. chromium, fluorine and selenium).

The dietary needs of specific groups (e.g. pregnant and breast-feeding women, vegetarians and the sick and convalescent) is an important issue on which pharmacists are often asked for advice. A further issue that has achieved national prominence in recent years is food safety. This covers such diverse topics as microbial contamination and food additives and contaminants.

Closely allied to the issues of diet and health is **Chapter 3 – Dental healthcare**. With an initial section on dental anatomy and physiology, it goes on to give a detailed explanation of the most common dental diseases. This covers plaque, calculus, dental caries, periodontal disease, gingival recession and halitosis. Of especial interest are the ways in which dental disease can be prevented. Issues ranging from plaque control, minimising the occurrence of dental caries, the involvement of dentists and the prevention of dental disease in children are described. Advice that can be given in the care of dentures is also explained.

One topic on which pharmacists are often called to give advice is that described in **Chapter 4 – Contraception**. Following a detailed explanation of the concepts of fertility and contraception, different types of contraception are described. The section on hormonal contraception explains the use of, and problems with, combined oral contraceptives, progestogen-only oral contraceptives, progestogen-only injectable contraceptives, progestogen-only intra-uterine contraceptives and other progestogen-only devices.

Other types of contraception are discussed: intra-uterine devices; barrier methods and spermicides; and so-called 'alternative' methods of contraception (e.g. coitus interruptus and natural family planning). Fertility devices and sterilisation are also considered. The demand for emergency contraception has also increased over recent years, and the use of hormonal methods and intra-uterine devices in such instances is described. It is also important for pharmacists to be aware of the availability of contraceptive services.

One of the most common situations in which pharmacists can make an invaluable contribution is in the national annual 'No smoking day'. The benefits derived from stopping smoking (or not starting) are illustrated in **Chapter 5 – Smoking**. Following a discussion of the prevalence of smoking, trends and behaviour, the different forms in which tobacco is smoked are described and the harmful nature of tobacco smoke is explained. Smoking-related diseases have multitudinous effects on the body (e.g. on the cardiovascular system, the respiratory system and the gastro-intestinal system) in the development of malignant disease and oral disease, and in inducing obstetric disorders and effects on the foetus. The dangers of passive smoking are described as are ways in which smoking can be prevented (including aversion and group therapy and nicotine replacement therapy).

Chapter 6 – Excessive alcohol consumption reports on the causes of excessive alcohol consumption, how alcohol consumption is measured and the limits and habits of alcohol consumption. In describing how alcohol is metabolised, the acute effects of alcohol consumption are clearly illustrated. Excessive alcohol consumption does not affect just the individual concerned: there are alcohol-related social problems and alcohol-related diseases (e.g. anaemias, endocrine disorders, hypertension and nervous system disorders). Alcohol also has especial effects on children, the elderly and pregnant and breast-feeding women. The symptoms of alcohol-dependence syndrome and ways in which sensible alcohol consumption can be promoted are described.

Drug abuse (Chapter 7) is a major social problem in which pharmacists can play an important role in helping to combat. The types of drug dependence (physical and psychological), the social factors which influence dependency, and the ways in which it is managed are explained. Dependence can arise from various routes of administration: inhalation, injection and oral. There is a detailed description of the identification and 'street names', methods of administration, actions, side-effects, and dependence and management for all of the commonly used drugs of abuse. These include alkyl nitrites, amphetamines, 'Ecstasy' and related stimulants, benzodiazepines, cannabis, 'designer' drugs, opioids and volatile substance abuse. Needle exchange schemes, dispensing for drug users, and the problem of forged prescriptions are also described.

Chapter 8 – Sport and exercise highlights the benefits of sport and exercise for health and explains why people participate in sport. The physiology of exercise and the effects on physiological systems (e.g. the cardiovascular system, muscles and the respiratory system) are also described. Sport and exercise also exert beneficial effects on the management of disease (e.g. arthritis, coronary disease, obesity and osteoporosis), although pharmacists should also be aware of the risks of sport and exercise. Specific problems include anaemia, asthma and breathing difficulties, gastro-intestinal symptoms, and hormonal problems in women. There are also risks in various medical conditions (e.g. infections, pregnancy and respiratory disease). Pharmacists need to know the effects of medication on sport and exercise, and the risks from AIDS.

Involvement in sports medicine is a potentially very important role for pharmacists, and the general principles of treating sports injuries (e.g. blisters, bursitis, haematomas, strains, and tendinitis and tenosynovitis) are illustrated. The treatment of exercise and sports-related conditions are also described (e.g. anxiety and stress, fungal infections, headache and verrucae). There are a plethora of sports nutrition and sports drinks products on the market, and understanding the ways of selecting appropriate products is important. The use and abuse of drugs in sport to enhance performance, and the use of illicit and therapeutic drugs are also areas in which pharmacists can give advice. Finally, participation in sports and exercise – covering the effects of training, fitness tests and the involvement of special groups (e.g. the elderly and disabled) – is explained.

The general population has become increasingly mobile over the past 30 years, travelling to parts of the world previously deemed completely inaccessible. **Chapter 9 – Health and travel** highlights the action to be taken before travelling. This includes immunisation and precautions for special groups of travellers (e.g. those with diabetes mellitus and HIV infection). Measures to prevent and manage conditions associated with travel (e.g. motion sickness and jet lag) and illnesses that might arise at the destination (e.g. infectious diseases, bites and stings, and sunburn) are described.

Chapter 10 – Contact lens care describes the types of lenses available and their cleaning, rinsing and disinfection, wetting, rewetting and comfort solutions, and protein removal. Complications related to contact lens wear are also explained.

A completely new chapter for this edition of the book is **Chapter 11 – Companion animals and human health**. It explains what a pet is, why it is kept and the benefits and disadvantages of keeping pets. Of particular importance for pharmacists is the ability to discern conditions associated with pets: ectoparasites (e.g. fleas, lice and ticks) and non-infective conditions (e.g. allergies, cancer, toxins and venoms). Infective conditions (zoonoses), endoparasitic infection, fungal infections, protozoal infections, rickettsial infections, spirochaete infection and viral infections are also described.

About the editor

Robin J Harman PhD, MRPharmS has been an Independent Pharmaceutical and Regulatory Consultant, based in Farnham, Surrey, England, since 1998. He launched and was Editor-in-Chief, from 1990–98, of *The Regulatory Affairs Journal* and *The Regulatory Affairs Journal (Devices)*, which provide information to the pharmaceutical and medical devices' industries respectively. Previously, he was an Editor in the Department of Pharmaceutical Sciences at the Royal Pharmaceutical Society of Great Britain. He edited the *Handbook of Pharmacy Health-care: Diseases and Patient Advice* (Pharmaceutical Press, 1990), and authored *Patient Care in Community Practice: A Handbook of Non-medicinal Health-care* (Pharmaceutical Press, 1989).

Contributors

Claire Anderson PhD, MRPharmS
Director of Pharmacy Practice and Social Pharmacy, The Pharmacy School, University of Nottingham, Nottingham

Alison Blenkinsopp PhD, MRPharmS
Professor, Department of Medicines Management, Keele University, Staffordshire

Derrick Garwood BDS
Dental Practitioner and Editorial Consultant, Royston, Hertfordshire

Larry Goodyer PhD, MRPharmS
Director of Pharmacy Practice Research, Department of Pharmacy, King's College, London

Robin J Harman PhD, MRPharmS
Independent Pharmaceutical and Regulatory Consultant, Farnham, Surrey

Steven Kayne PhD, FRPharmS, DAgVetPharm
Independent Pharmaceutical Consultant, Glasgow

Pamela Mason PhD, MRPharmS
Independent Pharmaceutical Consultant, London

Susan Shankie MSc, MRPharmS
Independent Pharmaceutical Consultant, Glasgow

Simon Wills PhD, MSc, MRPharmS
Head of Wessex Drug and Medicines Information Centre, Southampton University Hospitals NHS Trust, Southampton

1

Health, disease and health education

Claire Anderson and Alison Blenkinsopp

Health and ill-health

The profession of pharmacy has always been intimately involved with illness and its treatment, the management of medicines, and the promotion of health. A fundamental role of pharmacists is as advisers on all aspects of drug treatment to health professionals and to the public. However, in recent years, there has been a greater awareness that illness continues to place ever-increasing demands on national resources, and upon the healthcare systems of many developed nations. In the UK, this has led to a gradual change in government policy, leading to the recognition of the value of activities and programmes to prevent ill-health and thus to encourage health promotion. Emerging new structures in the National Health Service (NHS), including Health Improvement Programmes (local plans) and Health Action Zones (areas where new initiatives are being tested) allow for a more strategic approach to service provision and tackling inequalities in health. Pharmacists are already taking up opportunities to provide input and advice to these new developments.

What is health?

In order to understand the potential value of pharmacists' input to health promotion, it is important to consider the concept of health and peoples' perceptions of illness. Health is an imprecise and elusive concept. Each society and each generation develops its concepts of health based on common experience. In modern usage, health has come to mean the absence of illness or disease, or a state of well-being. Health is also used to describe physical fitness (e.g. the terms 'health club' and 'healthy living'). The word 'health' is related to concepts of wholeness, haleness and healing, implying that health concerns the whole person. Individuals tend to hold several, often conflicting, views of what health is at the same time. These views arise from many different influences; the medical model appears to be dominant in the west, but social concepts play a part. Lay concepts of health, derived from cultural factors, lie alongside medical concepts for most people, including healthcare professionals.

Researchers have proposed that health consists of physical, mental, emotional, social, spiritual, sexual, societal and environmental dimensions; the last two are largely outside the control of the individual. The medical view of health has been said to be the dominant one for healthcare professionals in the UK. Healthcare professionals, including pharmacists, acquire a particular view of health through their training and subsequent practice. However, some researchers have stressed the importance of professionals' lay health beliefs and how they also draw on these beliefs when advising people about their health.

The World Health Organization (WHO) has played an important role in debating definitions of health. It has defined health as a social as well as an individual factor:

> The extent to which an individual or group is able, on the one hand, to realise aspirations and satisfy needs, and, on the other hand, to change or cope with the environment. Health is therefore, seen as a resource for everyday life, not an

object of living; it is a positive concept, emphasis is on social and personal resources, as well as physical capacities.

WHO, 1984

Factors affecting health

A number of related factors contribute to an individual's health status. These may be fixed, or related to social and economic conditions, lifestyle, environment, or access to services (Table 1.1).

Fixed factors

Age, sex and genetic makeup have a major influence on health. However, there is little that can be done about them. Within a few years, developments in genetic science may make it possible to do much more than at present.

Social and economic factors

Poverty

People's health is affected by their circumstances. A sense of well-being, the feeling of having control over life, and optimism about the future all have positive effects on health. Low income can make it hard for people to afford even basic necessities (e.g. being able to keep the house warm, or to protect themselves and their family from accidents in the home by buying smoke alarms or replacing faulty wiring). Low income, deprivation, and social exclusion also affect health in other ways (e.g. through their association with smoking). One study found that, overall, one-third of children in the UK lived with at least one adult smoker; for low-income families, the figure rose to 57%. Other aspects sometimes taken for granted by the better off (e.g. car ownership) also make a dramatic difference for those relying on public transport. If the nearest supermarket is miles away and the bus does not go there, it is difficult for people to buy food which is both healthy and cheap. The food available from local shops is often relatively expensive, of poorer quality and with fewer choices. On some housing estates where local shops have closed, there may be no food shops other than 'fast food take-away' outlets. These areas have been described as 'food deserts', because it may be necessary to travel long distances to obtain fresh, healthy food.

Employment

Joblessness has been clearly linked to poor physical and mental health: those in work tend to live longer than the unemployed. Unemployed men and women are more likely than people in work to die from cancer, heart disease, accidents and suicide. Losing his job doubles the chances of a middle-aged man dying within the next five years.

Social exclusion

When social problems (e.g. poor housing, unemployment or low pay, fear of crime and isolation) are combined, as they often are, people's health can suffer disproportionately. Social exclusion involves not only social, but also economic and

Table 1.1 Factors affecting health

Fixed	Social and economic	Lifestyle	Environment	Access to services
Genes Sex Ageing	Poverty Employment Social exclusion	Diet Physical activity Smoking Alcohol Sexual behaviour Drugs	Housing Air quality Water quality Social environment	Education NHS Social services Transport Leisure

psychological, isolation. Although people may know what affects their health, it is often difficult for them to act on what they know. The best way to make a start on helping them live healthier lives is to provide help and support to enable them to participate in society, and to help them improve their economic and social circumstances. One study found that, compared with people with many social ties, the socially isolated were over six times more likely to die from a stroke and more than three times more likely to commit suicide. Neighbourhoods where people know and trust each other, and where they have a say in the way the community is run, can be a powerful source of support in coping with the day-to-day stresses of life which affect health.

Environment

The way in which the environment affects health often involves a complex mix of factors. Clean air and water and good quality housing are important for good health and well-being. People need to know that, if they do not smoke or they are giving up smoking, the government, local authorities and businesses are also taking action to ensure that general pollution is not harming their health and that the quality of the air they breathe is good. A recent study has suggested, for example, that high levels of ozone in the air in the summer months leads to increased hospital admissions for respiratory disorders.

Lifestyle

Whether people smoke, whether they are active, what and how much they eat and drink, their sexual behaviour and whether they take illicit drugs can have a dramatic and cumulative influence on how healthy people are and how long they will live.

Access to services

Education

A good education gives children the confidence and capacity to make healthier choices and the ability to better themselves and their future families. Poor educational achievement, and pregnancy in early teenage years, are closely linked. Research suggests that education, and particularly nursery education, can have an important impact on health in later life.

Health services

Health services which genuinely meet people's needs mean that people know how to seek help quickly and to obtain timely advice and treatment. Equal access to, and uptake of, health services is far from a reality. The 'inverse care rule' has been used to describe how those most in need of services and support may not have access to them. For example, some areas where there is the greatest need for heart bypasses actually have the lowest numbers of such operations carried out.

The inverse care rule also applies to the uptake of services designed to prevent ill-health. There is a lower uptake of health checks, and breast and cervical cancer screening, among some disadvantaged groups. Areas of relatively high deprivation tend to have a relatively low uptake of immunisation. Low expectations of health and health services, and a low propensity to complain, may perpetuate poor service standards. There are concerns about the quality of the primary care services available in some deprived areas.

Social services

Social services play a key role in people's health. They provide support for older people, whether at home or in residential care, the protection and care of vulnerable children and young people, support for people with mental health problems, and helping people with disabilities to live more independent lives. The importance of the close relationship between health and social care needs is now better recognised, and there will be greater liaison and co-ordination in the future.

Transport and leisure

Good transport planning allows people to access health and leisure facilities. Affordable, local leisure services make it easier for people to be physically active.

Inequalities in health

For many of the factors with the potential to affect health, the extent to which people's health is actually affected depends on their relative poverty or affluence, their gender, where they were born and brought up and their ethnic background.

Ill-health is not spread evenly: there are large differences in coronary heart disease deaths in people who live in the UK, but who were born elsewhere (e.g. people of Afro-Caribbean and South Asian ethnic origin). Children in the lowest social class are five times more likely to die from an accident than are those in the highest. Deaths from suicide amongst women have fallen through the 1980s and early 1990s; conversely, suicide deaths amongst young men rose substantially during the same period. There is a clear link between poverty and ill-health: the highest incidence of ill-health is nearly always experienced by the worst-off social classes. Income affects the quantity and quality of resources that can be purchased, the type of housing, stress levels, access to services and social mobility. Poor housing can cause ill-health due to overcrowding, damp, disrepair, poor bathroom and cooking facilities, increased stress and accidents. Homelessness is an increasing problem in the UK and has brought many health problems, including a marked rise in the number of cases of tuberculosis after many years of steady reduction. Many diseases occur more commonly in particular parts of the country. For example, more people die of lung cancer in the north of England than in the south. This, too, is related to social status, although geographical differences play a part.

The meaning of health and ill-health

A further important point to consider in determining health is the wide divergence in the interpretation of health and ill-health by healthcare professionals on the one hand, and by members of the public on the other. When individuals seek advice from healthcare professionals, the application of a disease label by the professional is the result of considering the symptoms reported by the patient and signs noted by the doctor, pharmacist or nurse. All too often, the term used to describe the diagnosed disease is incomprehensible to the patient who suffers from it. Nevertheless, the patient's condition can be conveniently and neatly categorised; and this labelling commonly suggests appropriate measures to be taken by the healthcare professional.

Conversely, the symptoms experienced by the patient can be termed an illness. The willingness on the part of the sufferer to take action to relieve the illness is determined partly by their ability to cope; and the severity of the illness is subjectively related by the sufferer to past experiences. People may report symptoms and have an illness (e.g. general malaise) but not suffer from a disease; equally, they may be diagnosed as having a disease (e.g. hypertension) but not perceive any symptoms that they would consider indicates the presence of an illness. Social class and gender difference in people's concept of health have also been identified. Men tend to see good health as 'being fit'; women are likely to see it as the absence of illness and being able to carry out everyday tasks.

Another facet of ill-health, sometimes used to indicate levels of morbidity (*see below*) in a population, is sickness; this describes an action by a patient that may be taken to indicate ill-health. Individuals may seek medical advice, take time off work or curtail their social activities of their own accord. Sickness may occur in the absence of disease or illness; conversely, the presence of disease or illness does not necessarily imply that any action suggestive of sickness will be taken.

Measuring health and disease

Valid measurements of health and disease, and application of the data in determining priorities and establishing effective health promotion programmes, have often been based upon assessment of large populations, rather than individuals. The study of disease in relation to populations is termed epidemiology, and the mortality data (*see below*) that have contributed to the development of this science have been collected in the UK since 1838.

It is not usually possible to monitor an entire population in specific studies of health and disease. Usually, the population under study is a defined group and includes both those that are healthy and those that are unwell. The possible causes of a disease may be determined by comparison of disease rates in different population groups; further comparisons may identify those members of the population at a higher risk of developing a disease than the general population.

More importantly for health promotion, epidemiology permits trends in health and disease to be monitored. Determination of trends identifies those diseases that are declining in importance, and highlights those that may require special attention in the future. One problem, however, in identifying trends, and in particular associated with disease monitoring over several decades, is that the criteria for reporting a particular disease may change with time. This can lead to false optimism (e.g. about the success of a particular form of treatment), when in fact the disease is currently being recorded under a new or different name.

Similarly, as awareness of certain disease states increases (e.g. AIDS), so too does the incidence of diagnosis. The most commonly quoted statistics to identify trends are morbidity and mortality data. These and other terms commonly used in epidemiology are defined in Table 1.2. Mortality statistics are produced by extracting and coding the causes recorded on the death certificate.

In the UK, measurements of morbidity are collected as part of the General Household Survey, conducted and published annually. This survey determines ill-health by seeking information on people's own opinion of their health, details of consultations with general practitioners, attendance at hospital out-patient clinics and in-patient data. In assessing chronic ill-health, people are asked to indicate whether they have a long-standing illness, infirmity or disability.

All epidemiological methods of measuring disease have disadvantages. Measurements of the prevalence of a disease are only valid if the condition is chronic, persistent and stable. However, some chronic sufferers will be omitted from the count if the condition is chronic but intermittent, because the prevalence indicates people that actually have the disease at any one point in time. Similarly, prevalence of acute conditions will be underestimated.

The incidence of a disease is often assumed to reflect the actual number of cases. However, in epidemiology, it is the number of new cases expressed as a proportion of the defined population at a stated point in time. As the incidence measure only counts the number of new cases, it

Table 1.2 Definition of terms used in epidemiology

Term	Definition
Birth rate	Number of live births expressed as a proportion of the population
Fertility rate	Number of live births expressed as a proportion of the number of women aged between 15 and 44 years of age
Incidence rate	Proportion of a defined group developing a condition within a stated period of time
Infant mortality rate	Number of infant deaths (under one year of age) expressed as a proportion of the number of live births
Mortality	Frequency of death
Morbidity	Frequency of illness and disability
Perinatal mortality rate	Number of stillbirths and deaths in the first week of life expressed as a proportion of the total births
Prevalence rate	Proportion of a defined group having a condition at one point in time
Standardised mortality rate	Number of deaths actually occurring in a given year expressed as a proportion of the number of deaths that would have been expected in that year had the conditions of a period of reference years prevailed
Stillbirth rate	Number of intra-uterine deaths after 28 weeks expressed as a proportion of the total births

does not take into account those cases that already exist, and therefore underestimates the number of chronic sufferers.

Historical perspectives and trends in disease

There has been ready availability of comprehensive health services in the UK for more than a generation. As a result, many people have come to accept without question that the apparent improvements in general health, and the increased numbers of people living to old age, are a direct consequence of developments in healthcare. The public observes a wide range of hospital services that can be readily and freely used in the event of acute emergencies as well as a primary care doctor service that can be accessed at any time of the day or night free of charge. In addition, there is a bewildering array of medicines promoting the image of 'a pill for every ill'; and a high profile in the media for 'high technology' medicine that promotes an image of successful management of many formerly untreatable conditions.

However, careful analysis of mortality and morbidity statistics collected throughout this and the last century has shown that the greater proportion of the improvements in life expectancy, and the decreased mortality, can be attributed to:

- improved standards of living, particularly nutrition
- developments in standards of hygiene
- control of the physical environment
- measures to limit population growth
- introduction of preventive and therapeutic measures.

The early improvements in health in the second half of the nineteenth century were primarily a consequence of:

- public health measures to cover open sewers
- provision of better quality drinking water
- long-term changes in agricultural production and distribution of food supplies.

These social developments led to a significant decline in the mortality from infectious diseases. The single largest cause of death in the mid-nineteenth century was tuberculosis. Although the tubercle bacillus was identified by Koch in 1882, the first effective drug treatment with streptomycin did not become available until 1947, and widespread BCG vaccination did not commence until 1954. Although the introduction of additional antituberculous drugs has further reduced the mortality, 57% of the initial reduction occurred before 1900. The resurgence of TB among homeless people and those living in overcrowded conditions in poverty and malnourishment brings echoes of the last century.

A pattern of decreased mortality before the introduction of effective therapeutic measures was also observed for other airborne infectious diseases (e.g. pertussis, measles and scarlet fever) and in infections carried by food and water (e.g. cholera and dysentery).

The reduced incidence of infectious diseases generated the greatest impact on the health of the population by significantly increasing the life expectancy of people under 45 years of age. In 1850, the life expectancy at birth was 40 years for men and 42 years for women; by 1996, this had risen to 74.6 and 79.7 years respectively.

Although these trends also reflect reduced infant mortality rates, even today the death rate during the first year of life still remains higher than at any time below 55 years of age in males and 60 years of age in females. The predominant causes of death in the first four weeks of life, and in the remaining period up to the end of the first year of life, are summarised in Table 1.3. The measurement of infant mortality rate is important because it is widely accepted as an indicator of a country's quality of healthcare and standard of living.

Unfortunately, the advances in the prevention and management of infectious diseases of the past have not produced continued improvements in the overall health of the population (as shown by mortality and morbidity statistics). Epidemics of the past have been replaced by the so-called epidemics of the 'industrial' or 'modern' era.

Health may also be measured as a positive variable, such as dental health status, assessed in terms of numbers of decaying, missing and filled teeth (DMF index) routinely recorded by dentists.

Table 1.3 Main causes of death in the first year of life

Neonatal period (under 4 weeks)	Post-neonatal period (4 to 52 weeks)
Complications of childbirth	Accidents
Complications of pregnancy	Congenital malformations
Congenital malformations	Infections
Low birth-weight	Respiratory diseases
	Sudden infant death syndrome

Health behaviour indicators are increasingly common measurements of people's behaviour, which are then used as a measure for health. Examples include smoking, drinking alcohol, using drugs, practising safe sex or planned fertility, immunisation status and screening for cervical cancer.

Measuring health from the individual's perspective

Measures of health from the individual's perspective are becoming increasingly important in assessing health status and are seen as 'subjective' measures (the factual statistical measures outlined above being seen as 'objective'). These include functional reports, involving self-reporting of physical activity (e.g. the ability to perform everyday tasks). Peoples' rating of their fitness level has also been used. The Nottingham health profile is an example of a broader measure of health status. It arose from examining the most important aspects of health cited by the general public. It is used extensively and claimed to be both reliable and valid. Six different dimensions are scored independently: physical mobility, pain, sleep, social isolation, emotional reactions and energy level. All these items are scored by respondents on a standard questionnaire. The profile is a subjective assessment of people's health status and places equal emphasis on physical and mental health.

Psychological well-being scales have measured the presence or absence of symptoms such as anxiety or depression. More positive measures (e.g. happiness and life satisfaction) have been also used. 'Life satisfaction' refers to the dimension of mental health; 'happiness' refers to feelings. Other measures include self-esteem, a sense of coherence and perceived control over one's life. Quality of life is used by some researchers to encompass the broader notion of health and is also increasingly used when evaluating the effect of health services, including the use of medicines. It includes both objective and subjective evaluations of life circumstances. Four domains are examined:

- psychological (e.g. depression)
- social (e.g. engagement in social and leisure activities)
- occupational (e.g. ability to carry out paid or domestic work)
- physical (e.g. pain, sleep, mobility).

The 'modern' epidemics

In data collected between 1946 and 1948, circulatory diseases (incorporating ischaemic heart disease and cerebrovascular disease) and cancer accounted for approximately 50% of all deaths in people over 35 years of age; by 1982, the proportion had increased to 73%. The dramatic increase in numbers of deaths from cancer and circulatory diseases in people over 35 years of age during the past 40 years has resulted in little overall change in the mortality rate, particularly for men.

Unfortunately, the advances in the prevention and management of infectious diseases of the past have not produced continued improvements in the overall health of the population (as shown by mortality and morbidity statistics). Epidemics of the past have been replaced by epidemics of the present. Among the most common causes of mortality and morbidity at the beginning of the twenty-first century are:

- coronary heart disease
- cerebrovascular disease
- cancer
- mental health problems (including stress)
- accidents
- chronic bronchitis and emphysema
- diabetes mellitus
- arthritis
- asthma.

There were 16 000 deaths a year from coronary heart disease in people under 65 years of age in 1997: this equates to one-fifth of all deaths. Men from the lowest social class are more than 50% more likely to die from coronary heart disease than are those from the highest. Treatment costs for coronary heart disease, stroke and related problems are estimated at £3.8 billion a year. The most important factors predisposing to coronary heart disease are smoking, raised plasma-cholesterol concentrations, a high-fat diet and hypertension; other contributory factors are obesity and lack of exercise. However, risk is also determined by social factors (e.g. ethnicity, gender and social class) and environmental factors (e.g. housing, the region of the country a person lives in, and access to health services and leisure facilities). Many of these factors are interrelated: obesity is commonly associated with a lack of exercise, raised plasma-cholesterol levels, obesity and high blood pressure can be related to poor diet, and a high dietary salt intake, excessive alcohol consumption and obesity can all cause hypertension.

Highlighting specific important facts serves to illustrate the scale of the health problems facing the population at the start of this century:

- 28% of males and 27% of females are smokers: 35% of women aged 16 to 24 are smokers
- a recent study funded by the European Union estimated that passive smoking kills more than 20 000 people each year in Europe
- the proportion of men drinking above 21 units a week has remained stable between 1986 and 1996 at around 27%. The proportion of women drinking above 14 units a week increased from 10% in 1986 to 14% in 1996. Younger people were more likely to drink above these levels than older people
- England has the worst record in Europe for teenage pregnancy (90 000 a year), 8000 of whom are under 16 years of age
- 18 000 drug addicts were registered in the whole of 1990. In the six months to March 1998, 23 916 were registered with drug misuse agencies, 57% of whom were using heroin.

What is health promotion?

The Ottawa Charter for Health Promotion (WHO, 1986) describes health promotion as:

> . . . the process of enabling people to increase control over, and to improve, their health. Health is seen as a resource for daily life not the object of living. It is a positive concept emphasising social and personal resources, as well as physical capacities.

The five Ottawa strategies for success were: to build healthy public policy, create supportive environments, strengthen community action, develop personal skills and re-orient health services.

The Jakarta Declaration on Health Promotion (1997) offers a vision and focus for health promotion into the twenty-first century. It recognises that 'health is a basic human right and is essential for social and economic development', and states that case studies from around the world provide convincing evidence that health promotion works. There is now clear evidence that comprehensive approaches to health promotion using a combination of the five Ottawa strategies are the most effective. Settings such as cities, local communities, schools, the workplace and healthcare facilities (e.g. pharmacies) offer practical opportunities for the implementation of comprehensive strategies. Participation is essential to sustain efforts; people have to be at the centre of health promotion action and decision-making processes for it to be effective. Access to education and information is essential to achieving effective participation and the empowerment of people and communities.

As with the debate about the meaning of health, there is much philosophical debate about the meaning of health promotion and how, or whether, it differs from health education. Until the 1980s, most interventions were termed 'health education', and health education was seen as part of preventative medicine. The term 'health promotion' was not mentioned in the *Pharmaceutical Journal* until the 1980s. Health promotion is increasingly used as the generic term and, although some try to distinguish health promotion and health education as separate entities, many see health education as part of health promotion.

The aims of health promotion interventions in pharmacy are not simply to provide a clinical outcome, but to achieve health gain encompassing an effect on quality of life, user's satisfaction and user empowerment (increased control over health or illness – concordance, as well as clinical outcomes). Health promotion is more than illness prevention; it is also about health protection, providing services that promote health-protecting lifestyles and about health development. The latter incorporates the creation of structured environments that are conducive to health and which support the development of disease-preventing and health-protecting lifestyles.

One way to conceptualise health promotion is provided by Beattie's structural grid (Beattie, 1990) (*see* Figure 1.1). This presents a taxonomy of health promotion that attempts to incorporate the spectrum of activities conducted. The framework identifies four discrete areas of health promotion:

1 *health persuasion*: interventions directed at individuals led by professionals (e.g. encouraging a pregnant woman to stop smoking)
2 *legislative action*: interventions led by professionals intended to protect individuals (e.g. lobbying for emergency contraception to be made more widely available)
3 *personal counselling*: interventions led by individuals; the health promoter acts as a facilitator not an expert (e.g. smoking cessation clinics for individuals)
4 *community development*: interventions, like those in personal counselling, seek to empower a group or a local community (e.g. working with the local community to develop services for menopausal women).

The grid provides a means of comparing different philosophies of health promoters through analysis of the quadrant where their work originates.

authoritative form of intervention

individual focus of intervention		*collective focus of intervention*
Health persuasion techniques (1)		Legislative action for health (2)
Personal counselling for health (4)		Community development for health (3)

negotiated form of intervention

Figure 1.1 Strategies of health promotion. (Reproduced from Beattie, 1990).

Methods of health promotion

A wide variety of methods are used to transmit information used for promoting health. The methods vary in the:

- size of their target audience
- level of involvement between health promoters and their audience (and thus the degree to which the message can be personalised or tailored to the individual)
- degree of feedback that can be obtained to monitor the effectiveness of the process.

The mass media reaches a significant proportion of any target population but, by definition, its messages are largely impersonal. Information will be relayed to all members within a defined population, not just those who may be at high risk of developing a particular condition.

Posters, television, radio, the Internet, newspapers, magazines and books are the most commonly used channels of the mass media. These can be extremely influential in drawing attention to particular issues. Appropriate sales promotion, advertising and sponsorship can highlight a link with a healthy activity. To be effective, messages conveyed by the mass media must be simple and non-stressful; they should also be enjoyable and interesting. Because of the potential audience and effect, it is vital that the message conveyed is accurate and responsibly portrayed. Endorsement by an authoritative personality (e.g. a well-known doctor or a government minister) may reinforce the positive nature of the message. Recent examples of the effect of the media on behaviour change include the decline in eating beef caused by the BSE scare in the late 1990s and the effects of the contraceptive pill scare of 1996, which resulted in a rise in the number of abortions after women stopped taking the pill. The mass media can also have positive effects. The TV soap 'Eastenders' has successfully increased the number of women seeking breast screening as a result of a character having breast cancer. The same series has also recently addressed the issue of schizophrenia and introduced the subject of folic acid and the prevention of neural tube defects.

More personal messages can be conducted in specific environments and targeted towards particular groups. The importance of providing health education at as young an age as possible has been recognised by the inclusion of health topics (e.g. smoking, sexual health and contraception) in the curricula of schools and colleges, and in activities at other centres where young people gather socially.

The greatest level of involvement and the maximum degree of feedback can be obtained with discussions between health promoters and individuals on a one-to-one basis, with the information being tailored to the individual. Ideally, the opportunities for education should be grasped by adopting an interactive approach. A much greater response will be obtained from individuals if they actively participate in the discussion, rather than merely being told what is good for them and what they should do. By adopting such a stance, individuals can be guided to develop a much greater responsibility for their own health.

Research indicates that interactive multimedia are more likely to be acted upon and remembered than other media. Research has also shown that interactivity enhances interest, active information processing, and satisfaction with a message which, in turn, contributes to the effectiveness and persuasiveness of educational materials. Health promotion materials that present information through multiple modalities (e.g. computers and videotapes) are more effective than those that rely on a single channel (e.g. leaflets).

The most important setting for pharmacists to carry out health promotion is in the pharmacy, although pharmacists can and do extend their health promotion role by giving presentations to small meetings of local people outside normal working hours. In the pharmacy, pharmacists work face to face with individuals and can tailor the information and responses to the specific needs of the individual. No one method of imparting information about health is appropriate for all situations. The most effective measures are usually a combination of impersonal mass media messages reinforced by inter-personal or personal information.

The role of the pharmacist

The influence of government and professional policy

During the 1990s, the health promotion role of pharmacists has become increasingly reported, researched and accepted by the profession and policy makers. In 1985, The Nuffield Committee proposed health promotion as part of an extended role for pharmacists (Nuffield Foundation, 1985). The 1992 Pharmaceutical Care report of the Royal Pharmaceutical Society (RPSGB) and UK Department of Health (DoH) further encouraged involvement in health promotion (RPSGB and DoH, 1992). Among its recommendations were that pharmacists should be encouraged to set aside areas for displaying material and providing advice and counselling, pharmacists to participate more widely in health promotion activities and campaigns, and to contribute to health promotion by offering diagnostic testing and screening.

The DoH publication, *Primary Care: The Future* (1996) listed health promotion in pharmacy as an area where innovative local practices existed, and called for national development of these initiatives. It proposed that pharmacists should be the first port of call for both advice and over-the-counter (OTC) medicines for treatment of common ailments, arguing that this would increase pharmacists' health promotion role. The report also said that pharmacists should be actively promoting the health of people, contributing to the local achievement of health targets, and encouraging the principle of self-care and individual responsibility for health.

The White Paper, *The New NHS: Modern, Dependable* (DoH, 1997) emphasised the need for local working in the NHS to reduce inequalities in health and to improve health. It highlighted the need for health promotion and introduced the idea of Health Improvement Programmes, which are joint plans to improve health and healthcare locally. Health Action Zones are now being formed, targeting areas where greatest inequalities in health exist.

The White Paper, *Saving Lives – Our Healthier Nation* (DoH, 1998a) focuses on improving the health of the population as a whole by increasing the length of people's lives and the number of years people spend free from illness. It seeks to improve the health of those who are worst off in society and to narrow the health gap. Four major target areas are included, namely coronary heart disease (CHD) and stroke, cancer, mental health and accidents. (*See* Table 1.4 for areas where pharmacists' health promotion activities could contribute.) The paper called for local areas to develop health improvement plans and to develop services to effectively deliver appropriate healthcare. Healthcare providers, including pharmacists, are held responsible for their contribution in making people healthier. The Scottish Green Paper, *Working Together for a Healthier Scotland* (DoH, 1998b), explicitly mentioned pharmacies as important settings for health promotion.

In September 1996, the RPSGB published *New Horizons*, a summary of the largest ever consultation on the future of the pharmacy profession. It gave a summary of the views of more than 5000 pharmacists. Health promotion was ranked second, after advice to patients, as the most important new or expanded service for patients that pharmacists should be providing. Building the future, the RPSGB's response to *New Horizons* stated that pharmacists help people to maintain good health by providing health screening, advice on healthy living and other services. It acknowledged that both ill and well people visit pharmacies, and that pharmacists are thus uniquely placed to offer health information and advice. The report suggested that, in future, pharmacists will be in demand by other healthcare professionals as centres for health advice sessions, and that pharmacists will also provide advice sessions in other settings. Pharmacists, it said, will also be involved in interpreting the increasing amount of health-related information available, for example, on the Internet.

The year 1998 saw further development of professional policy when the RPSGB and the DoH published *Guidance for the Development of Health Promotion by Community Pharmacists* (RPSGB, 1998). The guidance stated that health promotion is something that all pharmacists should do and the basic philosophy of health promotion is something all pharmacists should espouse. Health promotion, said the document, is not just about changing lifestyle, neither is it simply about providing information. It is also about providing services that improve the health of individuals and communities, and empowering people to have increased control over and to improve their health. Pharmacists, it argued, should work for health gain and not just for lifestyle changes, aiming to improve the health of the people they come into contact with, helping to increase the number of years that people spend free of illness.

Two levels of health promotion were proposed in the guidance: level one for all pharmacists; and level two for those who wished to specialise. Level one focuses on pharmacists encouraging healthy behaviour. Ideally, pharmacists will set aside an area for health promotion literature and information, and they and their staff will use leaflets to highlight health issues. Pharmacists will also respond to requests for advice and actively give simple health promotion advice when giving out prescriptions, making sales and advising about treating symptoms. In addition to these level one activities, in level two pharmacists will actively seek opportunities to promote health. Where appropriate, they will identify how ready a person is to change their behaviour and offer individualised advice and ongoing support.

Influence of the community pharmacy setting

It is clear that there are two distinct modes of health promotion operating in community pharmacies. Pharmacy staff are more likely to raise health promotion issues with regular customers, with whom they have an established rapport and feel comfortable. 'Passing trade', on the other hand, are those customers with whom pharmacy staff have incidental and occasional encounters without context, and so are unsure of the response to unsolicited advice. These customers may be more appropriately reached through

Table 1.4 How pharmacists can contribute to the key target areas in 'Saving Lives – Our Healthier Nation'

Health target areas	Pharmacist's contribution
Accidents	Health and safety in premises Provide access for disabled, prams, etc. Many falls in elderly are related to the adverse effects of medicines Provide information on how to avoid osteoporosis, so accidents do not lead to broken bones. Information about diet, vitamin D and sunshine, exercise and Hormone Replacement Therapy Encourage regular eye tests (e.g. South Hampshire RNIB project) Know emergency and first aid routines Provide first aid kits, encourage people to update them Discourage driving under the influence of prescription and non-prescription medicines.
Cancer	Advice, information and support about early detection and diagnoses of cancer Refer people for cancer screening Encourage covering up in sun, encourage effective, adequate use of sunscreens (pharmacies in New Zealand only sell sunscreens of factor 15 plus), special advice for children Provide reliable and up-to-date information about the risks of smoking, poor diet and too much sun
CHD and stroke	Pharmacists can target their messages to groups most at risk using their knowledge of their local community; using knowledge of ill-health and other problems gleaned from prescriptions and patient medication records, and customers' requests for advice about symptoms and treatments. Pharmacists can identify those at risk of CHD and stroke and provide high-quality services Give advice on all areas of healthy living Provide simple advice, more concentrated advice and ongoing support for those who wish to stop smoking, and supply and promote the use of nicotine replacement therapy Learn how to recognise a heart attack and resuscitation skills Blood pressure testing Concordance support to ensure people take medicines as prescribed, e.g. 50% of people stop taking statins after six months Audit use of aspirin as prevention post myocardial infarction, stroke etc. Warfarin clinics Smoke-free pharmacies Decrease stress at work for pharmacists and staff. Have an adequate number of staff, with adequate breaks, because pharmacies are open for long hours
Mental health	Support and advise people with anxiety, depression, phobias and panic attacks Help to tackle the problem of suicide in Sri Lankan, Indian and E. African women. Pharmacists in some areas with large ethnic populations are often of same racial origin as customers and patients Pharmacists are part of the support network Increase public understanding of mental health Reduce access to means of suicide, e.g. medicines such as paracetamol and antidepressants Provide supervised on-site administration of antidepressants using daily instalment dispensing Promote other ways of reducing stress, e.g. massage, aromatherapy, exercise, etc. Provide information about self-help groups Advise on effective treatment Concordance support

window displays, posters, leaflets and the Internet to stimulate awareness.

Pharmacists operate in a commercial environment and do not always use that to their advantage in health promotion. The sale of medicines and other health-related goods can incorporate health promotion and offer opportunities for business development. Pharmacists might also take advantage of the market for health and wellbeing, recognising in particular that people from the higher social classes are willing to spend money to maintain and support health.

Research and the evidence of effectiveness of pharmacy-based health promotion

As Health Authorities and individuals have begun to develop the health promotion role of the community pharmacist, the topic has become increasingly researched. Many of the studies were small, involving only a few pharmacies. Most studies have been conducted by pharmacists themselves, with perhaps inevitably very positive conclusions about a future role for pharmacists in health promotion, sometimes beyond that which could be justified on the basis of the study findings. There has been very little work on the quality, acceptability or effectiveness of the role of pharmacists in health promotion. Notable exceptions are the work of Maguire and colleagues in Belfast and Sinclair and colleagues in Aberdeen (Sinclair *et al.*, 1995), which showed that pharmacists can be involved in effective health promotion campaigns, health screening and smoking cessation services while running a busy dispensing pharmacy.

The seminal Barnet High Street Health Scheme (HSHS) was launched in 1991, and involves seven days of accredited training in health promotion knowledge and skills, together with ongoing support for the health promotion role. The scheme was evaluated in a number of ways, including in-depth interviews, customer surveys, audit and participant research. The main findings were that the HSHS has changed the attitudes and practice of participating pharmacists, with data from both interview and covert observational research. The findings showed that pharmacists were more likely to:

- be involved in health promotion than they were previously
- make informal and opportunistic interventions, linked to the sale or supply of medicines
- be involved in health promotion in the areas of diet, smoking cessation and asthma
- have moved away from a product-orientated role to a more patient-orientated one
- spend less time dispensing medicines and more time talking to and advising patients
- give social and psychological care to their patients; and to use health promotion leaflets more appropriately.

Lack of remuneration was found to be the largest barrier to involvement in health promotion perceived by the HSHS pharmacists; prior to training, time and lack of training were the largest barriers perceived by both these pharmacists and controls. Other studies have concluded that the main constraints to pharmacist involvement in health promotion are lack of time, space, finance, training and a perceived conflict between the professional and commercial roles of the pharmacist.

Following the Barnet scheme, a number of Health Authorities provided pharmacist training, with more than half of English Health Authorities saying in later research that they had been influenced by the Barnet scheme. Other published studies evaluating the effect of training in health promotion come from Aberdeen, Somerset and Wiltshire. Sinclair *et al.* (1995) in Aberdeen showed that trained pharmacists had a positive effect on smoking cessation compared with controls. Customers who were counselled by trained pharmacists were significantly more likely to have stopped smoking at the nine months follow-up.

The public's view of pharmacy health promotion

The published work to date suggests that the public are broadly sympathetic to the idea of pharmacists providing health advice, but that many do not perceive pharmacists as an obvious source of general health advice, and few would take the initiative in approaching pharmacists and asking for such advice. Face-to-face advice is perceived to be preferable, and consumers have said that they want to receive tailored advice. In the Barnet research, those consumers with prescriptions were more likely than others to regard the pharmacist as someone to consult for advice about staying healthy. Those Barnet consumers who had taken health promotion leaflets from the pharmacy were significantly more likely to be those who had asked the pharmacist about general health and those who thought it was the usual job of the pharmacist to give health advice. Consumers who were aware that leaflets were displayed in pharmacies were also those who were more likely to think that the media was the most convenient place to get advice about staying healthy. Many of the consumers interviewed in Barnet did not perceive that there was a role for community pharmacists in health promotion.

The Pharmacy Healthcare Scheme (PHS)

The Pharmacy Healthcare Scheme (formerly known as the Healthcare in the High Street campaign) was launched in 1986 in England and Scotland and later joined by Wales and Northern Ireland. The scheme provided pharmacists with a leaflet stand and a monthly supply of health education leaflets on one topic free of charge, thus enabling national co-ordination for the first time. In 1989, the Government allocated £250 000 to support the scheme and continues to allocate funding on an annual basis. In 1992, a limited company was formed to administer and develop the scheme, which was then renamed the Pharmacy Healthcare Scheme (PHCS).

Those organisations whose leaflets were featured in PHCS reported a strong response from the public. A leaflet on Alzheimer's disease resulted in 1200 inquiries to the Alzheimer's Disease Society within three weeks. The British Heart Foundation reported 14 000 requests for further information in the three months following a leaflet on coronary heart disease.

In 1993, the first national evaluation of the PHCS was commissioned. A total of 92% of pharmacists said they had heard of the scheme. The majority said that 'all' or 'most' of the leaflets were 'just picked up' by people; only a few were taken on the pharmacist's recommendation. This suggests that pharmacists' role in the scheme was largely the passive enabling of leaflet distribution, rather than a more active input. The NPA and a group of management consultants have been working with the PHCS to develop the role of pharmacists in health promotion and have recently made a number of recommendations about the scheme's future.

Since 1994, community pharmacist contractors have been remunerated through the professional allowance (part of the NHS contract for community pharmaceutical services) for displaying such health promotion leaflets, posters and publications as their Health Authority may approve. The pharmacy is required to display up to eight leaflets at any one time, although pharmacists may stock more if they wish to do so. The incorporation of this requirement into the criteria for the professional allowance ensured its wide application in practice, as well as providing a mechanism for more liaison between the Local Pharmaceutical Committee and the Health Authority.

Working with others

Health Action Zones are a key part of the government's drive to target areas with high levels of ill-health, improving the health of the worst off at a faster rate than the general population, thus attempting to reduce inequalities in health. These are long-term initiatives (up to seven years) targeted at the most deprived areas of the country. Health Action Zones (HAZs) have three main aims:

- to identify and address the health needs of local people
- to increase the effectiveness, efficiency and responsiveness of services
- to develop partnerships for improving health and health services, bringing together the work of different agencies.

The government has invested considerably in this initiative and there is money available to develop services. Areas in which pharmacists have become involved include:

- counselling people about the management of medicines
- tackling coronary heart disease and stroke by providing smoking cessation clinics and warfarin clinics
- providing information and advice about emergency contraception and teenage sexual health
- providing information and advice about the early detection of skin cancer and use of sunscreens
- reducing accidents by providing information about storage of medicines and avoiding driving while under the influence of certain medicines (e.g. antidepressants).

Case study – a scenario considering one model of the extent to which a community pharmacist could be involved in health promotion

Healthlines Pharmacy is much more health-orientated than it used to be. The pharmacist has stopped selling the products that supermarkets can sell more cheaply and is concentrating on health-related merchandise; she also no longer sells confectionery or jewellery. She has refitted her pharmacy, creating a special advice area. She is involved in the Health Authority accreditation scheme. She currently has a window display about stroke prevention organised by her local health improvement programme as part of National Stroke Week. She was paid to put the display up and audit customers' responses to it. She tries to talk about health to all her customers and patients even if it is only a brief mention (e.g. about smoking cessation to a pregnant mother, or a smoker buying a cough mixture). She believes this is encouraging them to ask her for advice about staying healthy.

While Mr G is waiting for his prescription, he picks up a booklet about healthy eating from a display rack and starts to read it. He notices that there are a number of leaflets in foreign languages for the local ethnic population. He looks around at the posters she has displayed about local exercise classes and her smoking cessation services. While her dispenser gets his prescription ready, Mrs P tells a customer about the importance of taking folic acid if she is trying to conceive and another about using insect repellents containing DEET, as well as taking anti-malarials, during her visit to India.

Two days later Mr G returns to the pharmacy and asks for a quiet word. He is worried about the effects that his 'water tablets' might have on his bladder as he often has to attend long board meetings and does not want to always be excusing himself. The prescription was for bendroflumethiazide (bendrofluazide) 2.5 mg. She tells him that it should not cause too many problems and that he should take his tablets on rising in the morning. He then confides that he is really more worried about impotence, because he has read in his Sunday newspaper that blood pressure drugs can cause such problems. She tells him that it can be a problem for some men and that, if it is, he should consult his GP as there are other appropriate treatments for him. He also tells her that his cholesterol level was raised and the GP has told him to change his diet. The pharmacist reinforces this advice and asks him if he is taking any exercise. He plays golf once a month, but that is all he can manage now, owing to pressure of work and so on. She discusses with him some simple things he can change, like walking instead of always going short distances by car, and using the stairs instead of lifts. She encourages him to think about taking up another sport, or playing golf once a week.

She asks him to let her know if he has any problems with his tablets. He returns a month later with a repeat prescription. He tells her that his tablets do not seem to be causing him any problems and that he has lost half a stone; he has been cutting down on business lunches and he is walking a bit more. His blood pressure has come down too.

He says he wants to encourage the other men in his company to stop smoking. She says she is willing to run a smoking clinic at a charge of £30 per person and that she is already doing this for a local department store and a bank. He says that he will put it to his colleagues.

The pharmacist developed her interest in health promotion when she was involved in a Health Authority training scheme for health promotion in community pharmacy. She is involved with a local audit group, which is developing standards for health promotion in community pharmacy. She goes to her local comprehensive school to talk about health promotion issues on a regular basis. She has been lobbying her local council about smoking in public places and has also written to her MP and the Prime Minister about tobacco policy. She is also lobbying her Health Authority to provide realistic remuneration for health promotion, especially when it does not involve a sale or a prescription.

References

Beattie A (1990). Knowledge and control in health promotion. In: Gable J, Calman N, Bury M, eds. *Sociology of the Health Service*. London: Routledge.

Department of Health (1996). *Primary Care: The Future*. London: HMSO.

Department of Health (1997). *The New NHS, Modern, Dependable*. London: HMSO.

Department of Health (1998a). *Our Healthier Nation*. London: HMSO.

Department of Health (1998b). *Working Together for a Healthier Scotland*. London: HMSO.

Nuffield Foundation (1985). *Report of the Inquiry into Pharmacy*. London: Nuffield Foundation.

RPSGB (1998). Guidance for the development of health promotion by community pharmacists. *Pharm J* 261: 771–775.

RPSGB, Department of Health (1992). *Pharmaceutical Care*. London: RPSGB.

Sinclair H K, Bond C M, Lennox A S, *et al.* (1995). Nicotine replacement therapies: smoking cessation outcomes in a pharmacy setting in Scotland. *Tob Control* 4: 338–343.

Further reading

Anderson C (1996). Community pharmacy health promotion activity in England: a survey of policy and practice. *Health Educ J* 55: 194–202.

Anderson C (1998). Health promotion by community pharmacists: consumers' views. *Int J Pharm Pract* 6: 2–12.

Anderson C (1998). Health promotion by community pharmacists: perceptions, realities, and constraints. *J Soc Admin Pharm* 15: 10–22.

Anderson C, Greene R (1997). The Barnet High Street Health Scheme: health promotion by community pharmacists. *Pharm J* 259: 223–225.

Black D, *et al.* (1982). *Inequalities in Health: The Black Report*. Harmondsworth: Penguin.

Blenkinsopp A, Panton R, Anderson C (1999). *Health Promotion for Pharmacists*, 2nd edn. Oxford: Oxford University Press.

Calman M (1987). *Health and Illness: The Lay Perspective*. London: Tavistock Publications.

Ewles L, Simnett I (1998). *Promoting Health: A Practical Guide*, 4th edn. London: Scutari Press.

Maguire T A (1995). The development of a community pharmacy based successful service model. *Int J Smoking Cess* 1: 27–32.

Maguire T A, Morrow N, Orr R (1987). Foot care as a focus for health promotion in the community pharmacy. *Pharm J* 239: 465–467.

Naidoo J, Wills J (1994). *Health Promotion Foundations for Practice*. London: Baillière Tindall.

Raeburn J, Rootman I (1998). *People-centred Health Promotion*. Chichester: Wiley.

Sharma S, Anderson C (1998). The impact of using pharmacy window space for health promotion about emergency contraception. *Health Educ J* 57: 42–50.

Todd J (1993). Community pharmacies: The High Street Health Scheme. *Health Educ J* 52: 34–36.

2

Dietary management

Pamela Mason

Food is essential to ensure growth, maintenance and repair of tissues, correct functioning of metabolic processes, and to provide energy to enable all these functions to be carried out. In addition, food has a social function and is a means of getting people together. Food is also used as a means of comfort or reward.

A great deal is written and spoken about nutrition by the lay press, professional bodies, government departments and the food industry itself. The result is a plethora of conflicting information which can, at times, be highly controversial. It is not surprising that there is a lot of confusion about what constitutes a good, well balanced, nutritious diet. Some people take an extreme standpoint and indulge in faddish diets in an effort to eliminate totally certain components. In doing so, their diet becomes unbalanced and they run the risk of both excesses and deficiencies. Others attempt a more rational approach, but quickly run into trouble because they do not have the background knowledge to assess the contradictory information objectively. They either struggle on, labouring under a variety of misconceptions, or revert to their original habits in the belief that 'nobody knows what they are talking about anyway'. At the other extreme, there are those who refuse to give any thought to dietary matters and indulge in dietary excesses, possibly at the expense of other, more nutritious, alternatives.

Diets in affluent societies contain a high proportion of fats and sugars. It has been recommended by many authorities that both of these should be reduced, and a greater emphasis placed on starchy foods as a means of providing energy. Conversely, people in developing countries are likely to be undernourished, and should increase their intake of proteins and fats, and aim for consumption of a greater variety of foods.

The modern diet has changed drastically in other respects too. Busy lifestyles and a steady reduction in the time spent in planning, shopping for, and preparation of food has led to reliance on a vast array of 'convenience' foods. The public now expects products with a long shelf-life, coupled with minimal preparation and cooking. In addition, choice is commonly linked to certain standards of appearance (e.g. good colour and texture). Consequently, a whole multitude of substances are added as preservatives, stabilisers, emulsifiers, binders, colouring and flavouring agents, and flavour enhancers. Salt and sugar are also added in large amounts (sometimes to the most unlikely products) to improve flavour.

Some modern food processing methods and prolonged storage also reduce the levels of valuable vitamins, although it is not often appreciated that losses also occur from fresh foods on storage and preparation. Fresh foods are not without risks of contamination, and the skins of fruit and vegetables may be coated with chemicals (e.g. insecticides and herbicides). Ready-to-eat salads are widely available and, if improperly prepared, have proved to be a source of *Listeria monocytogenes*. Cook-chill foods provide a fertile growing medium for bacteria, notably *Salmonella* spp. and *Listeria monocytogenes*, and may cause food poisoning if not reheated thoroughly. Modern intensive farming methods have also increased the level of bacteria in food (e.g. *Salmonella* spp. in poultry and eggs), and meat may contain residues of veterinary drugs.

During the mid-1990s, there was concern about bovine spongiform encephalopathy (BSE) ('mad cow disease') and the possibility that it could be transmitted to humans. The infective agent responsible for BSE was acquired through incorporation of animal products into cattle feed, and it was the consumption of tissue from bovine brain and spinal cord, used in products such as beefburgers, meat pies and sausages, which was considered to pose the greatest risk to humans. At the end of 1989, the UK government stated that UK beef products should not contain any brain, spinal cord or lymphoid tissue. However, there still exists the possibility that individuals who consumed large quantities of beef products prior to 1989 could be at risk. More research is required to assess the risk to humans and to develop methods of early detection in humans before the onset of clinical symptoms.

Genetically modified (GM) food has also become an area of concern. Genetic modification allows for more rapid breeding of plants to select desired characteristics (e.g. resistance to pesticides and frost) than traditional methods and therefore offers advantages, especially in farming and food production. No GM crops are yet grown commercially for food in the UK, although several trials are underway. GM foods available in the UK are made mainly from crops grown in the US and include tomato puree, soya, maize, cheese and a variety of enzymes used to make a large variety of products (e.g. fizzy drinks, baked goods and dairy produce). There is no evidence that GM foods on sale at the moment pose any risk to human health, although there is not enough evidence yet to state categorically that all GM foods are 100% safe. Consumers clearly want to know whether they are eating these products.

Pharmacists have an important role as providers of healthcare, and are in an effective position to advise on nutrition. Counselling may be required in various cases, including:

- advice about basic nutritious diets to maintain health and prevent diet-related diseases
- objective interpretation of the information available from different sources
- recommendations about vitamin and mineral supplements
- consideration of the needs of specific groups (e.g. vegetarians, infants and children, pregnant and lactating women, the elderly and the sick and convalescent)
- assessment of the potential risks associated with food additives and other chemicals used by the food industry and in agriculture
- counselling on food preparation and hygiene to reduce the risks of food-borne infections.

Diet-related diseases

Some diseases can be directly related to food or its lack and these are well documented. Such disorders were common in the UK until comparatively recently, and still are in developing countries. Undernourishment results in poor growth and repair of tissues, and specific deficiency syndromes are caused by lack of some vitamins (*see* Vitamins *below*).

Fungal contamination may occur during growth of crops or on subsequent storage. Ergotism (St Anthony's fire) is caused by ingestion of rye contaminated with *Claviceps purpurea*, and formerly occurred as epidemics but is now rarely seen. Aflatoxins, which have been implicated in the development of liver cancer, are potent toxins produced by *Aspergillus flavus*, which grows on many vegetables, particularly peanuts. Helminthic infections have always been a problem, and still are in areas where raw or undercooked meat or fish form part of the traditional diet. Bacterial or protozoal contamination of food is responsible for cholera, dysentery, giardiasis and salmonellal infections in areas where poor sanitation results in contamination of the water supply or human excrement is used as a fertiliser. Brucellosis is caused by the ingestion of unpasteurised milk and milk products obtained from cows infected with *Brucella* spp.

Improvements in agricultural yields, hygiene, health education and the increased availability of a wide range of foods to all income levels of society have eliminated most of these diseases in industrial nations. However, the incidence of other diseases has increased, and this has been linked to the increase in consumption of sugars, fats and salt. In some cases, poor diet is not necessarily the sole aetiological factor. Other factors include smoking (*see* Chapter 5), excessive alcohol consumption (*see* Chapter 6), lack of exercise (*see* Chapter 8) and emotional stress. The diet-related disorders referred to in this chapter are those considered to be caused or precipitated by the long-term consumption of the traditional diet of industrial nations. It is felt by many authorities that the incidence of these diseases would be significantly reduced if overall dietary adjustments were made. The role of diet in the development of dental caries is discussed in Chapter 3.

Obesity is becoming increasingly common in the western world and is caused by consumption of food in excess of an individual's energy requirements. Being overweight may affect a person psychologically: obesity is not considered attractive. Obese people are also at a physical disadvantage because they do not possess the suppleness or stamina of a person of desirable body-weight. Obesity also predisposes an individual to various diseases (e.g. cardiovascular disease, diabetes mellitus and joint disorders). Cardiovascular disease and gallstones are directly attributed to a high fat intake; hypertension may be associated with excessive salt consumption. Insufficient non-starch polysaccharides (*see* Carbohydrates *below*) in the diet has been linked to the development of several gastro-intestinal and related disorders (e.g. appendicitis, colorectal cancer, constipation, diverticulitis and irritable bowel syndrome). Poor diet may also cause or precipitate diabetes mellitus, and diet has been linked with some forms of cancer.

Symptoms of some disorders are produced as a direct reaction to certain components in the diet, but the underlying aetiology may involve immunological mechanisms or inappropriate biochemical reactions. Such conditions include food allergies and food intolerance, malabsorption syndromes and inborn errors of metabolism. Treatment usually involves removal of the offending food, and may require substitution with some other component. For more detailed information on dietary products for specific disorders, *see* Harman (1989).

Energy requirements

Energy values

The unit of energy in the International System of Units (SI) is the joule (J). This is the work done when a force of 1 Newton is displaced through a distance of 1 metre in the direction of the force. In nutrition, the kilojoule (1 kJ [1000 J]) and megajoule (1 MJ [10^6 J]) are used as more convenient units.

Energy values were formerly expressed in units of heat, employing the calorie. One calorie is the amount of heat required to raise the temperature of 1 g of water by 1°C at a specified temperature (i.e. from 14.5 to 15.5°C). This was formerly known as the 'small calorie' (cal) and distinguished from the 'large Calorie' (Cal) used in nutrition, which is equivalent to 1000 calories or 1 kilocalorie (kcal). Although, it is preferable to use the SI unit, the kilocalorie is widely used in nutrition.

In food, fats form the most concentrated source of energy: 1 g of fat provides 0.037 MJ (8.8 kcal). Other sources of energy are carbohydrates (expressed as monosaccharides), providing 0.016 MJ (3.8 kcal), and proteins 0.017 MJ (4 kcal). Energy values can therefore be calculated when the proportion of these constituents in food is known. Alcohol is also a source of energy: 1 g provides 0.029 MJ (7.0 kcal). Vitamins and minerals do not contribute any energy. Additional heat is provided by hot food cooling to the body's temperature of 37°C, and although this amount of energy is very small compared with the overall contribution, the effects are felt immediately and may be of considerable psychological benefit in producing feelings of comfort and warmth. There is, however, no nutritional advantage of hot food compared with cold food.

Individual requirements

Human energy requirements are variable and depend upon a number of different factors (e.g. age, sex, and body composition and size). Climate, environment and the state of a person's health must also be considered, but it is the amount of physical activity that has the greatest effect on individual energy requirements.

The basal metabolic rate (BMR) is the rate at which the body uses energy when the body is at complete rest. Values depend on age, sex, and body-weight. Examples of BMRs are:

- 7.56 MJ/day (1800 kcal/day) for a 65 kg man
- 5.98 MJ/day (1424 kcal/day) for a 55 kg woman.

The proportion of lean tissue (i.e. the fat-free mass, FFM) dictates the energy needed, and the BMR is therefore lower in the elderly or during starvation.

Additional energy requirements above the BMR occur when food is eaten and for any sort of activity. More energy is required for strenuous activity than light exercise, and heavier people need more energy than light people to carry out the same amount of activity. The Estimated Average Requirement (EAR) for energy is an estimate of the average requirement or need, and is equivalent to the BMR multiplied by the Physical Activity Level (PAL). PAL is the ratio of overall daily energy expenditure to BMR, and values range from 1.4 to 1.9. Most people in the UK have a PAL of 1.4, which represents very little physical activity.

Dietary reference values and food tables

The control of dietary energy intake is dictated by appetite; nutrient consumption is not. However, a good, regular, mixed diet should provide all the nutrients required and, in theory, in-depth nutritional knowledge is not necessary. However, in practice, the correct balance of nutrients may not be achieved. In many parts of the world, deficiencies occur because there may be a general shortage of food or a lack of variety. In developed nations, where these problems do not exist, overt clinical deficiencies are uncommon. However, there may still be a poor balance of nutrients in the diet as a result of over-consumption of fats and refined carbohydrates (especially sugars) at the expense of other foods.

The diets of adults are largely determined by what was eaten during childhood and reflects the nutritional knowledge of their parents, which, in turn, would have been based on the level of general health education available at the time. In addition, restrictions may have been imposed by culture, ethics or religion. In order for individuals to assess the adequacy of their diets and to make any appropriate adjustments, an awareness of nutritional needs is necessary.

Dietary reference values

A knowledge of the disease states produced by deficiencies of some nutrients has enabled the compilation of a list of nutrients that are essential to maintain health and activity. Furthermore, controlled scientific studies have been able to assess the minimum amounts of some nutrients required to prevent clinical deficiency syndromes (e.g. 10 mg per day of ascorbic acid prevents scurvy). However, solely preventing a deficiency disease does not necessarily guarantee health. This is because the actual amount needed to maintain health may exceed that required to prevent a deficiency disease. There are other nutrients for which clinical deficiency states are unknown, presumably because they are required in such small amounts or are widely distributed throughout foods, or both. Nevertheless, research has highlighted essential roles of such nutrients in metabolic pathways and, consequently, they too are considered necessary to maintain health. Various authorities have made recommendations regarding the amounts of essential nutrients necessary to maintain health. However, the amounts suggested may differ because different criteria are used as the basis for the recommendations.

In 1979, the then UK government Department of Health and Social Security (DHSS) set Recommended Daily Amounts (RDAs) of food energy and nutrients for groups of people in the UK. The definition of the RDA for a nutrient was 'the average amount of the nutrient which should be provided per head in a group of people if the needs of practically all members of the group are to be met'. Therefore, to ensure that everyone received adequate amounts, RDAs were higher than the average amount required by the group. This was widely misinterpreted as the minimum amount required by individuals to maintain health. Individuals vary in their needs: some may consume less than the RDA without any apparent ill effects, and problems may not arise until the intake falls significantly below the RDA. RDAs were intended to be used when planning food supplies for groups of people, or when interpreting data obtained from surveys of food supplies or dietary intake.

The UK Department of Health (DoH) issued a new set of guidelines in dietary reference values for food energy and nutrients for the UK (DoH, 1991). It has been recognised that nutritional reference values are required in a variety of applications, including assessment of the adequacy of individual diets. Consequently, four standards have been defined to replace the former RDAs. All four standards are covered by the term Dietary Reference Values (DRVs).

- **EAR**
  Estimated Average Requirement of a group of people for energy or a nutrient. About half will usually need more than the EAR, and half less.
- **LRNI**
  Lower Reference Nutrient Intake for a nutrient. An amount of the nutrient that is enough for only the few people in a group who have low needs. Most people will need more than the LRNI if they are to eat enough, and if individuals are habitually eating less than the LRNI they will almost certainly be deficient.
- **RNI**
  Reference Nutrient Intake for a nutrient. An amount of the nutrient that is enough, or more than enough, for about 97% of people in a group. This level of intake is, therefore, considerably higher than most people need. If individuals are consuming the RNI of a nutrient, they are most unlikely to be deficient in that nutrient.
- **Safe intake**
  A term used to indicate intake or range of intakes of a nutrient for which there is not enough information to estimate EAR, LRNI, or RNI. It is an amount that is enough for almost everyone but is not so large as to cause undesirable effects.

EARs of energy are the average values of energy required by various groups. Consequently, some people within a group will require more, and others less, than this amount. The exact amount of energy required by an individual is equal to the amount of energy expended, and therefore varies with the level of physical activity.

Fats, sugars and starches are major contributors to energy intake, and an inadequate intake results in weight loss. There are, however, no deficiency signs or symptoms specifically associated with a low intake of these nutrients, and there is no EAR, LRNI or RNI. Research has shown that health is affected by the proportions in the diet of fats, starches and sugars, and it was deemed by the DoH (1991) that some guidance was required on the desirable intakes of these nutrients. DRVs are quoted as representing the average contribution that fats, sugars and starches should make to dietary energy for groups of people.

The DoH (1991) has emphasised that all DRVs for proteins, vitamins and minerals should be treated with caution. They are only indications of the ranges of requirements likely to be found within the UK population, and the values for energy, fats, sugars and starches are intended only to be indications of appropriate intakes.

DRVs have been assessed for healthy groups, including those with extra needs (e.g. infants, children, and pregnant and breast-feeding women), but have not taken into account the increased demands made by illness and convalescence (*see* Dietary needs of specific groups *below*). Specific deficiency syndromes or disorders requiring specialised dietary management are clinical problems and should be treated by specialists. Table 2.1 lists EARs for energy and RNIs for nutrients for adults aged 19 years and over.

Food tables

Tables that list the composition of nutrients and energy provided by various foods are available, and may help to assess the adequacy of a diet. They may also be useful in highlighting those foods that contain a specific nutrient needed by an individual (e.g. the requirement for calcium increases during lactation and may not be met by

Table 2.1 Daily EARs for energy and daily RNIs for nutrients for adults of 19 years of age and over

	Men	Women[a]
Energy (PAL = 1.4)	8.77–10.60 MJ[b]	7.61–8.10 MJ[b]
Protein[c]		
19 to 50 years of age	55.5 g	45.0 g
over 50 years of age	53.3 g	46.5 g
Ascorbic acid	40 mg	40 mg
Vitamin A (retinol equivalents)	700 µg	600 µg
Vitamin B group		
total folate	200 µg	200 µg
nicotinic acid equivalent	16 to 17 mg[b]	12 to13 mg[b]
pyridoxine[d]	1.4 mg	1.2 mg
riboflavin	1.3 mg	1.1 mg
thiamine	0.9 to 1.0 mg[b]	0.8 mg[b]
vitamin B_{12}	1.5 µg	1.5 µg
Vitamin D	[e]	[e]
Calcium	700 mg	700 mg
Chloride	2.5 g	2.5 g
Copper	1.2 mg	1.2 mg
Iron	8.7 mg	8.7 to 14.8 mg[f]
Magnesium	300 mg	270 mg
Phosphorus	550 mg	550 mg
Potassium	3.5 g	3.5 g
Iodine	140 µg	140 µg
Selenium	75 µg	60 µg
Sodium	1.6 g	1.6 g
Zinc	9.5 mg	7.0 mg

[a] The requirement for many nutrients increases during pregnancy and lactation and, where appropriate, these are discussed under Dietary needs of specific groups.
[b] The actual value depends on age, the level of physical activity, or both.
[c] Milk or egg protein. These figures assume complete digestibility. For diets based on high intakes of vegetable proteins, correction may need to be applied.
[d] Based on protein providing 14.7% of EAR for energy.
[e] No dietary sources may be necessary for people who are sufficiently exposed to sunlight, but the DoH recommends that the RNI after 65 years of age is 10 µg/day for men and women; supplements may be required by children and adolescents during the winter (*see* Dietary needs of specific groups), and housebound adults.
[f] This intake may not be sufficient for women with large menstrual losses and iron supplements may be required.
The figures for this table are derived from DoH (1991).

the individual's regular diet, *see* Dietary needs of specific groups *below*). Tables may be arranged as a list of foods under each nutrient, or as an alphabetical list of foods with analysis of composition. The Further reading section (*see below*) lists publications which contain food tables.

The actual values quoted are based upon laboratory analysis of several samples. Tables from different laboratories, particularly in different countries, will not necessarily show the same figures because there are many factors that may influence the nutrient levels. These include the variety of plant or animal used for analysis, the season or climate, the level of minerals in the soil, and other growing and feeding conditions. The level of nutrients also falls after harvesting. For example, some vitamins are destroyed by heat, light or prolonged storage (especially if allowed to dry out), or if the flesh of fruits and vegetables is bruised. Losses during cooking must be taken into account if the tables quote values for raw food only. Nutrients may also be lost in preparation because the skins of many fruit and vegetables are discarded.

Food tables are not intended to be used to calculate the exact amount of nutrients ingested; this is time-consuming and the final result would be very inaccurate. However, they are useful as a means of comparing the composition of foods, and they may help to introduce new foods into the diet when attempting to increase the variety. Food tables are also useful in assessing the energy provided in the diet and will be familiar to those attempting to reduce weight. Tables may also be used to estimate the contributions to total dietary energy made by carbohydrates, fats and proteins, and to assess the extent of adjustment required to comply with the recommendations made by the UK DoH (*see* Dietary constituents *below*).

Dietary constituents

Carbohydrates

Carbohydrates contain carbon, hydrogen and oxygen, and are based upon a chemical structure consisting of sugar units (usually glucose) linked together in a variety of ways. They may be classified as monosaccharides or disaccharides (sugars) and polysaccharides. Dietary sugars are further classified as 'intrinsic', which comprises sugars contained within the cell walls of fruits and vegetables, and 'extrinsic', which are not found in the cell walls of food. Extrinsic sugars include lactose, honey and sucrose used in baking or added at the table.

Monosaccharides

Monosaccharides are the simplest sugars. Glucose (dextrose) occurs naturally in some foods (e.g. fruit and vegetable juices) as free glucose, or is obtained from other carbohydrates following digestion. Fructose (laevulose) occurs in honey and also in some fruits and vegetables, and is the sweetest sugar. Galactose does not occur freely, but is a constituent of lactose.

Disaccharides

Disaccharides may be hydrolysed to yield two monosaccharide units. Sucrose is a combination of glucose and fructose, and occurs naturally in sugar cane, sugar beet, and some fruits and root vegetables (e.g. carrots). Lactose is less sweet than sucrose, and is a combination of glucose and galactose; it occurs in the milk of all animals. Maltose is a combination of two molecules of glucose and is formed during digestion of starch.

Polysaccharides

Polysaccharides (complex carbohydrates) ultimately yield a number of monosaccharide units on hydrolysis. Those that can be digested by man are starches, which are broken down in the body to the simplest sugar unit, glucose. Any glucose not immediately required by the body is converted into glycogen, which acts as a reserve glucose supply (*see* Participation in sports and exercise in Chapter 8). Further excesses are converted into fat and deposited in adipose tissue. Starch is the form in which energy is stored in the seeds and roots of many plants. It is enclosed within granules and cannot easily be digested until treated with moist heat, which allows the granules to swell, burst and release the starch. Good food sources of starch include baked beans, bread, cereals, potatoes and yams.

Non-starch polysaccharides (NSP) (formerly called roughage and dietary fibre) is present in food that has undergone minimal processing. NSP include plant polysaccharides that are water-insoluble (e.g. cellulose) and water-soluble polysaccharides (e.g. pectins, gums, mucilages and other hemicelluloses). The latter are abundant in barley, oats, fruits and legumes, although most sources contain both types of NSP. Good sources of NSP include whole grain cereals, nuts, and fruits and vegetables (especially legumes). The NSP content of fruits is increased if the skins are consumed, although the beneficial effects are diminished if the fruit is pulped or puréed.

The role of carbohydrates in the diet

Sugars
When the general term 'sugar' is used, it usually means sucrose, which is the most common sugar

consumed in the modern diet. Sucrose is a relatively recent addition to man's diet and has only been widely used in the last 150 years. Before that, it was only available in small quantities for the wealthy, and the only sugars ingested in the general diet were those occurring naturally in foods. Sugars are purely a source of energy and are often referred to as 'empty calories' because they do not contain proteins, vitamins, minerals or NSP. If sugar is consumed in large amounts, it may replace more nutritious foods as a source of dietary energy.

Increased use of sugar has been linked to many diseases (e.g. behaviour disorders, cancer, cardiovascular disease, diabetes mellitus and gallstones), although there are many conflicting reports. Excessive consumption of sugar may, however, cause obesity which, in turn, is associated with many of these diseases.

All authorities agree that the intake of non-milk extrinsic sugars should be reduced, as they are not an essential form of dietary energy. Indeed, they could be eliminated from the diet completely, but this is probably impractical in a western diet. The DRV for non-milk extrinsic sugars is about 60 g/day, representing 10% of total energy intake. This is an average figure for the UK population, and is based on a contribution by protein of 15% to dietary energy (which is above the RNI) (*see* Proteins *below*) and by alcohol of 5%. If alcohol is excluded from the diet, then the DRV increases to 11% of total energy. A substantial proportion (about 66%) of the sugars consumed are present in processed foods, including savouries (e.g. tomato soup, tomato sauce and baked beans). In some cases, the sugars could be removed or reduced, as their function is merely to improve a product's flavour. A re-educated palate would soon adapt to less sweet alternatives. However, in many cases, the sugar in a recipe has a specific function (e.g. as a preservative in jams, to lower the freezing point in ice-creams or to influence the texture of biscuits and cakes). The only alternative in such cases would be to select more nutritious alternatives.

Food or drink rich in sugars is used by many people as an immediate source of energy in the belief that the feelings of fatigue, commonly attributed to 'low blood sugar levels', will be relieved. In healthy, well-nourished individuals, the plasma-glucose concentration is maintained within very narrow limits, relying on the body's own stores of glycogen and fat to make up any deficit. This does not, however, alter the fact that there are some people who report hypoglycaemic symptoms that are immediately relieved by consumption of food. The condition has been labelled 'functional hypoglycaemia' as blood testing produces no evidence of chemical hypoglycaemia. Such individuals, once diabetes mellitus has been excluded, should be advised to substitute NSP-rich complex carbohydrates (particularly legumes, fruits and vegetables) for sugar-rich foods. Frequent small meals and snacks may help prevent the symptoms, although the intake of total dietary energy must be carefully controlled to avoid weight gain.

There is nothing to be gained by substituting white sugar with any of the other forms available (e.g. brown sugar, raw cane sugar, glucose syrups, honey and molasses). There is no difference between them, apart from flavour and appearance, and all have the same effects on metabolism. There are alternative methods of sweetening available (*see* Sugar substitutes *below*), but it should be borne in mind that substitutes do not play a part in reducing the basic desire for sweet foods.

Sugar substitutes

These may be derived from sugars which have been chemically altered so that they can no longer be classified as sugars, or they may be totally unrelated to sugars (artificial sweeteners) and are many times sweeter than sucrose. Artificial sweeteners possess no nutrient value at all.

Sorbitol Sorbitol is half as sweet as glucose, from which it is prepared by reduction, and has the same energy value. It also occurs naturally in some fruit and vegetables. It is used as a bulk sweetener (i.e. when a large quantity is required for cooking or sprinkling on foods) and a carbohydrate source. It is converted in the liver to fructose by the enzyme sorbitol dehydrogenase or to glucose by aldose reductase. It is absorbed slowly and incompletely from the gastro-intestinal tract and does not directly need insulin for metabolism. It is, therefore, a useful sweetener in diabetic products. Mannitol is an isomer of sorbitol used as a bulk sweetener, and has no energy value because most of it is eliminated from the body unmetabolised.

Aspartame Aspartame is 200 times as sweet as sucrose. It is derived from the amino acid phenylalanine and, therefore, should not be used by patients with phenylketonuria. Aspartame is mainly used as a table-top sweetener. As its sweetness is lost at high temperatures, its use in cooking is restricted. Aspartame is also present in soft drinks, although poor stability in solution may limit the shelf-life of products sweetened with this agent alone. It is consequently often mixed with saccharin.

Acesulfame potassium Acesulfame potassium is 130 to 200 times as sweet as sucrose, and may be used in cooking. There may be a slight after-taste when used alone.

Cyclamates Cyclamates (usually sodium cyclamate) are 30 times as sweet as sucrose, stable at high temperatures and have a good shelf-life.

Saccharin Saccharin is 200 to 500 times as sweet as sucrose. It has, on rare occasions, caused allergic or photosensitivity reactions. It has a characteristic bitter after-taste and some of the salts (e.g. saccharin sodium) are considered more palatable.

Thaumatin Thaumatin is 2000 to 3000 times as sweet as sucrose, and is the sweetest natural substance known, although it has a liquorice-like after-taste. It is a polypeptide obtained from a West African fruit, katemfe (*Thaumatococcus daniellii*). It is not used as a table-top sweetener, but is usually found in combination with other sweetening agents in processed food and drinks. It is also used in very small amounts as a flavour enhancer.

Starch

Foods with a high starch content have, in the past, been considered 'fattening' and were often avoided in weight-reducing diets. In fact, weight for weight, starch provides about the same amount of energy as proteins, and less than half the amount provided by fats. Starch is only fattening if quantities in excess of individual energy requirements are consumed. In the UK, the DoH has recommended the reduction of the contribution to dietary energy made by fats (*see* Fats and cholesterol *below*), and this may be effected by a simultaneous increase in the starch contribution. The DRV for starch, intrinsic sugars, and lactose in milk and milk products is 37% of total energy; separate individual values do not exist. The percentage total energy is based on a contribution by protein of 15% to dietary energy, and by alcohol of 5%. If alcohol is excluded from the diet, the DRV increases to 39% of total energy.

Non-starch polysaccharides

Epidemiological studies show that populations in rural Africa and other non-industrialised communities that consume a diet rich in NSP are less likely to develop certain gastro-intestinal diseases (e.g. appendicitis, constipation, diverticular disease, haemorrhoids and irritable bowel syndrome) than those in industrialised nations, where the NSP intake is substantially lower. Absence of disease has been related to large stool size, and epidemiological studies show that stool weights below 150 g/day are associated with increased risks of bowel cancer and diverticular disease. In the UK, the average stool weight is about 100 g/day. Stool consistency is equally important, and colonic disorders may be related to the increased difficulty experienced in passing small, hard stools. This is a well accepted cause of constipation and diverticular disease, and treatment of both conditions involves an increase in NSP.

Diet appears to be an important aetiological factor in the development of appendicitis, although the exact mechanism is unknown. NSP reduces colonic transit time, and this may reduce the contact time of potential carcinogens with the mucosal surface. Increased intestinal bulk may have the effect of diluting the effect of any carcinogenic elements, or there may be an anti-carcinogenic component present in the NSP.

Several trials have shown a correlation between an increase in NSP and a reduction in plasma-LDL-cholesterol concentrations, although some workers claim that it is only those foods rich in soluble NSP that have this effect. Other trials, however, have shown that there is no difference between oat bran (which contains soluble fractions) and wheat bran (which contains partly soluble fractions) in their cholesterol-lowering effect. The actual mechanism is not clear, and the reduction in concentrations may simply be a result of the replacement of saturated fats in the diet by NSP-rich foods. In general, insoluble NSP (e.g. cellulose) decrease colonic transit time and also absorb water, resulting in the production of soft stools with an increase in volume and frequency; they have little effect on plasma-cholesterol concentrations. Conversely, soluble NSP (e.g. guar gum and pectins) appear to lower plasma-cholesterol concentrations, but have little effect on bowel function. There are, however, exceptions: ispaghula and xanthan gum (both soluble NSP) have a good laxative action as well as a beneficial effect on plasma-cholesterol levels; conversely sterculia (karaya gum) has no effect on either.

The DoH (1991) proposes an average intake of NSP of 18 g/day for adults (range 12 to 24 g/day) from a variety of foods whose constituents contain it as a naturally integrated component. Young children should eat proportionately less because there is a small risk that, if eaten to excess, high-bulk NSP-rich foods may prevent sufficient energy-rich foods being eaten to ensure adequate growth. No increase in stool weight occurs with intakes of NSP above 32 g/day. Although there is no evidence of adverse effects above this level, the DoH sees no virtue in exceeding this value. Too rapid an increase in NSP intake can cause abdominal pain, flatulence and diarrhoea. The increase should be made gradually with plenty of fluid taken at the same time.

Phytic acid, present in all grains, reduces the absorption of some important minerals (e.g. calcium, magnesium, manganese, phosphorus and zinc). This may need to be taken into consideration when increasing the NSP intake in diets low in mineral content, although NSP-rich foods are usually higher in mineral content than their more refined counterparts. Increased NSP intake, therefore, usually leads to an increased intake of minerals. There is eight times the level of phytic acid in wholemeal flour when compared with white flour. However, when flour is used to make bread, phytase present in yeast destroys up to one-third of the phytic acid content of wholemeal flour and nearly all that in white flour. Yeast phytase also occurs in the gastro-intestinal tract, and there is some evidence to suggest that the body can adapt to a large intake of phytic acid. However, vegetarians (*see* Dietary needs of specific groups *below*) may experience deficiencies of those minerals (e.g. iron and zinc) bound by phytic acid for which the best dietary source is animal products.

Fats and cholesterol

Fats, like carbohydrates, are composed of carbon and hydrogen, but contain less oxygen. Chemically, they are esters of glycerol (glycerin) and fatty acids. Most are triglycerides (i.e. one molecule of glycerol is combined with three fatty acid molecules), and this is the form of most dietary fats. The essential fatty acids (formerly called vitamin F) are unsaturated linoleic acid and alpha linolenic acid; they cannot be synthesised in the body and must be obtained in the diet. Fatty acids are classified as saturated (no double bonds), monounsaturated (one double bond), or polyunsaturated (two or more double bonds). Myristic acid, palmitic acid and stearic acid are saturated fatty acids; oleic acid is a monounsaturated fatty acid that occurs in all fats. Polyunsaturated fatty acids are derived from two sources: linoleic acid (the omega-6 series) from plants, meat and poultry; or linolenic acid (the omega-3 series) from marine mammals and fish, and some plants (e.g. evening primrose oil, obtained from *Oenothera biennis*). The main source in western diets is the omega-6 series. Arachidonic acid is a polyunsaturated fatty acid present in animal fats and synthesised in the body from linoleic acid.

All natural fats contain both saturated and polyunsaturated fatty acids, but the nature and proportion of the constituent fatty acids dictate the properties of the fat. Polyunsaturated fatty acids are less stable than saturated fatty acids and react gradually with air, turning the fat rancid. Products made with polyunsaturated fats therefore have a short shelf-life. A high polyunsaturated content renders a fat liquid at room temperature, although it will generally solidify at low temperatures (e.g. in a refrigerator). In everyday terms, fats that are solid at room temperature are referred to as 'fats'; those that are liquid at room temperature are termed 'oils'. In reality, however, they are all fats. Polyunsaturated fatty acids can be converted by hydrogenation (reduction) into saturated fatty acids and *cis*- and *trans*-monounsaturated fatty acids. This process is used during the manufacture of some products to increase the shelf-life or alter the physical properties (e.g. to make hard margarines). Animal fats generally contain a higher proportion of saturated fatty acids than plant oils, although there are some exceptions (e.g. the semi-solids – coconut oil, palm kernel oil and palm oil – contain a high proportion of saturated fatty acids).

Dietary fat occurs in two forms: visible fat, which includes butter, margarine, lard, vegetable oils and the fat that can be seen on meat; or invisible fat, which includes that contained in lean meat, milk and nuts.

Cholesterol is a fat-like steroid alcohol. An essential substance, it is involved in the formation of bile acids and some steroid hormones, and is a component of cytoplasmic membranes. Most of our requirements are synthesised in the liver, and dietary sources of cholesterol have a more limited influence. Cholesterol is present in many animal products, especially in those containing saturated fats: particularly high levels are found in egg yolk, shellfish and offal (e.g. brain, liver and kidney). About half of the dietary cholesterol is absorbed. Eggs provide the main dietary source of cholesterol in the UK, of which an average of three to four are consumed per person each week.

The role of fats in the diet

The amount of energy derived from all fats is roughly equivalent. Some animal fats may contain vitamins A and D and cholesterol; vegetable fats may contain carotene (a precursor of vitamin A) and vitamin E. Fats are a more concentrated source of dietary energy than carbohydrates or proteins, and are the form in which most of the energy reserve is stored in animals and some plant seeds. Fats are the slowest of the food types to pass through the stomach (carbohydrates are the fastest), and as a consequence are said to have a 'high satiety value'.

Essential fatty acids have a variety of functions, including maintaining the function and integrity of cellular and sub-cellular membranes, the regulation of cholesterol metabolism, and as precursors of prostaglandins and arachidonic, eicosapentaenoic (EPA), and docosahexaenoic acids (DHA).

A high intake of saturated fatty acids raises plasma-cholesterol concentrations, especially LDL levels, which in turn is linked to an increased risk of cardiovascular disease. Monounsaturated fatty acids probably have no effect on plasma-cholesterol concentrations; however, linoleic acid and its derivatives reduce cholesterol levels. Linolenic acid and its derivatives inhibit clot formation and reduce plasma triglycerides. A high-fat diet has also been implicated as a risk factor for cancer (e.g. breast cancer and colorectal cancer), although there is insufficient evidence to support this. However, on the evidence that is available, it would seem prudent to moderate intake of saturated fatty acids and total fat.

Epidemiological studies show that populations consuming diets with a high ratio of dietary polyunsaturated to saturated fatty acids (P:S ratio) do not indicate a high incidence of cardiovascular disease, breast cancer or colorectal cancer. Reports that diets high in polyunsaturated fatty acids increase the risk of gallstones and pancreatic cancer have not been substantiated, and there is little evidence of association with any human disease. The effects of *cis*- and *trans*-isomers of fatty acids on the body remain to be elucidated. Several studies have shown that *trans* fatty acids, found in many margarines and products made from them (e.g. pies, cakes and biscuits) also increase plasma cholesterol levels. It would be prudent not to exceed the current estimated average level. DRVs for adults for fatty acids and total fat are given in Table 2.2.

To achieve the proposed dietary modifications, the following changes are suggested:

- use semi-skimmed or skimmed milk
- reduce consumption of fatty meat (e.g. red meat) and replace with poultry or white fish (consumption of fatty fish will increase the amount of polyunsaturated fatty acids in the diet, but will not aid the reduction of total fat intake)
- grill or microwave instead of frying

Table 2.2 Dietary Reference Values (DRVs) for fatty acids and total fat for adults as a percentage of daily total energy intake

Fatty acid	DRV	Total fat (%)
saturated fatty acids	10	11
cis-monounsaturated fatty acids	12	13
cis-polyunsaturated fatty acids[a]	6	6.5
including:		
linoleic acid	1.0	
linolenic acid	0.2	
trans-fatty acids	2	2
total fatty acids	30	32.5
total fat (i.e. the sum of fatty acid intake and glycerol)	33	35

These figures are the average intake for the population and assume that the contribution by protein to food energy is 15% and that of alcohol is 5%. Figures in parentheses indicate DRVs as a percentage of food energy excluding alcohol.

[a] Cis-polyunsaturated fatty acids should provide an average of 6% of total dietary energy for the population but individual intake should not exceed 10%.

- replace butter and lard with low fat spread and margarine and cooking oils low in saturated fatty acids.
- limit consumption of pastries, pies, cakes, biscuits, chocolate and cream.

These recommendations are not intended for children under five years of age. When a household elects to change from whole milk to low-fat forms, whole milk should still be provided for the under-fives (*see* Dietary needs of specific groups *below*).

Most nutrition labels on foods state the content or composition of fats. As a general guide, however, butter contains 59 to 63% saturated fatty acids (including *trans* fatty acids), and lard up to 48%. The amount in margarine varies according to the type of oil used and the method of production. Hard margarines can contain between 39 and 57% saturated fatty acids; soft margarines can contain between 21 and 49%. Vegetable oils vary widely in composition, and by no means are they all low in saturated fatty acids. Tropical oils have very high levels of saturated fatty acids; some of them (e.g. coconut oil and palm kernel oil) contain even more than butter. The lowest levels are found in corn oil, olive oil, peanut oil, rapeseed oil, safflower oil, soyabean oil and sunflower oil. Rapeseed oil and olive oil are the best sources of monounsaturated fatty acids (62 and 72% respectively). Total fat intake will also be reduced if food is grilled, poached, steamed or baked rather than fried.

The role of cholesterol in the body

The link between high plasma-cholesterol concentrations and ischaemic heart disease is now well established. A reduction in plasma-cholesterol concentrations by dietary modification (*see below*) appears to reduce the risk for developing atherosclerosis. In established disease, there is evidence that reducing plasma-cholesterol concentration decreases the rate of progression of atheromas and stimulates regression. High plasma-cholesterol concentrations may also contribute to the formation of gallstones. The British Hyperlipidaemia Association has recommended that adults with a plasma-cholesterol concentration between 5.2 and 6.5 mmol/litre should receive advice on diet (*see below*). Other risk factors (e.g. smoking, *see* Chapter 5, and lack of exercise, *see* Chapter 8) and those with higher levels may, in addition, require drug therapy.

Fats are water insoluble and are carried in the circulation, by various fractions of lipoproteins, to muscles for utilisation as an energy source, or to adipose tissue for storage. Very low-density lipoproteins (VLDLs) are produced in the liver, and transport endogenous triglycerides and cholesterol. Hydrolysis of VLDLs produces low-density lipoproteins (LDLs), which transport about 70% of the cholesterol in the circulation.

Most of the cholesterol utilised for various functions in the body is synthesised in the liver. When sufficient cholesterol is stored to meet these requirements, further synthesis is inhibited. There is also a mechanism that can alter the number of active LDL receptors (the uptake site) on cell membranes, so that cholesterol taken into the cells from the bloodstream is regulated. LDLs are catabolised in the liver, but if the LDL receptors are suppressed, cholesterol remains in the circulation. This process contributes to the deposition of cholesterol on the arterial walls and the formation of atheromas.

High-density lipoproteins (HDLs) are synthesised in the liver, and carry about 25% of the circulating cholesterol. They take cholesterol away from the tissues, including the arterial walls, and transport it to the liver for catabolism. Thus, a high plasma-concentration of LDL-cholesterol is harmful, whereas a high concentration of HDL-cholesterol may be beneficial. A low plasma-concentration of HDL-cholesterol may be harmful independent of the LDL-cholesterol concentration. Measurement of the total plasma-cholesterol concentration may not be a useful indicator of risk because total cholesterol includes the HDL fraction, which is protective. It is thought by some that the ratio of LDL-cholesterol to HDL-cholesterol is a more important determinant of risk for ischaemic heart disease. A high HDL level appears to be particularly beneficial in women. In addition, research work indicates that LDL-cholesterol needs to be oxidised prior to its deposition in the arteries. It is for this reason that the anti-oxidant status of the body is thought to be important, and an adequate intake of dietary antioxidants (e.g. vitamins A, C and E) can help to ensure this.

Age and sex have an effect on plasma-cholesterol concentrations. In men, the plasma concentration of LDL-cholesterol increases steadily until it peaks between 40 and 50 years of age. Women have lower plasma concentrations of LDL-cholesterol initially, but these rise after the menopause until about 60 years of age, and the final plasma concentration in women is higher than in men. This is reflected in the difference in ages between men and women at which ischaemic heart disease may occur.

Plasma-cholesterol concentrations are influenced by saturated fatty acid intake rather than dietary cholesterol, which has only a small effect. Adoption of a low-fat, high-NSP diet, increasing the polyunsaturated fatty acid content, should not necessitate any further reduction in dietary cholesterol. The DoH (1991) does not give any specific recommendations about the dietary intake of cholesterol. The average daily intake in adults is 350 to 450 mg, which would fall without any further dietary adjustment if the above guidelines were followed.

Saturated fatty acids increase plasma-cholesterol concentrations, particularly the LDL fraction, whereas polyunsaturated fatty acids lower plasma concentrations when substituted for saturated fatty acids. However, the exact mechanism of action and role in the diet of polyunsaturated fatty acids is not clear. Plasma concentrations are lowered to a greater degree by reducing saturated fatty acid intake than by increasing polyunsaturated fatty acid intake. Indeed, increasing polyunsaturated fats would increase total fat, and hence energy, intake and should not be recommended in the light of the increasing incidence of obesity.

Marine fish oils form a high proportion of the diet of Eskimos and appear to protect them from developing ischaemic heart disease. There are two omega-3 polyunsaturated fatty acids implicated, eicosapentaenoic acid (EPA) and docosahexaenoic acid (DHA). They reduce platelet numbers and aggregation. They have also been shown, in some studies, to lower the plasma concentrations of LDLs, although this is disputed, but they do appear to reduce plasma levels of triglycerides. They may also slightly raise the plasma concentrations of HDLs. The presence of EPA and DHA is rare in the average UK diet, which has a greater bias towards meat than fish. Trials in which western men were given regular supplements of fatty fish or fish oil have shown a beneficial effect on plasma-cholesterol concentrations and clotting factors. Oily fish (e.g. herring, mackerel and salmon) are good sources of these fatty acids, although those reared on fish farms are not because they do not feed on plankton, which is the original source in the food chain. Not all fish represent good sources: fatty acids are not found in freshwater fish, and only very small amounts are found in white fish. However, a regular diet of lean fish has been shown to be protective, although the mechanism of action is not clear. It has been suggested that eating fish two to three times a week may reduce the risk of ischaemic heart disease.

Fish oil supplements may be beneficial, but they should not be recommended without supervision in patients with cardiovascular disease or diabetes because there are insufficient data available on long-term use. Their antiplatelet action may cause an interaction with aspirin or anticoagulants. There may also be potential adverse effects from the long-term ingestion of excessive quantities of fatty fish. This is a particular problem in those fish derived from areas associated with problems of marine pollution, because lipophilic toxins may concentrate in the fish oils. It should also be borne in mind that the overall lifestyle of Eskimos is somewhat different from that of western people, and this may also be a significant factor in their relative freedom from ischaemic heart disease.

Proteins

Proteins are made up of carbon, hydrogen, oxygen and nitrogen; some also contain sulphur. Proteins are made up of chains of amino acids, some of which may be synthesised by the body using any excess of other amino acids available. These are the non-essential amino acids:

- alanine
- arginine
- aspartic acid
- cysteine
- glutamic acid
- glycine
- histidine
- proline
- serine
- tyrosine.

Arginine and histidine are required in infant growth and are therefore considered essential amino acids for infants. Histidine may also be essential in adults.

The eight amino acids that must be provided in the diet and are classified as essential are:

- isoleucine
- leucine
- lysine
- methionine
- phenylalanine
- threonine
- tryptophan
- valine.

Amino acids are found in both animal and plant foods, but the types and proportion vary widely. The quality of a protein is dependent on the content of essential amino acids. Animal proteins are rich in the essential amino acids and are therefore described as having a high biological value. Plant foods have a low biological value because each individual source does not provide all the essential amino acids in sufficient quantities. However, mixing several plant foods together provides the total complement required, a fact that must be borne in mind by vegetarians (*see* Dietary needs of specific groups *below*).

The role of proteins in the diet

Proteins are required for growth and repair of tissues, and any excess is used as a source of energy. However, if the diet is deficient in other energy-producing foods, proteins will be used instead, and this function supersedes their main function of tissue regeneration. It is, therefore, essential that sufficient carbohydrates and fats are provided with proteins.

In the average UK diet, one-third of the proteins ingested are derived from plant sources; the remainder comes from animal foods. Animal products (and some plant sources) also contain saturated fats, and this should be borne in mind when selecting foods. Proteins from vegetable sources are commonly associated with NSP.

The UK DoH (1991) estimates that the protein RNI for all adults of 19 years of age and over is 0.75 g/kg/day. Additional requirements are necessary during pregnancy and lactation, and for children (*see* Dietary needs of specific groups *below*). The RNI for the elderly is the same as for younger adults, but because of the small amount of lean body mass per kg body weight in the elderly, the resultant figure per unit lean body mass is higher than in younger adults. There is some evidence that very high protein intakes may aggravate poor or failing kidney function, and because there is no proven benefit of protein intakes in excess of the RNI, the DoH concludes that intakes should not exceed twice the RNI.

Vitamins

Most vitamins cannot be synthesised in the body but must be provided in the diet. They are organic compounds required by the body in small amounts for a variety of metabolic functions. They do not, however, provide any energy. They are often grouped together with minerals (*see* Minerals *below*), which are inorganic elements also essential in small amounts.

Vitamins are classified as water-soluble or fat-soluble. This property is important in consideration of their food source, stability (especially during cooking) and storage in the body. Fat-soluble vitamins (A, D, E and K) may be found in foods with a high fat content (e.g. vitamins A and D in oily fish). They are stored in the body, and ingestion of excessive quantities over a long period may be toxic. Water-soluble vitamins (the vitamin B group and ascorbic acid) are less stable than fat-soluble vitamins, particularly in boiling water. They do not accumulate in the body, and must be provided in the diet on a regular basis. Most are less toxic in large doses than fat-soluble vitamins because they are rapidly excreted in urine; nevertheless, adverse effects can occur following ingestion of large quantities over a prolonged period (*see* Vitamin and mineral supplements *below*).

Ascorbic acid

Ascorbic acid (vitamin C) is a water-soluble vitamin essential for the formation of collagen and intercellular material. It is, therefore, required for the development of bone, cartilage, and teeth, and for wound healing. Ascorbic acid is important in the maintenance of capillaries and is also involved in the regulation of intracellular oxidation-reduction potentials. Ascorbic acid is an antioxidant and is one of several dietary antioxidants that appears to be protective against a range of diseases, including cardiovascular disease, some cancers, cataract and Parkinson's disease. Man cannot synthesise ascorbic acid and must provide it in the diet.

Ascorbic acid occurs mainly in fruits and vegetables, but exists in only small amounts in milk and other animal products. It is readily absorbed from the gastro-intestinal tract. Valuable food sources include blackcurrants, Brussels sprouts, citrus fruits, green peppers and mangoes. Potatoes (especially new potatoes) contain relatively little ascorbic acid, but nevertheless represent a good source in the diet because of the amount commonly eaten. There is no ascorbic acid in whole grain cereals. The amount present in food can vary considerably depending upon the season, and large amounts are lost during cooking, storage and on exposure to light. Cutting or bruising fruits and vegetables activates the destructive ascorbic acid oxidase enzyme. The minimum amount of ascorbic acid necessary to prevent clinical scurvy is 10 mg/day; the RNI is 40 mg/day for adults, 50 mg/day for pregnant women, and 70 mg/day during lactation. High costs of seasonal foods in the winter may price foods rich in ascorbic acid out of the reach of low-income households. Supplements may be required, particularly during the winter, for vulnerable groups (e.g. the very young and the elderly, those with chronic illnesses, cigarette smokers, and pregnant and breast-feeding women).

Vitamin A

Vitamin A is a fat-soluble vitamin obtained from animal and plant sources. It is essential for growth, vision (especially night vision), and for maintenance of epithelial tissue. Deficiency of vitamin A causes xerophthalmia, a progressive disorder characterised by night blindness, corneal drying, corneal ulceration and keratomalacia. There are two main forms of vitamin A. Retinol is the form found in animal foods (e.g. liver, kidney, eggs and dairy products) and accounts for two-thirds of the vitamin A intake. The remainder is supplied by carotenoids such as beta-carotene, which are found in plants (e.g. carrots and other green or yellow vegetables). These are converted in the body to retinol, although they are less effectively utilised than animal sources. Carotenoids are antioxidants and appear to be protective against a range of diseases, including cardiovascular disease, some cancers, cataract and Parkinson's disease. There is a legal requirement in the UK to fortify all margarine with vitamin A to provide the same amount as in butter. Vitamin A is readily absorbed from the gastro-intestinal tract, although absorption may be impaired if fat or protein intake is low and in the presence of fat malabsorption. There is little lost from food during cooking, except when high temperatures are used (e.g. in frying), but vitamin A is unstable in the presence of light and oxidising agents. The RNI of vitamin A for adult males is 700 μg/day and for females 600 μg/day. Requirements increase during pregnancy and lactation although it is important not to consume excessive amounts during pregnancy (*see* Dietary needs of specific groups *below*). Excessive doses of vitamin A over a long period are toxic; acute toxicity may also occur with ingestion of high doses.

Vitamin B group

There are several water-soluble vitamins in this group which, although chemically unrelated, all act as cofactors in various enzyme reactions. They occur together in similar foods and can lead to multiple deficiency disorders in cases of low dietary intake.

Biotin

Biotin (vitamin H) is an essential coenzyme in fat metabolism, and may be supplied in sufficient quantities by bacterial synthesis in the colon. Good dietary sources of biotin are egg yolk and offal; other sources include cereals, dairy products, fish, fruits and vegetables. Deficiency is unlikely, except in the unusual circumstance of excessive consumption of raw egg-white. Egg-white contains a protein, avidin, which binds with biotin and prevents its absorption. Deficiency may also occur in long-term parenteral nutrition. No RNI has been set in the UK, although 10 to 200 mg/day has been assessed as a safe intake for adults.

Folic acid

Folic acid is a coenzyme in several metabolic processes, including nucleic acid synthesis (*see also* Vitamin B_{12} *below*). Deficiency causes megaloblastic anaemia, and may arise as a result of low dietary intake or malabsorption. Additional amounts are also required in pregnancy. Folic acid is present in liver, nuts, pulses, fresh green leafy vegetables and yeast, and is well absorbed from the gastro-intestinal tract. It is, however, readily destroyed by cooking. The RNI is 200 μg/day total folate for adults, increasing to 300 μg/day during pregnancy and 260 μg/day during lactation. However, studies have demonstrated that taking a folic acid supplement before and during pregnancy reduces the incidence of neural tube defects. The DoH recommends that all women from the time when they start to plan a pregnancy and until the 12th week of pregnancy should take a daily supplement containing 400 μg of folic acid. Women who are at particular risk of having a baby with a neural tube defect (e.g. they or their partner have parented such a child before or the woman suffers from epilepsy) should take a folic acid supplement providing 5 mg a day and this should be obtained on prescription.

Nicotinic acid and nicotinamide

Nicotinic acid and nicotinamide are both called niacin (vitamin B_3). They are converted in the body to coenzymes that are involved in electron transfer reactions in the respiratory chain, and thus play a part in the utilisation of energy from food. Deficiency causes pellagra. Nicotinic acid is formed in the body from tryptophan (an essential amino acid); food that contains tryptophan but little nicotinic acid (e.g. eggs and milk) does therefore provide the body with nicotinic acid. The RNI is calculated as nicotinic acid equivalents: it is 6.6 mg/1000 kcal for all ages, increasing to 8.9 mg/1000 kcal during lactation. RNIs in mg/day based on DRVs for energy are given in Table 2.1 above. Good dietary sources (including tryptophan-containing foods) are Cheddar cheese, eggs, fish, meat, milk, pulses and potatoes; absorption from the gastro-intestinal tract is good. Nicotinic acid and nicotinamide are heat-stable and little is lost during cooking.

Pantothenic acid

Pantothenic acid (vitamin B_5) is a component of coenzyme A involved in the metabolism of carbohydrates, fats and proteins, and thus in the release of energy from foods. Pantothenic acid is also involved in the synthesis of sterols (including cholesterol) and acetylcholine in the body. It is widely distributed in foods, including egg yolk, fresh vegetables, liver, kidney, milk, whole grain cereals and yeast, and is readily absorbed from the gastro-intestinal tract. Some may be lost during cooking. There is no RNI in the UK as deficiency is unlikely, but the current dietary intake of 3 to 7 mg/day has been assessed as a safe intake for adults.

Pyridoxine

Pyridoxine is one of three similar compounds that are referred to as vitamin B_6; the other two are pyridoxal and pyridoxamine. These compounds are converted in the body to the active forms, pyridoxal phosphate and pyridoxamine phosphate. The main function of pyridoxine is in amino acid metabolism, although it also plays a part in carbohydrate and fat metabolism. Two metabolic functions of particular note are the conversion of tryptophan to nicotinic acid and the formation of haemoglobin. Pyridoxine is also involved in enzyme reactions that control the synthesis and metabolism of most neurotransmitters (e.g. dopamine and noradrenaline). Good sources include fruits, eggs, fish, meat, potatoes and other vegetables, and whole grain cereals, although there may be some losses during cooking. Pyridoxine is readily absorbed from the gastro-intestinal tract. The dietary requirement depends on protein intake and the RNI is 15 μg/g protein per day. Absolute RNIs are given in Table 2.1 and are based upon protein providing 14.7% of dietary energy. Certain people may, however, need supplements (e.g. people who consume excessive amounts of alcohol and those taking certain drugs, including isoniazid). Excessive supplementation for long periods can cause peripheral neuropathies.

Riboflavin

Riboflavin (vitamin B_2) is involved in oxidation–reduction reactions in tissues, and therefore in the utilisation of energy from food. Deficiency results in ariboflavinosis, a disorder characterised by angular stomatitis, cheilosis, glossitis and seborrhoeic keratosis. Good sources of riboflavin include Cheddar cheese, eggs, green leafy vegetables, kidney, liver, milk and yeast extract; riboflavin is well absorbed from the gastro-intestinal tract. In the UK, about one-third of the average intake of riboflavin is derived from milk. There is some loss of riboflavin during cooking, but exposure to light causes greater losses. The RNIs for riboflavin are 1.3 mg/day for men and 1.1 mg/day for women, increasing to 1.4 mg/day during pregnancy and 1.6 mg/day during lactation. It is considered that a good mixed diet will provide the required amounts, and deficiency of this vitamin is rare in the western world.

Thiamine

Thiamine (vitamin B_1) is principally involved in the metabolism of carbohydrate, and the dietary requirements are consequently related to the carbohydrate intake and metabolic rate of an individual. Deficiency of thiamine causes beriberi. Thiamine is also involved in the metabolism of alcohol, which puts people with chronic alcohol dependence at risk of developing a deficiency syndrome (*see* Chapter 6). Valuable sources include cereals, peanuts, peas, pork, potatoes, soya beans and rice. In the UK, all flour (except wholemeal) is fortified with thiamine because so much is lost during processing. Thiamine is well absorbed from the gastro-intestinal tract. An average of 20% is lost during cooking; this percentage is even greater if the medium is alkaline. The RNI for thiamine is 0.4 mg/1000 kcal for most groups of people. Absolute RNIs for adults are given in Table 2.1.

Vitamin B_{12}

Vitamin B_{12} refers to a group of cobalt-containing compounds called cobalamins, and includes cyanocobalamin and hydroxocobalamin. Together with folic acid, vitamin B_{12} is involved in nucleic acid synthesis and is required by rapidly dividing cells, particularly those involved in erythropoiesis. It is also involved in the metabolism of amino acids and fats. Deficiency causes megaloblastic anaemias and nerve cell degeneration. The best source is liver, although vitamin B_{12} is also present in other forms of meat, dairy products, fish, fortified cereals and yeast extract. The RNI is 1.5 μg/day for adults, increasing to 2.0 μg/day during lactation. It is not found in any plant products, which puts vegetarians (*see* Dietary needs of specific groups *below*), particularly strict vegans, at risk of deficiency. Other people at risk are those who do not secrete intrinsic factor in gastric juice and are therefore unable to absorb vitamin B_{12}.

Vitamin D

Vitamin D refers to several related fat-soluble sterols that possess the common property of preventing or curing rickets. Deficiency causes rickets in children and osteomalacia in adults. The natural form is cholecalciferol (activated 7-dehydrocholesterol, or vitamin D_3), which is produced by the action of ultraviolet light on 7-dehydrocholesterol present in the oily secretions of the skin. The main commercial form is ergocalciferol (calciferol, or vitamin D_2). Active metabolites of vitamin D, produced in the liver and kidneys, regulate calcium and phosphorus homoeostasis by action in the bones, gastro-intestinal tract and kidneys.

Vitamin D is not widely distributed in foods, but is readily absorbed from the gastro-intestinal tract. Oily fish are a good source (especially fish liver), and other sources, which contain much smaller amounts, include dairy products, eggs and liver. There is a legal requirement in the UK to fortify all margarine with vitamin D. Vitamin D is not destroyed by cooking. The form present in animal products is cholecalciferol, which was formed in the living animal by the action of sunlight on its skin or obtained from its food. There are therefore seasonal variations in the quantity present. In the UK, exposure of the skin to the sun's ultraviolet radiation during the summer months builds up liver stores of vitamin D to last through the winter months, and no dietary source is necessary. However, a dietary supply is required by people who cover up their skin during the summer, or by the housebound. This is particularly important for the elderly, and the RNI for people over 65 years of age is 10 μg/day. The RNI for pregnant and breast-feeding women is also 10 μg/day (*see* Dietary needs of specific groups *below*). Vitamin D deficiency is a risk in people with dark skins, particularly those that live in Northern Britain, where exposure to sunlight can be limited. Vitamin D is the most toxic of all the vitamins in excessive doses, and results in more calcium being absorbed than excreted. The excess is deposited in the kidneys, which consequently become damaged.

Vitamin E

Vitamin E (alpha-tocopherols) refers to fat-soluble compounds, of which alpha tocopheryl acetate has the highest vitamin E activity. Vitamin E acts as an antioxidant and helps to protect cytoplasmic membranes from damage by free radicals; it is one of several dietary antioxidants which may help to protect against various diseases (e.g. cardiovascular disease, some cancers, cataract and Parkinson's disease). It also assists the absorption of fatty acids. It is essential in the diet, and neurological deficiency syndromes can occur in patients with malabsorption syndromes, genetic blood disorders or in malnourished premature infants. Good sources are cereals, eggs, peanut butter and vegetable oils (e.g. cottonseed oil, safflower oil, sunflower seed oil and wheat-germ oil). Absorption requires the presence of bile. Vitamin E is not destroyed by cooking, although it may be subject to oxidation reactions and may be destroyed by freezing. Vitamin E requirements are largely determined by the polyunsaturated fatty acid content of the diet, which varies widely, and so it is not possible to set DRVs. However, safe intakes have been assessed as above 4 mg/day for men and above 3 mg/day for women.

Vitamin K

Vitamin K refers to fat-soluble compounds essential for the formation of prothrombin and other clotting factors, and for the maintenance of a normal prothrombin concentration in the plasma. The clotting time of the blood is prolonged and spontaneous haemorrhage may occur in vitamin K deficiency. Phytomenadione (vitamin K_1) is the naturally occurring form and is found in cauliflower, cereals, egg yolk, green leafy vegetables (e.g. cabbage and spinach), peas and vegetable oils. A series of compounds called menaquinones (vitamin K_2) are synthesised by bacteria in the colon and can provide sufficient vitamin K. Absorption of vitamin K depends on the presence of bile. Losses may occur on exposure to light but little is lost during cooking. Too little information exists to establish accurate DRVs for vitamin K, but an intake of 1 μg/kg/day appears to be safe and adequate for adults. Deficiency may occur in obstructive jaundice, severe liver disease, or as a result of inadequate absorption. Oral anticoagulants (e.g. warfarin) act by antagonising the actions of vitamin K.

Minerals

There are a number of minerals that are essential for life, and all must be obtained from the diet. The major minerals are needed in relatively large amounts, whereas the trace elements, although still essential, are only required in small amounts and may be toxic in excess.

Major minerals

Calcium

The greatest proportion (99%) of calcium in the body is in the bones and teeth, where it provides strength and support. It also acts as a reserve supply that may be drawn on to fulfil its other functions, which include roles in blood clotting, enzyme activity, muscle contraction (e.g. in the heart) and nerve function. Calcium is present in bread, dairy products, dried figs, eggs, peanuts, sardines and some vegetables (e.g. aubergines, cabbage, onions and watercress). The amount of calcium absorbed from dietary sources is generally between 20 and 30%, although this varies with requirements. Absorption may be impaired by phytic acid present in NSP (*see* Carbohydrates *above*). The RNI of calcium is 700 mg/day for adults, with increased requirements during infancy, childhood, and lactation (*see* Dietary needs of specific groups *below*). There is also some evidence that additional amounts of calcium (up to 1200 mg/day in total with 800 iu of vitamin D) may help to reduce the risk of hip fracture in elderly people. Vitamin D is essential for calcium absorption, and, in British diets, calcium deficiency is more likely to be caused by vitamin D deficiency rather than dietary deficiency of calcium.

Iron

Most of the iron in the body is present in haemoglobin; the rest is in myoglobin and the cytochrome enzymes, or stored as ferritin and haemosiderin. Iron in haemoglobin is principally involved in the transport of oxygen from the lungs to the tissues. A lack of iron eventually causes iron-deficiency anaemia because the body's stores become depleted. Dietary sources include meat (especially kidney and liver), eggs, figs, dried apricots and cocoa. Small amounts may also be found in some vegetables (e.g. aubergines, cabbage, potatoes and watercress). Only about 5 to 15% of the iron in the diet is absorbed, although this increases when body stores are low or when needs are greatest (e.g. in children, or in pregnant and breast-feeding women). It is absorbed most readily from meat, which accounts for 20% of the total dietary intake. The overall absorption is increased in the presence of ascorbic acid but decreased in the presence of tannins (e.g. in tea). The RNI is 8.7 mg/day for men and postmenopausal women and 14.8 mg/day for premenopausal women. Women suffering regular heavy menstrual losses may require even more.

Magnesium

More than half the magnesium content of the body is in the skeleton. It is also present in all cells and acts as a cofactor in many enzyme systems. Magnesium is involved in muscle contractility, neuronal transmission and phosphate transfer. It is an essential constituent of chlorophyll and is found in green vegetables. Other sources include bread, eggs, meat, milk and peanuts. The average amounts ingested in the diet are 237 mg/day (women) and 323 mg/day (men). Deficiency is rare, although it may occur in chronic alcoholic dependence or in severe diarrhoea. The RNIs for magnesium are 270 mg/day for women and 300 mg/day for men, and for breast-feeding women, 320 mg/day.

Phosphorus

Phosphorus (as phosphates) has many functions in the body, ranging from provision of strength and support in bones and teeth (calcium phosphate) to liberation and utilisation of energy from nutrients. Phosphates are constituents of cells, nucleic acids, carbohydrates, some fats, and proteins, and are essential in activating some of the B-group vitamins. The RNI for phosphorus is 550 mg/day for adults and increases to 990 mg/day during lactation. Phosphorus is present in many foods and deficiency is not known.

Potassium

Potassium is the principal cation of intracellular fluid, and is involved in carbohydrate metabolism, enzyme reactions, muscle contraction and nerve conduction. Potassium is present in a wide range of foods (e.g. bread, cauliflower, cheese, eggs, meat, milk, oranges, potatoes, raisins and tomatoes). The average amounts ingested in the diet are 2.43 g/day (women) and 3.19 g/day (men), of which most is absorbed. Dietary deficiency of potassium is unlikely to occur, but losses may arise during diuretic therapy or in chronic diarrhoea, and must be corrected clinically rather than nutritionally. The RNI for potassium is 3.5 g/day for adults.

Sodium

Sodium is the principal cation of extracellular fluid, and is involved in maintaining the fluid and electrolyte balance, and in muscle and nerve activity. The sodium content is low in unprocessed foods, but high in many processed foods, especially smoked foods. Particularly high levels are found in bacon, baked beans, cornflakes, Marmite, smoked fish and soy sauce; sodium is even present in instant coffee. The main dietary intake is in the form of sodium chloride (salt), although other food additives (e.g. sodium bicarbonate present in baking powder, sodium alginate, sodium ascorbate, sodium benzoate and sodium citrate) also contribute sodium to the diet. Sodium is readily absorbed from the gastro-intestinal tract. Average intakes of sodium in the British diet are 2.35 g/day (women) and 3.38 g/day (men), with individual intakes ranging from 2 to 10 g/day. The amount required in a temperate climate is considerably less than this. The amount of sodium lost in the urine is homoeostatically regulated by the kidneys to maintain the plasma concentration within narrow limits. The amount lost in sweat is less readily controlled, and extra sodium may be required in the diet during periods of strenuous work, particularly in high temperatures, to prevent muscular cramps (*see* Chapter 8, The risks of sport and exercise). However, adaptation does occur so that the sodium concentration in sweat decreases and sodium requirements return to normal. The RNI for sodium is 1.6 g/day for adults.

Several epidemiological studies across different populations have shown a correlation between high sodium intake and hypertension. Populations with a low sodium intake do not show as marked an increase in blood pressure with age as seen in western nations. These results have been difficult to reproduce within populations, which may be a result of the difficulty in obtaining consistent blood pressure readings from individuals since these can be subject to considerable personal variation. There may also be certain inherent factors that make some people susceptible to developing hypertension in the presence of a high sodium intake. Other factors (e.g. excessive alcohol intake, lack of exercise, obesity, smoking and stress) influence the development of hypertension and need to be considered when interpreting data. People moving into areas with a high average intake of sodium do show an increase in blood pressure, although other factors may also be responsible, since a change in culture inevitably results in overall social and nutritional changes. In some studies, restriction of sodium intake has not shown significant changes in blood pressure in normotensive individuals and only a marginal improvement in mildly hypertensive subjects.

Although quantitative information on high sodium intakes is lacking, the DoH (1991) advises that intakes of more than 3.2 g/day may lead to raised blood pressure in susceptible adults.

The functions of salt in industrial food processing are similar to those of sugars (i.e. it is used as a preservative, to influence texture or to enhance flavour). Salt from this source can only be reduced if processed foods are largely avoided. There is no justification for adding salt to food during home cooking or at the table other than one of personal taste, and this source can be reduced immediately. Salt substitutes (usually potassium salts) may be used to flavour food after cooking, although these are contra-indicated in renal disease and in patients taking certain drugs (e.g. ACE inhibitors) because of the risk of hyperkalaemia. Alternative means of flavouring foods are varied and include herbs, spices, garlic, onion, pepper, vinegar, lemon juice and yoghurt. Increasing carbohydrate and NSP consumption (*see* Carbohydrates *above*) may cause a slight increase in salt consumption because it is added to bread and some breakfast cereals. However, provided that the recommendations to reduce overall consumption are followed, this should not represent a major source. For those who have to follow a low-salt diet as part of the management of a clinical condition, it is suggested that they regularly scan nutrition labels and select only those products claimed to be salt-free (although initially, professional advice from a dietician may be necessary).

Trace elements

Trace elements are widely distributed in foods and deficiency is rare because minute quantities are required. They have only recently been recognised as essential.

Chromium

Chromium is involved in carbohydrate metabolism and the utilisation of glucose, and acts as a cofactor for insulin. It is widely distributed and good food sources include liver, milk and vegetables, although the best source is brewers' yeast. A little is also present in chicken, fish, fruits and cereals. Deficiencies may arise in those consuming large quantities of sugars, fats and refined cereals. There is no RNI in the UK for chromium, but more than 25 µg/day has been assessed as a safe intake.

Cobalt

Cobalt forms part of the vitamin B_{12} molecule, and can only be utilised by man in this form.

Copper

Copper is a component of many enzyme systems, including cytochrome oxidase. It is involved in haemoglobin synthesis, nerve function, bone growth and connective tissue metabolism. The principal sources in the diet are bread, cereals, meat and vegetables. Shellfish and offal (e.g. heart, kidney and liver) are particularly rich in copper. An adequate diet provides sufficient copper and deficiency is rare, although premature infants may be at risk (*see* Dietary needs of specific groups *below*). The RNI for copper is 1.2 mg/day, increasing to 1.5 mg/day during lactation.

Fluorine

Fluorine is present in bones and teeth, and contributes to the prevention of tooth decay (*see* Chapter 3, Prevention of dental disease). The principal food sources are salt-water fish (especially those eaten whole) and tea. Small amounts may be found in cereal, meat, fruits and vegetables. Drinking water contains the ionised form, fluoride, but in variable amounts, and may be below the optimum level for temperate climates of 1 mg/litre (1 ppm). In warmer climates, where more water is likely to be consumed, the optimum level is lower. Some authorities undertake fluoridation of the water supply, and this should be borne in mind before recommending fluoride supplements for children, because excessive ingestion of fluoride can cause mottling of the teeth. No supplementation is required if the level of fluoride in the water exceeds 700 µg/litre. For levels below this, *see* Chapter 3, Prevention of dental disease. There is no RNI in the UK for fluoride, but 0.05 mg/kg/day has been assessed as a safe upper limit for infants and young children; there is no figure for adults.

Iodine

Iodine is essential for the formation of the thyroid hormones, thyroxine (T_4) and liothyronine (T_3, or tri-iodothyronine), and a deficiency may cause hypothyroidism. The best dietary source is seafood, but iodine is also found in cereals and vegetables grown in iodine-rich soil. Animal products are a source of iodine, but the amount depends on their dietary intake. In Britain, iodides are widely used in animal feeds, and thus milk and milk products are the main source; other important sources are meat and eggs. Absorption may be reduced by goitre-producing compounds present in some members of the cabbage family. Deficiency is rare, although it may occur in isolated parts of the world where the soil is iodine-deficient and the population relies totally on locally produced food. Deficiency may also occur in strict vegetarians (e.g. vegans) who consume no milk. Iodised salt may be used as a supplement if necessary. The RNI for iodine is 140 μg/day for adults. An upper intake of 17 μg/kg/day, or no more than 1000 μg/day, has been set.

Manganese

Manganese is a cofactor for the enzymes arginase and the phosphotransferases. Good sources include leafy vegetables, nuts, pulses, spices and whole grain cereals; tea is a particularly rich source. There is no RNI in the UK for manganese, but more than 1.4 mg/day has been assessed as a safe intake for adults.

Selenium

Selenium is a component of the enzyme glutathione peroxidase, and is involved in the removal of harmful peroxides. Sites of action include the blood vessels (endothelium), eye (lens), kidney, liver and erythrocytes. There is also an association with vitamin E, although the exact relationship is unclear. Selenium is an antioxidant and it is one of several dietary antioxidants which may help to protect against various diseases (e.g. cardiovascular disease, some cancers, cataract and Parkinson's disease); Good dietary sources include seafood and meat (particularly liver and kidney). Cereals also contain selenium, but the content depends on the level of selenium in the soil. In the UK, selenium intakes have fallen considerably in recent years, because bread is now made from European wheat rather than Canadian wheat, which contains a higher concentration of selenium. No deficiency disorders have been recognised in man, although a form of cardiomyopathy has been observed in children living in an area of China where the selenium content of grains and beans in the diet is low. The RNI for selenium is 75 μg/day for men and 60 μg/day for women. In high doses, selenium is toxic and a maximum safe intake from all sources has been set at 450 μg/day for adult males.

Zinc

Zinc is an essential component of many enzyme systems involved in a variety of pathways, including insulin synthesis, nucleic acid metabolism and spermatogenesis. It also has a role in wound healing and may be involved in taste sensation. Deficiency results in retarded growth in children. Most of the zinc in the body is in the bones, but this does not act as a reserve and zinc must be provided in the diet on a regular basis. Zinc is associated with proteins in foods and the best source is meat (especially liver). Other sources include cereals, cheese, eggs, milk, legumes and nuts. Absorption is poor (less than 50%), and this is further reduced in the presence of whole grain cereals and other foods with a high-NSP content, because of the presence of phytic acid. The RNI for zinc is 9.5 mg/day for men and 7 mg/day for women. In the UK, the average daily intake has been assessed as 9 to 12 mg, although vegetarians and vegans may ingest less, because of the lack of meat in their diet coupled with a high-NSP intake.

Vitamin and mineral supplements

A very popular question for pharmacists concerns the value of vitamin and mineral supplements, and their ability to boost energy and reduce the risk of disease. It must be stressed that vitamins and minerals contribute absolutely nothing to dietary energy. The only way they could possibly be of benefit is if fatigue is a symptom of a deficiency disorder, which is unlikely in a well-balanced diet. Similarly, emotional disturbances would benefit more from relaxation therapy than vitamin supplementation. However, in many instances, counselling alone may not be enough, and the value of a placebo effect should not be overlooked. For some groups, however, regular vitamin supplements are essential (*see* Dietary needs of specific groups *below*). People who consume excessive quantities of alcohol may also need vitamin supplements because alcohol provides energy and may therefore preclude the intake of more nutritious alternatives. Moreover, thiamine is required in the metabolism of alcohol, and excessive alcohol consumption causes thiamine deficiency. For a more detailed discussion on nutritional deficiency associated with excessive alcohol consumption, *see* Chapter 6.

It should, of course, be made clear to many of those requesting vitamin and mineral supplements that their best source is in a good diet. Pharmacists may offer guidance on food sources, and could also offer the following advice as to how vitamin losses from foods may be reduced:

- eat raw fruits and vegetables whenever possible
- use the minimum amount of water for cooking and avoid overcooking
- eat food as soon as possible after cooking and avoid reheating
- store fruits and vegetables in a cool dark place and use as soon as possible after purchasing
- do not use sodium bicarbonate when cooking vegetables
- cook frozen vegetables without prior thawing and for as little time as possible
- use vegetable water in stocks or gravies.

Clinical deficiency syndromes should not be treated by self-medication with vitamin supplements or by diet alone. These pathological states must be referred to medical practitioners.

There is little justification for megadoses of dietary supplements, and, in some cases, this can prove harmful. However, it is important to be aware that DRVs could change, and that amounts of vitamins and minerals recommended in the future may not be easily obtainable from the diet alone. For example, there is increasing evidence that calcium in amounts of about 1200 mg/day may be helpful in preventing hip fracture in the elderly. It would be difficult for most people to obtain this amount from the diet alone. Fat-soluble vitamins in excess of requirements are stored in the body and may produce toxic effects. Although water-soluble vitamins are not stored, megadoses may still cause adverse effects by exacerbating existing conditions or interacting with drugs. Large doses of nicotinic acid may precipitate asthmatic attacks, aggravate peptic ulceration or produce hepatotoxicity. Nicotinic acid also raises the plasma-urate concentration and may therefore aggravate gout. Folic acid supplementation is advised for the prevention of neural tube defects in pregnancy, but should otherwise not be undertaken without supervision. This is because taking the supplement could mask the clinical symptoms of megaloblastic anaemia caused by vitamin B_{12} deficiency. Patients treated with levodopa for Parkinson's disease should not be given pyridoxine supplements, even at low doses, because of an interaction with the drug unless a dopa decarboxylase inhibitor is also given. Long-term supplementation with high doses of pyridoxine has been shown to cause peripheral neuropathies.

Some water-soluble vitamins have been shown to induce a state of dependency and produce withdrawal symptoms. Megadoses increase the efficiency of the elimination pathways and, consequently, if the supplementation is stopped abruptly, the vitamin obtained naturally from dietary sources may be eliminated too quickly. For example, clinical scurvy may follow abrupt withdrawal of megadoses of ascorbic acid, and convulsions have been seen in some infants born to mothers who ingested large doses of pyridoxine during pregnancy.

Non-nutritive constituents

There are some substances present in foods and drinks that have no nutritional value at all and, indeed, may actually have adverse effects.

Caffeine

Caffeine is the most common non-nutritive constituent and has been the subject of many studies. It has been suggested as an aetiological agent for many conditions, including benign mammary dysplasias, cancers, ischaemic heart disease, spontaneous abortion and teratogenic effects. The evidence to support these claims is, in many cases, inconclusive or conflicting. Moderate consumption is not a significant risk to health. However, caffeine is known to be a central nervous system stimulant and in moderate doses (200 to 300 mg) it elevates mood. In larger doses, caffeine produces anxiety, diarrhoea, insomnia, irritability, headache, nausea and tremor. Tolerance and physical dependence occur, and withdrawal may cause symptoms of anxiety, irritability, headache, lethargy, poor concentration and restlessness.

Caffeine is automatically associated with coffee, but it is, in fact, contained in other beverages and also in chocolate. Some analgesic preparations, particularly headache tablets, contain caffeine. Boiled coffee contains considerably more caffeine than filtered or percolated coffee. The amount of caffeine present in plants varies according to species, and the final amount contained in drinks depends on the method and length of time of brewing. Average amounts of caffeine present in a mug (about 300 mL) of some drinks are:

- ground coffee 230 mg
- instant coffee 130 mg
- tea 80 mg
- cocoa or drinking chocolate 8 mg
- decaffeinated coffee or tea 6 mg
- cola 36 mg

Chocolate bars contain some caffeine, although the amount is well below that likely to cause stimulation. Dark chocolate contains about 80 mg of caffeine per 100 g bar; milk chocolate contains only about 20 mg per 100 g bar; white chocolate contains almost none.

No firm conclusions have been reached to suggest that caffeine should be avoided by the general population, although in view of its stimulant properties, only moderate intake should be recommended. Caffeine in tea and coffee has been shown to reduce the absorption of iron from food. Decaffeinated coffee may produce problems as a result of its other constituents and should also be drunk in moderation.

The biological half-life of caffeine is increased in pregnancy. It crosses the placenta and low concentrations are found in breast milk. Although no conclusive evidence suggests that caffeine has an adverse effect on the foetus, it may be prudent for pregnant women to reduce their intake. Oral contraceptives also increase the half-life of caffeine.

Theobromine

Theobromine is a muscle stimulant, and about 200 mg is present in a cup of drinking cocoa; it is also present in tea and coffee. Chocolate bars also contain theobromine, but the concentrations are unlikely to cause problems in the average amounts ingested.

Herbal teas

Herbal teas are frequently considered to be 'healthy' because claims are made that they do not contain caffeine or tannins; they are therefore considered by some as substitutes for tea or coffee. However, they too may present problems if ingested in large quantities, and the constituents should be examined critically. For example, maté contains caffeine, and blackberry contains tannins. Some herbs (e.g. juniper, pennyroyal and raspberry) stimulate the uterus and, if ingested in large quantities during pregnancy, may induce abortion. Volatile oils that may cause kidney damage are present in juniper and pennyroyal. Lovage and yarrow contain coumarins, which may potentiate the action of anticoagulants. Chamomile, golden rod, marigold and yarrow have been associated with hypersensitivity reactions in susceptible people. Comfrey, larkspur, hawthorn and uva-ursi all contain potentially toxic compounds.

Dietary needs of specific groups

Infants, children and adolescents

Infants obtain most of the nutrients they require from milk alone during the first few months of life. Those nutrients present in only small amounts in milk (e.g. iron and copper) are stored in sufficient quantities in the liver to last until the infant is weaned. Milk may be either breast milk or an infant formula milk (modified cows' milk or one derived from soya protein). It is generally considered that breast milk is the preferred option, provided the mother herself is well nourished. Unmodified cows' milk has very little copper in it and, occasionally, copper deficiency may occur in infants fed on this alone once their initial reserves have been depleted. Boiling cows' milk to render it sterile for infant consumption was formerly responsible for infantile scurvy. However, this is rarely now reported in the UK because all infant formula milks are supplemented with ascorbic acid. The energy requirements of infants increase with age (*see* Table 2.3) and, in proportion to body size, the need is greater than that of adults.

As the kidneys of very young infants are unable to cope with excessive amounts of sodium, salt should not be added to their feeds. Sugar in any form should also be used conservatively, because it has no nutritional value other than as a source of energy. Excessive sugar consumption either causes malnourishment because the child is satiated and does not feel the need for more nutritious foods, or paves the way for obesity in later life by laying down early fat deposits. Dietary sugars are also the cause of dental caries (*see* Chapter 3, Dental disease). Added salt and sugars are not necessary in a balanced diet, and the general recommendations for the population are to reduce consumption. As food taste is based largely on habit, parents may help their offspring considerably by restricting the availability of these items in the diet.

The digestive system of infants takes several months to develop, and solid weaning foods should not be introduced until the child is around four months of age. Weaning is a gradual process and infants should continue to receive milk. This may be breast milk or infant formula milks. Follow-up milks can be used from the age of six months, but whole cows' milk should not be given as a main drink until the infant is 12 months old. Whole cows' milk is a valuable energy source for young children and should not be replaced with skimmed milk in the diets of children under five years of age (*see* Fats and cholesterol *above*). However, it has been suggested by the DoH (1994) that the gradual introduction of semi-skimmed milk from two years of age onwards is acceptable, provided that sufficient energy and fat-soluble vitamins are derived from other dietary sources. From two years of age, the infant should be able to digest and metabolise a diet similar to the rest of the family. A special diet is not necessary for young children provided that they receive sufficient nutrients and dietary energy for growth. Inadequate nutrition during infancy and childhood results in stunted physical growth and possibly mental retardation, although this is more of a problem in developing countries than western nations. The demand for most nutrients increases with age up to adult levels, and should be adequately provided by a varied diet. Some nutrients are required in greater amounts during childhood and adolescence.

The RNI for calcium for infants up to 12 months of age is 525 mg/day. Thereafter, 350 mg/day (1 to 3 years), 450 mg/day (4 to 6 years), and 550 mg/day (7 to 10 years). Adolescents have the greatest requirement of all: 1000 mg/day (males) and 800 mg/day (females). Vitamin D deficiency, leading to rickets, may occur, particularly in children living in northern hemisphere countries because of inadequate exposure to sunlight during the winter months;

Table 2.3 EARS for energy and RNIs for protein for infants

Age range in months	EAR for energy MJ/day (kcal/day)	RNI[a] for protein (g/day)
Boys		
0 to 3	2.28 (545)	12.5
4 to 6	2.89 (690)	12.7
7 to 9	3.44 (825)	13.7
10 to 12	3.85 (920)	14.9
Girls		
0 to 3	2.16 (515)	12.5
4 to 6	2.69 (645)	12.7
7 to 9	3.20 (765)	13.7
10 to 12	3.61 (865)	14.9

[a] These figures, based on egg and milk protein, assume complete digestibility.
The figures for this table are derived from DoH (1991).

infants and children with dark skins are at particular risk. Rickets was a severe problem in industrial towns in the UK around 1900. As a result of the dense smog that filled the air, further reducing the available sunlight, 70% of children living in such areas developed rickets This led to the current practice of fortifying margarine and some milk products with vitamin D. Cows' milk has less vitamin D than breast milk and, consequently, all infant formula milks, including follow-on milks, are also fortified. However, cows' milk is a valuable source of calcium and should be encouraged in the diets of children over 12 months of age and adolescents.

The RNI of vitamin D is 8.5 µg/day for infants under six months of age, and 7 µg/day for children up to three years of age. Supplements of vitamin D are recommended for weaned infants and children (especially vegans, *see below*), particularly during winter months. Vitamin D is toxic in excess (*see* Vitamins *above*) and the recommended dose should not be exceeded. In general, supplements are unnecessary for breast-fed babies under six months of age unless there is a risk of low levels in the mother's milk; neither are they necessary for infants receiving 500 mL per day or more of infant formula milks.

However, premature infants may need supplements of some vitamins because they have insufficient body stores to last until weaned. The DoH (1994) recommends the administration of children's vitamin drops, containing vitamins A and D, from six months to five years of age in all infants, unless adequate vitamin status can be assured from the diet and exposure to sunlight. It is considered that older children and adolescents do not need vitamin D supplements, provided that they have adequate exposure to sunlight. (For more detailed information on infant feeding, breast and formula milks, and feeding problems, *see* Child health and immunisation, in Harman (1990). For the effect of fluoride on prevention of dental caries, and the recommendation of fluoride supplements for infants and children, *see* Chapter 3, Prevention of dental disease.)

The RNI of iron for infants from 7 to 12 months is 7.8 mg/day, which is nearly as high as that for adult men. Iron deficiency is a risk in infants and young children, and particular emphasis should be put on including iron-rich sources of food in the diet from the time of weaning. For examples of foods rich in iron, *see* Minerals *above*. The RNI for iron for adolescent males is 11.3 mg/day, which is greater than that for adult men; female adolescents require 14.8 mg/day and even more if they suffer regular heavy menstrual losses. A well mixed diet should provide enough, although deficiencies may arise in vegetarian diets (*see* Vegetarians *below*). The requirements for some of the vitamin B group also increase above the adult level during adolescence. Again, these extra nutritional demands should be met by the diet, and deficiencies are unlikely. Problems may, however, arise out of bad eating habits (e.g. regularly missing meals and indulging in inappropriate snacks ('junk' food) rich in refined carbohydrates, fats and sugars, and deficient in proteins, vitamins and minerals).

Psychological problems may occur in some adolescents as a result of undesirable weight. Fat deposits are laid down at puberty, particularly in females, and may initially be the cause of severe distress. Reassurance and counselling on appropriate diets may be of benefit at this stage. The increased energy demands of adolescence, and a consequent increase in appetite, may cause excessive fat deposits if inappropriate foods are eaten. Dietary management is essential at this stage to avoid obesity in adulthood. Anorexia nervosa is a condition that may occur in adolescents, particularly in females, and reflects a distorted perception of body size. Undereating causes dramatic weight loss, and is a serious clinical problem requiring medical intervention and, in some cases, psychiatric counselling.

Pregnant and breast-feeding women

The total nutritional and energy requirements of a growing foetus must be supplied by the mother. If these extra demands are not met, the maternal body stores will be depleted.

It has been calculated that up to 293 MJ (70 000 kcal) of additional energy is required during the nine months of pregnancy. However, considerable reductions occur in physical activity during pregnancy, which may compensate for the increased needs. The DoH (1991) recommends an increase in EAR for energy of 0.8 MJ/day (200 kcal/day) for the final trimester. Women who were underweight at the start of pregnancy may need to eat more. Up to 4 kg of fat may remain at the end of the pregnancy to supplement the extra demands of lactation. A gain in weight above the extra weight contributed by the foetus is necessary during pregnancy for the well-being of both mother and child; for a non-obese woman, the increase in weight should be of the order of 12.5 kg.

For most women, the fat gained during pregnancy will be lost afterwards, particularly if they breast-feed. This may not be the case in obese women, and they do not need to provide as much extra energy in their diets as non-obese women. They do, nevertheless, have the same requirements for an adequate supply of essential nutrients. Slimming during pregnancy without medical supervision is to be discouraged because it may result in a low-birth-weight infant. Dieting too soon after parturition may prove stressful for the mother, and should preferably be delayed until she has stopped breast-feeding. The mother's diet during pregnancy and lactation should consist of foods rich in starch, vitamins and minerals. Foods containing sugars, fats and refined carbohydrates should be limited. A marginal increase in protein intake is recommended during pregnancy: an extra 6 g a day of mixed proteins should be added to the RNI for non-pregnant women (45 g/day), making a total of 51 g/day.

Women who have several pregnancies and breast-feed each infant may suffer large losses of calcium and develop osteomalacia. In developed countries, however, osteomalacia is more likely to be a consequence of vitamin D deficiency. Lack of calcium or vitamin D in the mother may also lead to rickets in the infant (*see above*). The RNI for vitamin D during pregnancy is 10 µg/day, and since dietary sources may not supply this amount, supplements are recommended. Calcium absorption increases during pregnancy, and no additional calcium is generally needed. Calcium is widely distributed in food, and a good balanced diet should therefore supply a sufficient quantity. For examples of good dietary sources of calcium, *see* Minerals *above*. The needs of the pregnant adolescent are, however, particularly high.

The RNI for vitamin A increases to 700 µg/day during pregnancy. The amount present in a good balanced diet is considered sufficient to meet the demands of the mother, and to lay down stores in the liver of the foetus. There is evidence to suggest that ingestion of excessive amounts of vitamin A during pregnancy may have an adverse effect on the foetus. Although there are, as yet, no reported cases of adverse effects in the UK, the DoH has advised that all women who are, or who may become, pregnant should not take vitamin A supplements except under medical supervision. The advice also extends to excluding liver or liver products (e.g. liver pâté and liver sausage) from the diet because animal liver contains extremely high levels of vitamin A. Good dietary sources of vitamin A include dairy products, eggs, margarine, carrots, green vegetables and tomatoes and other fruits. Vitamin A is generally combined with vitamin D in supplements, and often occurs naturally with vitamin D (e.g. fish-liver oils); this must be taken into consideration if vitamin D supplementation is required (*see above*).

There are marginal increases in the RNIs of some of the B-group vitamins, but these are likely to be met from the diet. However, folic acid supplementation is recommended to reduce the risk of neural tube defects. A supplement providing 400 µg/day should be recommended from the time when a pregnancy is planned until the 12th week of pregnancy; this should be taken in addition to increasing the dietary intake. For examples of good sources of folic acid, *see* Vitamins *above*. If the woman is at particular risk of having an infant with a neural tube defect (because of a previous history in herself or her partner, or because she suffers from epilepsy), she should take a folic acid supplement providing 5 mg/day and this should be prescribed by the doctor. In addition, folic acid deficiency may arise in pregnancy as a result of the increased demands made by erythropoiesis. Supplements are generally recommended to prevent megaloblastic anaemia. The RNI for folate during pregnancy is 300 µg/day.

The increased needs for iron caused by pregnancy should be met without a further increase in iron intake, because of cessation of menstrual losses and by mobilisation of maternal stores and increased intestinal absorption. Supplements may be required by women with low iron stores. Women who stop eating liver during pregnancy should be advised to substitute other types of lean red meat and meat products as good dietary sources of iron; other sources of iron include bread, vegetables and fortified breakfast cereals. It has been suggested that pregnant women may need supplements of pyridoxine, although there is no official recommendation. Megadoses may even be harmful to the foetus (*see* Vitamin and mineral supplements *above*). The amount of ascorbic acid ingested should be increased during pregnancy, and the RNI is 50 mg/day. This can readily be met from the diet by increasing the amount of fresh fruits and vegetables consumed, or by supplementation.

The surplus fat remaining at the end of pregnancy is used during the first weeks of lactation to meet some of the increased energy requirements. However, additional energy intake, over and above pre-pregnancy intakes, is needed during lactation. As soon as weaning begins, the mother's energy needs begin to return to their pre-pregnancy levels and two different groups are defined for the purpose of assessing EARs for energy: Group 1 mothers are those whose breast milk supplies all or most of the infant's food for the first three months, and Group 2 mothers, whose breast milk supplies all or nearly all the infant's food for six months. EARs during lactation are:

	MJ/day (kcal/day)	
up to 1 month	1.9 (450)	
1 to 2 months	2.2 (530)	
2 to 3 months	2.4 (570)	
	Group 1	*Group 2*
4 to 6 months	2.0 (480)	2.4 (570)
over 6 months	1.0 (240)	2.3 (550)

The actual amount will vary between women depending on the weight gained during pregnancy, and those nursing more than one infant have greater requirements. To meet the increased demands, the quantity of food consumed should be increased, taking into account the same recommendations for dietary adjustments during pregnancy (*see above*). Protein consumption should increase: the RNIs during lactation are 56 g/day for the first four months of breast-feeding, and 53 g/day for the next four months.

The RNI of vitamin D is the same during lactation as for pregnancy (*see above*). However, the requirement for calcium increases and the RNI during lactation is 1250 mg/day; the RNI for vitamin A increases to 950 µg/day. A further increase in some of the B-vitamins is necessary, and may be provided in the diet. The RNI of folate is 260 µg/day, which is less than during pregnancy, but still above the RNI for non-pregnant women. The RNI of ascorbic acid increases to 70 mg/day.

The elderly

The overall nutritional requirements of the elderly are the same as those of younger adults. However, the basal metabolic rate decreases with age as a result of the decrease in the fat-free mass, which together with a reduction in physical activity, generally results in a decrease in total energy requirements. In order to avoid an increase in weight, elderly people must decrease their total intake of energy, but without upsetting the recommended contributions made by the various components (i.e. carbohydrates, fats and proteins, *see* Dietary constituents *above*). The RNI for protein for the elderly is the same as for younger adults (*see* Proteins *above*), but because of the small amount of lean body mass per kilogram body weight in the elderly, the resultant figure per unit lean body mass is higher than in younger adults. Inexpensive protein sources include milk, eggs and pulses. The requirements for vitamins and minerals do not decrease with age and an adequate intake must be maintained.

Scurvy in the elderly is not common but many elderly people do have low reserves of ascorbic acid and, as a consequence, may have symptoms of depression, fatigue, myalgia, and weakness. Wound healing may be impaired and skin may bruise easily. The deficiency may arise as a result of poor understanding of dietary requirements, restricted income or an inability to chew fruits and vegetables. These problems could be overcome by explaining the necessity of ascorbic acid in the diet, and suggesting food sources that are inexpensive or require minimal or no chewing (e.g. soft, seedless fruits, and fruit juices). Vitamin D deficiency may arise in the elderly, especially the housebound. The DoH (1991) has set the RNI for vitamin D at 10 μg/day for all people over 65 years of age. As there are few dietary sources, supplements may be necessary to achieve this level.

Elderly people, particularly those with physical disabilities (e.g. poor vision, loss of teeth, or arthritis), may have difficulty in preparing and eating food. Those living alone may have little incentive to prepare food for themselves, and financial problems may make good food prohibitively expensive for some. Malnourishment may occur as a consequence of a monotonous and nutritionally incomplete diet. Those with difficulties should be encouraged to consume nutritious foods that require minimal preparation (e.g. bread, breakfast cereals, cheese, eggs, fruit, milk and salads). Consumption of NSP-rich foods should also be encouraged to help prevent constipation. If possible, there should be one cooked meal a day, and relatives may be able to help with the provision of this. Alternatively, it may be possible to arrange a daily visit from a meals-on-wheels service. Local luncheon clubs fulfil a dual role of providing a cooked meal and an opportunity for the lonely to meet other people.

Friends, relatives, neighbours or home-helps may be called upon to do the shopping of elderly housebound or disabled people, and this provides a good opportunity to directly influence their diets. Helping elderly people to make shopping lists, explaining why some foods should be added and others rejected, could increase their nutritional knowledge and interest in food, with a consequent improvement in nutritional status.

Vegetarians

A vegetarian diet in its most basic form is one that excludes meat; most vegetarians will also not eat fish. Lacto-vegetarians allow milk and milk-products in their diet, ovo-vegetarians allow eggs, and ovo-lacto-vegetarians allow both. A vegan diet totally excludes all animal products, but the most restrictive diet of all is that of fruitarians, which allows only raw fruit and nuts.

Vegetarian diets may be adopted for reasons of health, religion, or an aversion to using animals to satisfy human needs. Some studies undertaken to compare the health of vegetarians with non-vegetarians have shown a decreased incidence of cardiovascular disease, gallstones and gastro-intestinal disorders in the former group. However, these results may be attributed to an overall difference in lifestyle and a greater awareness of health issues among vegetarians, as much as to dietary differences. A parameter that can be scientifically measured is the plasma-cholesterol concentration, and this is generally lower in vegans than non-vegetarians; vegetarians either show no difference or an intermediate level. This may be attributable to the fact that, in a vegan diet, saturated fats contribute less than 10% to the total dietary energy, which is considerably less than that of the general population. Lacto-vegetarians consume more saturated fatty acids in dairy products, although the exact amount depends on whether whole or low-fat milk is used. High plasma-cholesterol concentrations are associated with an increased risk of ischaemic heart disease.

Meat contains much fat, which is a concentrated source of energy. Avoiding all meat, therefore, reduces total dietary energy, which must be compensated for by increasing the amounts of other foods eaten. Fruits and vegetables contain mostly water and supply little energy unless eaten in great quantity; cereals and dairy products are high in energy. A reduction in dietary energy may be beneficial to some adults, particularly if overweight, but it is not desirable in growing children. Consequently, a great deal of thought and planning must go into devising vegetarian diets (especially vegan diets) for the young (*see below*). Vegetarians and vegans generally consume less refined sugars than non-vegetarians, although their total sugar consumption may be similar as a consequence of the natural sugar content of fruits. Starch and NSP intake is also higher and reflects the reduction in fat consumption. Plant proteins have a lower biological value than animal proteins (*see* Proteins *above*), and are thus unable to supply all the essential amino acids unless a mixed variety, preferably from different food groups, is consumed. For example, baked beans on toast is a combination of a pulse and a cereal, and the combination of the constituent proteins has a high biological value.

Vegans may be at risk of reduced calcium intake because of the lack of milk in their diets. Many non-animal foods do contain calcium (e.g. leafy vegetables and nuts), and judicious selection should ensure adequate dietary intake. Problems may, however, arise because oxalic acid present in some plants, and phytic acid in nuts and cereals (particularly whole grain cereals), bind with calcium and reduce absorption. Phytic acid also binds with other minerals, including iron and zinc. These minerals may already be deficient in vegan diets as the principal dietary sources are meat, eggs, and dairy products. Ascorbic acid enhances iron absorption, and consequently consumption of foods rich in ascorbic acid at the same time as plant sources of iron increases the amount absorbed. In many cases, ascorbic acid and iron occur together in plant foods.

Vegans who have inadequate exposure to sunlight run the risk of vitamin D deficiency. The few available dietary sources are all animal products and are therefore denied to them. Supplements may be necessary, especially during the winter months. Similarly, as the only natural sources of vitamin B_{12} are meat, fish, and dairy products, vegans are advised to take supplements (which are of bacterial origin). Yeast extracts, meat substitutes (e.g. derived from soya) and a number of commercially produced vegan foods are fortified with vitamin B_{12}. Iodine deficiency may be a risk in vegans, as the best sources of iodine are milk and fish. Although vegetables contain iodine, the amount in them depends on the levels in the soil.

Well-planned vegetarian and vegan diets should not pose any threat to health, and are thought to reduce risks of some diet-related diseases common in the western world. Pregnant and breast-feeding women, and children on such diets, should not suffer any adverse effects provided that the extra requirements for energy and nutrients are met (*see above*). Some authorities consider that infants should not be fed vegan diets, although others disagree. A full understanding of how the particular nutritional needs of infants and young children may be met by a vegan diet is necessary. Weaning should start at the same age in vegan infants as non-vegetarians (*see above*), but the diet should be supplemented with breast or soya infant formula milks up to two years of age to avoid calcium deficiency. The high energy requirements of young children will not be satisfied by vegetable foods unless large amounts are eaten, and this may require an increase in the number of meals per day. Alternatively, fats may be added to the diet. Riboflavin and vitamins B_{12} and D are likely to be deficient and may need supplementation, and ascorbic acid with each meal should increase the absorption of iron from food. This vitamin is widely present in fruits and vegetables, but additional supplementation may be beneficial.

The elderly may safely continue with their chosen form of diet, although adjustments may have to be made in the actual foods eaten to take into account some of the feeding problems associated with old age (*see above*). This may be more of a problem for vegans because milk and eggs, which are inexpensive, nutritious and easy to eat, are not available in their diet.

The change from a meat diet to a vegetarian diet should be gradual. Red meat should be eliminated first, then white meat, fish and, finally, eggs and dairy products, if required, adding in sufficient vegetarian foods to compensate at each stage. A sound knowledge of the nutritional requirements of the body is essential, particularly if planning diets for vulnerable groups. A wide variety of foods must be consumed to ensure that the diet provides all the necessary amino acids, vitamins and minerals, and use of food tables (*see* Dietary constituents *above*) may be of help.

Immigrants

Immigrants to a foreign country may face dietary problems. They may have special needs dictated by habit, culture or religion, or the non-availability or expense of their traditional foods, or both.

Some non-Caucasian races do not consume milk after weaning, which results in the disappearance of lactase (the enzyme required to digest lactose) from the gastro-intestinal tract. Subsequent challenge with milk causes lactose intolerance, which is characterised by watery diarrhoea and abdominal discomfort. The only remedy is to avoid milk and milk products. However, gradual re-challenging with milk products will slowly restore some lactase activity.

Asian women and children are particularly at risk of developing osteomalacia and rickets. Vegetarian diets, sometimes coupled with inadequate exposure to sunlight, may lead to vitamin D deficiency. As dietary sources of this vitamin are largely unavailable in vegetarian diets, supplements are necessary and absolutely essential for pregnant and breast-feeding women. Some traditional non-meat diets may be low in iron, and children are particularly at risk if they develop iron-deficiency anaemia (*see also* Vegetarians *above*).

The sick and convalescent

Disease or trauma (e.g. burn injuries or surgery) may result in reduced nutritional status and, if long-term, malnutrition. Metabolic losses of nitrogen may occur, particularly during infections, and disorders involving the gastro-intestinal tract may cause malabsorption of some nutrients (e.g. vitamins and minerals). Repair of tissues increases the requirements for nutrients, especially proteins. However, appetite is often poor in illness, and this further reduces the levels of essential nutrients. Consequently, body stores are depleted and tissues may become wasted.

The requirements for all nutrients increase during convalescence and are similar to those needed for growth. However, a poor appetite may not allow these demands to be met in full. Foods must be selected with care in order to satisfy the criteria of low bulk, high levels of proteins, vitamins and minerals, and sufficient energy to meet the metabolic demands of repair and replenishment. Variety is also important to stimulate an interest in food. Convalescents may appreciate small but frequent meals, rather than being overwhelmed by individual large meals. Convalescents who do not appear to be regaining their normal appetite, and especially those continuing to lose weight, may need referral. Dietary supplements may be indicated, and are available for oral, nasogastric, and intravenous routes (BNF 9.3, 9.4, and BNF Appendix 7).

Slimmers

Ideally, the energy provided in the diet should match exactly the amount of energy expended, and this is controlled reasonably accurately by appetite. Problems arise when individuals fail to adjust their diets to take into account reduced requirements occasioned by reduced activity or increasing age, or both. Previous habits are maintained, resulting in a steady, and sometimes insidious, increase in weight. An intake in excess of requirements of only 0.042 MJ (10 kcal) per day for one year would cause a weight increase of 0.5 kg. Fat is laid down under the skin and around internal organs. The physiological function of fat deposits is to provide a reserve energy supply for times of increased need. In affluent nations, such episodes rarely occur, and therefore as long as energy intake exceeds energy expended, fat will continue to accumulate.

The degree of body fatness can be measured by calculating the Body Mass Index (BMI), which is expressed as:

$$\text{weight (kg)} \div \text{height (m)}^2$$

A BMI between about 20 and 25 represents the healthy range; between 25 and 30 may be described as overweight; and over 30 is recognised as obesity. Various authorities publish charts relating ideal weight to height. These are often used by life insurance companies to assess the risk of early death, as there may be a correlation between excessive weight and ischaemic heart disease, diabetes mellitus and hypertension. Correlations have also been made with conditions that may not prove fatal, but nevertheless decrease the quality of life (e.g. gallstones, gout, joint disorders and varicose veins). Being overweight may also increase the risk of complications in pregnancy or surgery. All these risks increase with excessive amounts of body fat. A heavy body-weight caused by build up of muscles (e.g. in athletes) does not appear to be associated with increased risks from these diseases, provided that body fat is not also increased.

Actual gain in weight will eventually cease if the individual's energy intake becomes equal to output, but no weight will be lost until the equation is reversed. There may be a variety of reasons to account for the initial weight gain, not the least of which may be bad eating habits begun during childhood. Many women blame pregnancy, but the fat laid down should be utilised during the third trimester and lactation (*see* Dietary needs of specific groups *above*). Once breast-feeding has ceased, there should be no significant gain in weight above the pre-pregnancy level, provided that consumption of the extra food required for pregnancy and lactation stops. In some people, compulsive overeating may have a psychological cause (e.g. anxiety, depressive disorders or emotional disturbances), and medical help may be necessary to treat such conditions before initiating a weight-reducing diet. If boredom is the reason, a change in lifestyle as well as diet is likely to be successful. Overweight people are generally physically inactive, and a gradual and programmed increase in exercise is often of benefit (*see* Chapter 8).

Weight will be lost by providing less energy in the diet than is expended. It has been estimated that each kilogram of excess weight represents 29.3 MJ (7000 kcal) of stored energy. Reducing the daily dietary energy intake by 4.2 MJ (1000 kcal) will result in a loss in weight of up to one kg/week. However, simply reducing the total amount of food eaten without any thought given to nutrient content is not recommended, and may be dangerous if drastic reductions are continued long term. Only the energy provided by food must be reduced; the requirement for all other nutrients remains the same. An increase in physical activity (*see* Chapter 8) is also beneficial for weight control, although exercise without dietary modification will not produce significant weight loss.

Any food is fattening if enough is eaten. The difference lies in the energy density: fat-rich foods have a high energy density; fruits and vegetables have a low energy density. The most effective way of retaining a nutritious balance in a weight-reducing diet is to cut out as many energy-rich foods as possible. Alcohol and non-milk extrinsic sugars should not be consumed at all because they may contribute a significant amount to total dietary energy. The amount of visible fats in the diet (e.g. butter, margarine, cooking oils and fat on meat) should be reduced as much as possible; foods with a high content of invisible fats (e.g. red meat and whole milk) should be avoided. As overweight people are at increased risk of developing ischaemic heart disease and hypertension, they are also advised to follow the general recommendations made by the DoH (1991) for reduction of saturated fatty acids and salt in the diet (*see* Dietary constituents *above*).

Some food energy is required, and this may be supplied by complex carbohydrates (e.g. bread, pasta, potatoes and rice). NSP-rich carbohydrates (e.g. whole-grain cereals and wholemeal bread) are particularly beneficial because some people on weight-reducing diets complain of constipation. It has been postulated that NSP is also of direct benefit because it has a high satiety value and reduces the craving for other 'filling' foods, although the evidence for this is inconclusive. Fruits and vegetables are a good source of vitamins and minerals, and some NSP, and contribute little energy. The protein requirement remains the same, but low-fat sources should be chosen (e.g. lean meat and fish, low-fat cheeses, and skimmed milk).

When there is a negative energy balance, fat stores are depleted, but there is also some loss of non-fat tissues. These tissues, referred to as the fat-free mass (FFM) (*see* Carbohydrates *above*), comprise the body organs, bones, and muscles. The amount lost from the FFM increases disproportionately to the degree of the energy deficit, and can be considerable in very low calorie diets (*see below*). The basal metabolic rate (BMR) is determined by the metabolic requirements of the FFM and consequently decreases as the FFM is reduced. In addition, the energy expended as heat in response to food intake decreases as intake decreases. The net result is a decrease in energy demands, which may be perceived by the individual as failure of the diet (i.e. despite strictly adhering to it, the rate of weight-reduction slows down or ceases). A further reduction in dietary energy intake is necessary to effect further weight losses. This may be offset to some extent by increasing the levels of physical activity.

Very low calorie diets (VLCDs) are used to reduce weight rapidly by severely restricting the daily energy intake to below 2.5 MJ (600 kcal), and are intended to be used as a complete replacement for all food intake. Early VLCDs were associated with sudden death, particularly as a result of ventricular arrhythmias. It has been suggested that the cause might have been a rapid loss of protein from vital tissues as a result of too drastic a reduction in the FFM (*see above*). Such diets require careful formulation to ensure adequate amounts of good quality proteins, vitamins and minerals. The DHSS (1987) laid down guidelines on VLCDs in obesity. VLCDs should provide a minimum of 1.68 MJ (400 kcal) and 40 g of protein per day for women, and 2.1 MJ (500 kcal) and 50 g of protein per day for men; the vitamin and mineral content should also be adequate. The use of VLCDs should be restricted to the severely obese. It is absolutely essential that the instructions for use of these products are strictly followed.

VLCDs should not be used as the sole nutritional source for longer than three to four weeks, and medical advice and supervision is necessary before prolonging this period or repeating the diet. People wishing to lose weight are recommended to try traditional methods first, and should consult their doctor before embarking on a VLCD. Medical supervision, perhaps under hospital conditions, is recommended for anyone suffering with cancer, cardiovascular disease (including hypertension), diabetes mellitus, kidney disease or any other major clinical condition. Extreme caution should be exercised for those with abnormal psychological states. VLCDs are not recommended for infants, children, adolescents, pregnant or breast-feeding women, or the elderly. All members of these groups should only undertake weight-reduction under medical supervision.

It should be emphasised that the use of VLCDs does not contribute to the changes in eating behaviour necessary to maintain the reduced weight once the programme has been completed. People become overweight by consuming excessive quantities of food at meal-times, eating a lot of snacks between meals, or both. Such habits must be broken, which may initially be difficult. Dividing the total daily food allowance into several small meals rather than eating one or two large ones may be of benefit. However, it must be emphasised that strict control of quantities consumed must be exercised. It may be helpful, particularly when first embarking on a weight-reducing diet, to calculate the food allowance for the day and then divide it into portions to be consumed throughout the day. This helps establish a new routine and educates the individual with regard to the quantities that may be consumed. Once the desired weight has been reached, it must be maintained, and former eating habits must not be resumed. Permanent weight reduction, therefore, involves a total change in eating habits.

Non-compliance with a weight-reducing diet or inappropriate diets are generally the reasons for failure to lose weight. It should be stressed, particularly to people taking part in group weight-reducing schemes, that comparisons between individuals of weight lost against daily calories should not be made. Individuals vary greatly in their requirements, and a good weight-reducing diet should be designed on a personal basis. The best guide to a successful diet is loss of weight; if this ceases, dietary energy must be further reduced, while still maintaining adequate levels of nutrients for health. Patience is also essential as learning new eating habits and reduction in weight takes time.

Food safety

Microbial contamination

Food may be responsible for illness by being the vehicle for transmission of pathogenic micro-organisms, and contamination may occur at any stage of its production. The most common infecting micro-organisms are *Salmonella* spp., *Staphylococcus aureus*, *Campylobacter* spp. and *Clostridium perfringens*.

Salmonella and *Campylobacter* spp. are present in the faecal flora of many animals, and intensive farming methods increase the likelihood of contamination of meat and other animal products. In the UK, there has been a dramatic increase in contamination of hen's eggs with *Salmonella enteritidis* DT4, which infects the genital tracts of hens. Although the actual proportion of contaminated eggs is still likely to be small, the risk of salmonellosis may be high because, nationally, a large number of eggs are consumed each day. This is a particular problem in vulnerable groups (e.g. the very young and old, pregnant women and the chronically sick). The chicken carcass itself may also be contaminated. Duck's eggs are also contaminated with *Salmonella* spp. *Listeria monocytogenes* is ubiquitous, and infections in humans have increased. People at risk include the elderly and immunocompromised. This micro-organism is particularly hazardous for pregnant women because of adverse effects on the foetus. Pigs may be an important source of *Yersinia enterocolitica*, although this micro-organism could potentially contaminate many other foods as it is widely distributed in environmental water. A toxin produced by *Clostridium botulinum* causes botulism; although rare, the condition may be fatal, and is associated with improperly canned or bottled food. Other micro-organisms implicated in food-borne infections include *Bacillus cereus* and *Vibrio parahaemolyticus*; *Escherichia coli* is often responsible for traveller's diarrhoea (*see* Chapter 9, Prevention and management of conditions associated with travel).

Animals may contract infections initially from feedstuffs, grazing on contaminated land or from water, and may show clinical symptoms or be asymptomatic carriers. Transmission from other infected animals, birds or humans may occur at any stage of production (e.g. on the farm, in transit to market or in the slaughterhouse). Subsequent bad practices in handling carcasses may cause cross-contamination or additional contamination with other micro-organisms right up to the time of purchase by the consumer. Thereafter, the consumer may introduce further micro-organisms or unwittingly cross-contaminate other foods if poor practices of storage and preparation of food are adopted (*see below*).

Pathogenic micro-organisms in the human gastro-intestinal tract may be transmitted by the faecal-oral route during illness or convalescence, to both animals or food. Some individuals may remain asymptomatic carriers for years. *Staphylococcus aureus* is present as part of the normal flora in the nares, skin and perianal area of many people. This micro-organism is also found in skin lesions (e.g. boils, carbuncles and ulcers). Animals may be responsible for direct transmission of micro-organisms to food if they are allowed in food preparation areas, or via humans who prepare food with unwashed hands after handling them. Insects (e.g. flies and cockroaches) may be responsible for transporting bacteria to food, and people may pick up bacteria from fomites (e.g. towels, door handles, taps or lavatory flush chains and handles). Poor sewage and rubbish disposal allows insects and scavenger animals to come into contact with many micro-organisms.

Food-borne gastro-intestinal infections are often referred to as food poisoning, although this term also refers to poisoning with non-bacterial toxins, such as solanine in badly stored potatoes, organophosphate contamination of food, and inherently toxic foods such as fungi (e.g. *Amanita* spp.). Conversely, some food-borne gastro-intestinal infections are not traditionally classified as food poisoning (e.g. dysentery and typhoid fever). Infective cases of food poisoning that are thought to have been caused by food bought or eaten from a public place must, by UK law, be notified to the Environmental Health Officer of the local council. Dysentery and typhoid fever must also be notified, although they are covered under a different Act of Parliament.

In many cases, the inoculum required to cause clinical symptoms is large. Therefore, contamination with a few micro-organisms is unlikely to have any adverse effect. However, if food is left to stand unrefrigerated for several hours, bacteria will rapidly divide and sufficient numbers will quickly result; under optimum conditions over two million bacteria could result after seven hours from one bacterium. Some sporing bacteria (e.g. *Clostridium perfringens* and *Bacillus cereus*) are even able to form spores at high temperatures. Cooking, therefore, will kill vegetative cells but not destroy spores. Subsequent storage at optimum growth temperatures allows the spores to germinate and multiply. *Bacillus cereus* favours warm, moist conditions, and has been found to be a particular problem in cooked rice left for long periods at room temperature.

Food hygiene

It is the responsibility of everyone concerned with the manufacture and preparation of food to ensure that the risk of its contamination at every stage of production is kept to an absolute minimum. Government legislation controls the food industry (including agriculture) and retail trade; the consumer also has a responsibility, and there are government guidelines to reduce the level of food contamination in the home. This is especially important for those groups most at risk (*see above*). The appearance, taste or smell of food is not usually changed by pathogenic micro-organisms (as opposed to spoilage micro-organisms). This makes the task of those responsible for preventing infections doubly difficult, and reinforces the need for scrupulous practices of hygiene.

Stringent controls are necessary to reduce the level of contamination of raw foods, and to prevent cross-contamination between foods and recontamination of cooked food. Commercial food handlers must be well trained, and should not be allowed to prepare food if suffering from a gastro-intestinal infection. Retailers must also lay down strict guidelines covering hygiene for their premises and staff. Consumers should avoid making purchases in those food stores that do not appear to be cleaned regularly, and where the staff have dirty overalls, hands and fingernails. Careful selection of food is essential, and damaged packages, dirty or cracked eggs and food from overfilled freezers should be avoided. Dents in cans may damage the inner lacquer and allow leaching of tin particles into the food. Rusty or faulty seams may disrupt the integrity of the can, and swollen ends indicate the presence of gas inside, which could indicate contamination with *Clostridium botulinum*. The batch code stamped on the can indicates the canning date. It consists of a four-figure number, of which the first three digits indicate the day of the year (i.e. out of 365) and the fourth digit is taken from the last figure of the year (i.e. 0599 is the code for 28 February 1999). Raw food should appear fresh and use-by dates for all foods observed.

The optimum temperature for growth of pathogenic bacteria is 37°C, although the range for most is 15 to 45°C. Some may grow at even higher temperatures, albeit at a reduced rate. Most bacteria are killed above 60°C, but this does not destroy spores or toxins. Bacteria are not killed by low temperatures or freezing, but most do cease multiplication below 5°C, and refrigerators should be kept below this temperature. A notable exception is *Listeria monocytogenes*, which can multiply slowly at 4°C. Freezers should be maintained at –18°C and defrosted regularly, because this helps them to run more efficiently and economically.

Food must be transported home after purchase as quickly as possible. This is particularly important for frozen food, which must not be allowed to defrost. Fresh food is also at risk, especially on warm days or if kept in hot cars or offices for any length of time before going home; bacteria may multiply to a significant level after only one hour. Cooked food and food intended to be consumed raw should be kept well away from raw meat and fish at all times. This point is particularly important when storing food in a refrigerator. Raw meat and fish should be stored on plates or drip trays at the bottom of the refrigerator, so that the juices cannot drip onto other food.

If cooked food is not intended to be eaten straight away, it must be cooled quickly and refrigerated or frozen to reduce the chances of recontamination or germination of spores. Not all bacteria are killed by cooking, and survivors start to multiply as soon as the optimum temperature is reached. Cooling to a temperature suitable for refrigeration must not take more than one hour. Warm food placed in a refrigerator will raise the internal temperature. Similarly, warm food should never be put straight into a freezer. Cooked food should not be kept for longer than one to two days, and it must be reheated thoroughly and once only. This is particularly important with purchased cook-chill food, which has been associated with *Listeria monocytogenes* contamination. All preserved foods, once opened, should be treated in exactly the same way as fresh food.

Some foods are intended to be cooked from frozen, but dense, bulky foods (e.g. meat) must thaw completely before cooking, to allow even temperature distribution to ensure that the centre is fully cooked. It is better to thaw food in a refrigerator than at room temperature, to limit bacterial multiplication. Once thawed, food must not be refrozen without first cooking it. Bacteria start to multiply during thawing, and the population reached will become dormant if refrozen. Multiplication continues during the second thaw, so that the final population could well approach the numbers required to cause illness.

It is essential to wash all vegetables and salads thoroughly, paying particular attention to those intended to be eaten raw. *Listeria monocytogenes* has been associated with ready-to-eat salads, and it is recommended that vulnerable groups avoid these. Consumption of raw meat and fish is not advised and, because of the increase in incidence of contamination of eggs with salmonella, it is also recommended that raw eggs, or products made with them, should not be consumed by anybody. Additionally, vulnerable groups should not consume any dish prepared with fresh eggs unless both the white and yolk are hard, which signifies that they are thoroughly cooked. This does not apply to pasteurised eggs. Some soft cheeses (e.g. Brie and Camembert) and blue-vein cheeses have been associated with contamination by *Listeria monocytogenes* and should be avoided by pregnant women and immunocompromised people. It is also recommended by the DHSS (1988) that unpasteurised milk should not be given to infants and young children.

A strict stock rotation system should be followed, and all food storage cupboards and shelves kept scrupulously clean. Bacteria can multiply in food spills and may be transferred to other food in the kitchen by flies or human hands. Pets may contaminate food by transferring bacteria from their coats, paws or saliva onto work surfaces, and they should be kept out of food preparation areas. Work surfaces should be cleaned regularly, and especially between preparing meat and other food. If possible, a separate chopping board and knife should be reserved for raw meat. All cleaning cloths and tea-towels should be regularly cleaned and kept solely for use in the kitchen. Separate cleaning cloths should be used for the floor, dustbin and work surfaces, and disposable cloths and scourers changed frequently. Scrubbing brushes used to clean crockery and cutlery should not be used to scrub vegetables. Hands should always be washed before preparing food, after touching the dustbin, pets or soiled nappies, and after visiting the lavatory. All cuts, grazes and open wounds should be covered with dressings.

Home-canning or bottling of meat and vegetables is discouraged because of the difficulties involved in generating the high temperatures required to destroy the spores of *Clostridium botulinum*. However, home-bottling of most fruits may be quite safe because spores do not survive in acidic environments less than pH 4.5.

For information on prevention of food-borne and water-borne infections during travel, *see* Chapter 9, Prevention and management of conditions associated with travel.

Food additives and contaminants

The safety of food may be compromised by the presence of additives used during commercial processing or residues of chemicals used during agricultural production. Legislation exists to control these factors.

Food additives

Food additives are used in commercial food processing for a variety of reasons. For example, preservatives and antioxidants are necessary for the safety and stability of the product; others are required to facilitate processing methods. Some are not absolutely necessary and merely serve to influence the appearance or enhance the flavour of the product. Many processed products available today would simply not exist without additives and, for many others, the appearance would be considered unappetising.

In the UK, only approved additives may be used in commercially processed foods, and it is illegal to add anything that is considered unsafe. Serial numbers have been given to many of the approved additives (*see* Table 2.4); the prefix 'E' means that they have also been approved by the European Union. Food additives must be listed on food labels by category, together with the serial number or chemical name, or both. UK-approved additives that have not been allocated a number must be listed on food labels by their chemical name. Unpackaged food, beer, spirits and wine are not covered by this legislation. Not all food additives are synthetic chemicals, and many natural substances have been given E-numbers. Thus, a statement on a food label implying that the product is free from artificial additives may still have E-numbers listed (e.g. E440(a) is pectin used in jam-making). Some additives may even have a nutrient value (e.g. E300 is L-ascorbic acid).

Studies have demonstrated a relationship between additives in food and some allergic conditions (e.g. asthma and urticaria). The claimed association with behaviour disorders in children, notably hyperactivity, has been well publicised. Wide coverage of these issues in the media has led to the erroneous belief that additives with E-numbers are unsafe. The reverse, in fact, is true, and additives with E-numbers are those that have been approved for use. However, it is accepted that some individuals may react to certain approved additives, and should avoid them. Some preservatives (e.g. sulphites, E220–E227) can precipitate attacks in asthmatics, and may also cause skin rashes. Colours and antioxidants may also induce skin rashes, and tartrazine has been linked with asthma. Large doses of colours have been associated with hyperactivity in children, although the evidence is conflicting because the aetiology of behaviour disorders is probably multifactorial. It is often assumed that natural products are safer than synthetic chemicals, but this is not always the case. One study has shown that annatto (E160b), a natural food colour, precipitates more adverse reactions than synthetic tartrazine (E102). People who must avoid a specific additive should be familiar with both its name and number as either may be used on a food label.

Food contaminants

Modern methods of agriculture and animal husbandry are designed to increase the yield of food in the most economic way. For crops, this may involve the use of fungicides, herbicides or insecticides. Residues may remain on the crop after harvesting, and possibly in the soil to contaminate future crops. Continued productivity relies on the use of artificial fertilisers, which have a tendency to seep away from fields and pollute water with phosphates and nitrates. This same water may eventually find its way back to other crops if used for irrigation, or may end up as drinking water. Fruits and vegetables may be treated with chemicals after harvesting to improve the appearance and increase the shelf-life.

Animals are exposed to similar chemical contaminants in their feeds or pasture, and this may represent an indirect route to humans who subsequently eat the animal products. Growth promoters (e.g. antibiotics) are used extensively in animal feeds because they can increase the body-weight by up to 5% and improve feed conversion efficiency. This is an important economic advantage, although much concern has been expressed over their use. Drugs used to treat farm animals may also be a source of contamination in the products intended for consumption. Legislation exists to control the use of chemicals and veterinary drugs in farming practices, and to minimise the levels of residues in food. A withdrawal period is sometimes specified for licensed veterinary preparations, to indicate the time after cessation of treatment before the animal or any of its products can be used as human food. However, there is still widespread concern about the long-term effects of chemical or drug residues in food, and there is a growing trend towards food produced by so-called 'organic' methods. These methods preclude the use of any synthetic chemicals or growth promoters. It takes time for an organic farm to become viable if starting on land that was previously farmed by conventional methods and, at present, the demand for 'organic' food exceeds the supply. It is difficult to avoid consuming food that is not contaminated in some way with residues of chemicals or drugs. Even home-grown 'organic' food may become contaminated by drift of chemical spray from neighbouring allotments or gardens. Control of any atmospheric pollutants that may contaminate food is out of the hands of the individual and can only be undertaken by government legislation on a national scale. International policies may be the only means of controlling the levels of some substances.

The role of the pharmacist

Diet has become a confusing issue to the public, and is a problem likely to be presented on many occasions and in different ways to pharmacists. Prevention of diet-related diseases and overall health improvements may be facilitated by following government recommendations to

Table 2.4 Serial numbers of food additives approved for use in the UK

Colours	
E100	curcumin
E101	riboflavin
E101a	riboflavin-5′-phosphate
E102	tartrazine
E104	quinoline yellow
E110	sunset yellow FCF
E120	cochineal
E122	carmoisine
E123	amaranth
E124	ponceau 4R
E127	erythrosine
E128	red 2G
E129	allura red AC
E131	patent blue V
E132	indigo carmine
E133	brilliant blue FCF
E140	chlorophyll
E141	copper complexes of chlorophyll and chlorophyllins
E142	green S
E150a	plain caramel
E150b	caustic sulphite caramel
E150c	ammonia caramel
E150d	sulphite ammonia caramel
E151	brilliant black PN, black PN
E153	carbon black (vegetable carbon)
E154	brown FK
E155	brown HT (chocolate brown HT)
E160a	alpha-carotene; beta-carotene; gamma-carotene
E160b	annatto; bixin; norbixin
E160c	capsanthin; capsorubin
E160d	lycopene
E160e	beta-apo-8′-carotenal
E160f	ethyl ester of beta-apo-8′-carotenoic acid
E161b	lutein
E161g	canthaxanthin
E162	beetroot red (betanin)
E163	anthocyanins
E170	calcium carbonate
E171	titanium dioxide
E172	iron oxides; iron hydroxides
E173	aluminium
E174	silver
E175	gold
E180	litholrubine BK

Table 2.4 continued

Preservatives	
E200	sorbic acid
E202	potassium sorbate
E203	calcium sorbate
E210	benzoic acid
E211	sodium benzoate
E212	potassium benzoate
E213	calcium benzoate
E214	ethyl 4-hydroxybenzoate (ethyl para-hydroxybenzoate)
E215	ethyl 4-hydroxybenzoate, sodium salt (sodium ethyl para-hydroxybenzoate)
E216	propyl 4-hydroxybenzoate (propyl para-hydroxybenzoate)
E217	propyl 4-hydroxybenzoate, sodium salt (sodium propyl para-hydroxybenzoate)
E218	methyl 4-hydroxybenzoate (methyl para-hydroxybenzoate)
E219	methyl 4-hydroxybenzoate, sodium salt (sodium methyl para-hydroxybenzoate)
E220	sulphur dioxide
E221	sodium sulphite
E222	sodium hydrogen sulphite (sodium bisulphite)
E223	sodium metabisulphite
E224	potassium metabisulphite
E226	calcium sulphite
E227	calcium hydrogen sulphite (calcium bisulphite)
E228	potassium bisulphite
E230	biphenyl (diphenyl)
E231	2-hydroxybiphenyl (orthophenylphenol)
E232	sodium biphenyl-2-yl oxide (sodium orthophenylphenate)
E233	2-(thiazol-4-yl) benzimidazole (thiabendazole)
E234	nisin
E235	natamycin
E239	hexamine (hexamethylenetetramine)
E242	dimethyl dicarbonate
E249	potassium nitrite
E250	sodium nitrite
E251	sodium nitrate
E252	potassium nitrate

Table 2.4 continued

E280	propionic acid
E281	sodium propionate
E282	calcium propionate
E283	potassium propionate
E284	boric acid
E285	sodium tetraborate (borax)
E1105	lysozyme
Antioxidants	
E300	L-ascorbic acid
E301	sodium L-ascorbate
E302	calcium L-ascorbate
E304	6-*O*-palmitoyl-L-ascorbic acid (ascorbyl palmitate)
E306	extracts of natural origin rich in tocopherols
E307	synthetic alpha-tocopherol
E308	synthetic gamma-tocopherol
E309	synthetic delta-tocopherol
E310	propyl gallate
E311	octyl gallate
E312	dodecyl gallate
E315	erythorbic acid
E316	sodium erythorbate
E320	butylated hydroxyanisole (BHA)
E321	butylated hydroxytoluene (BHT)
Emulsifiers and stabilisers	
E322	lecithins
E400	alginic acid
E401	sodium alginate
E402	potassium alginate
E403	ammonium alginate
E404	calcium alginate
E405	propane-1,2-diol alginate (propylene glycol alginate)
E406	agar
E407	carrageenan
E407a	processed euchema
E410	locust bean gum (carob gum)
E412	guar gum
E413	tragacanth
E414	gum arabic (acacia)
E415	xanthan gum
E416	karaya gum
E417	tara gum
E418	gellan gum
E432	polyoxyethylene (20) sorbitan monolaurate (Polysorbate 20)

Table 2.4 continued

E433	polyoxyethylene (20) sorbitan mono-oleate (Polysorbate 80)
E434	polyoxyethylene (20) sorbitan monopalmitate (Polysorbate 40)
E435	polyoxyethylene (20) sorbitan monostearate (Polysorbate 60)
E436	polyoxyethylene (20) sorbitan tristearate (Polysorbate 65)
E440	pectins: pectin; amidated pectin
E442	ammonium phosphatides
E444	sucrose acetate isobutyrate
E445	glycerol esters of wood rosins
E460	microcrystalline cellulose; alpha-cellulose (powdered cellulose)
E461	methylcellulose
E463	hydroxypropylcellulose
E464	hydroxypropylmethylcellulose
E465	ethylmethylcellulose
E466	carboxymethylcellulose, sodium salt (CMC)
E470a	sodium, potassium and calcium salts of fatty acids
E470b	magnesium salts of fatty acids
E471	mono- and diglycerides of fatty acids
E472(a)	acetic acid esters of mono- and di-glycerides of fatty acids
E472(b)	lactic acid esters of mono- and di-glycerides of fatty acids
E472(c)	citric acid esters of mono- and di-glycerides of fatty acids
E472(d)	tartaric acid esters of mono- and diglycerides of fatty acids
E472(e)	mono- and diacetyltartaric acid esters of mono- and diglycerides of fatty acids
E472(f)	mixed acetic and tartaric acid esters of mono- and diglycerides of fatty acids
E473	sucrose esters of fatty acids
E474	sucroglycerides
E475	polyglycerol esters of fatty acids
E476	polyglycerol esters of polycondensed fatty acids of castor oil (polyglycerol polyricinoleate)
E477	propane-1,2-diol esters of fatty acids
E481	sodium stearoyl-2-lactylate

Table 2.4 continued

E482	calcium stearoyl-2-lactylate
E483	stearyl tartrate
E491	sorbitan monostearate
E492	sorbitan tristearate
E493	sorbitan monolaurate
E494	sorbitan mono-oleate
E495	sorbitan monopalmitate
Sweeteners	
E420	sorbitol; sorbitol syrup
E421	mannitol
E953	isomalt
E965	maltitol; maltitol syrup
E966	lactitol
E967	xylitol
E950	acesulfame K
E951	aspartame
E952	cyclamic acid
E954	saccharin and its sodium, potassium and calcium salts
E957	thaumatin
E959	neohesperidine DC
Non-artificial sweeteners (e.g. hydrogenated glucose syrup) do not have a category name and are listed by chemical name only.	
Others	
Acids, anti-caking agents, anti-foaming agents, bases, buffers, bulking agents, firming agents, flavour modifiers, flour bleaching agents, flour improvers, glazing agents, humectants, liquid freezants, packaging gases, propellants, release agents, sequestrants and solvents.	
E170	calcium carbonate; calcium hydrogen carbonate
E260	acetic acid
E261	potassium acetate
E262	sodium acetate; sodium hydrogen diacetate
E263	calcium acetate
E270	lactic acid
E290	carbon dioxide
E296	malic acid
E297	fumaric acid
E325	sodium lactate
E326	potassium lactate
E327	calcium lactate
E330	citric acid
E331	sodium dihydrogen citrate (monosodium citrate); disodium citrate; trisodium citrate
E332	potassium dihydrogen citrate (monopotassium citrate); tripotassium citrate
E333	monocalcium citrate; dicalcium citrate; tricalcium citrate
E334	L-(+)-tartaric acid
E335	monosodium L-(+)-tartrate; disodium L-(+)-tartrate
E336	monopotassium L-(+)-tartrate (cream of tartar); dipotassium L-(+)-tartrate
E337	potassium sodium L-(+)-tartrate
E338	orthophosphoric acid (phosphoric acid)
E339	sodium dihydrogen orthophosphate; disodium hydrogen orthophosphate; trisodium orthophosphate
E340	potassium dihydrogen orthophosphate; dipotassium hydrogen orthophosphate; tripotassium orthophosphate
E341	calcium tetrahydrogen diorthophosphate; calcium hydrogen orthophosphate; tricalcium diorthophosphate
E350	sodium malate; sodium hydrogen malate
E351	potassium malate
E352	calcium malate; calcium hydrogen malate
E353	metatartaric acid
E354	calcium tartrate
E355	adipic acid
E356	sodium adipate
E357	potassium adipate
E363	succinic acid
E380	triammonium citrate
E385	calcium disodium ethylenediamine-NNN′N′-tetra-acetate (calcium disodium EDTA)
E422	glycerol
E431	polyoxyethylene (40) stearate
E450(a)	disodium dihydrogen diphosphate; trisodium diphosphate; tetrasodium diphosphate; dipotassium diphosphate; tetrapotassium

Table 2.4 continued

	diphosphate; dicalcium diphosphate; calcium dihydrogen diphosphate
E451	pentasodium triphosphate; pentapotassium triphosphate
E452	sodium polyphosphate; potassium polyphosphate; sodium calcium polyphosphate, calcium polyphosphates
E479b	thermally oxidised soyabean oil interacted with mono- and diglycerides of fatty acids
E500	sodium carbonate; sodium hydrogen carbonate (bicarbonate of soda); sodium sesquicarbonate
E501	potassium carbonate; potassium hydrogen carbonate
E503	ammonium carbonate; ammonium hydrogen carbonate
E504	magnesium carbonate; magnesium hydrogen carbonate
E507	hydrochloric acid
E508	potassium chloride
E509	calcium chloride
E511	magnesium chloride
E512	stannous chloride
E513	sulphuric acid
E514	sodium sulphate; sodium hydrogen sulphate
E515	potassium sulphate; potassium hydrogen sulphate
E516	calcium sulphate
E517	ammonium sulphate
E520	aluminium sulphate
E521	aluminium sodium sulphate
E523	aluminium ammonium sulphate
E524	sodium hydroxide
E525	potassium hydroxide
E526	calcium hydroxide
E527	ammonium hydroxide
E528	magnesium hydroxide
E529	calcium oxide
E530	magnesium oxide
E535	sodium ferrocyanide
E536	potassium ferrocyanide
E538	calcium ferrocyanide
E541	sodium aluminium phosphate
E551	silicon dioxide (silica)

Table 2.4 continued

E552	calcium silicate
E553a	magnesium silicate synthetic; magnesium trisilicate
E553b	talc
E554	aluminium sodium silicate
E555	potassium aluminium silicate
E556	aluminium calcium silicate
E559	aluminium silicate (kaolin)
E570	stearic acid
E574	gluconic acid
E575	D-glucono-1,5-lactone (glucono-delta-lactone)
E576	sodium gluconate
E577	potassium gluconate
E578	calcium gluconate
E620	L-glutamic acid
E621	sodium hydrogen L-glutamate (monosodium glutamate; MSG)
E622	potassium hydrogen L-glutamate (monopotassium glutamate)
E623	calcium dihydrogen di-L-glutamate (calcium glutamate)
E624	monoammonium glutamate
E625	magnesium diglutamate
E627	guanosine 5′-disodium phosphate (sodium guanylate)
E630	inosic acid
E631	inosine 5′-disodium phosphate (sodium inosinate)
E632	dipotassium inosinate
E633	calcium inosinate
E634	calcium 5′-ribonucleotides
E635	sodium 5′-ribonucleotide
E640	glycine and its sodium salt
E900	dimethylpolysiloxane
E901	beeswax
E902	candelilla wax
E903	carnauba wax
E904	shellac
E912	montan acid esters
E914	oxidised polyethylene wax
E920	L-cysteine hydrochloride
E925	chlorine
E926	chlorine dioxide
E927b	carbamide
E938	argon
E939	helium
E941	nitrogen

Table 2.4 continued

E942	nitrous oxide
E948	oxygen
E953	isomalt
E999	quillaia extract
E1200	polydextrose
E1201	polyvinylpyrrolidone
E1202	polyvinylpolypyrrolidone
E1404	oxidised starch
E1410	monostarch phosphate
E1412	distarch phosphate
E1413	phosphated distarch phosphate
E1414	acetylated starch
E1422	acetylated distarch adipate
E1450	starch sodium octenyl succinate
E1505	triethyl citrate
E1518	glycerol triacetate (triacetin)-propan-1,2-diol (propylene glycol)

Food additives must be listed on food labels by category, together with the serial number or chemical name, or both. There are other food additives approved for use in the UK which have not been assigned a serial number; these must be listed on food labels by chemical name.
Numbers prefixed with an E have also been approved by the European Union.

reduce the intake of fats (particularly saturated fats), salt, non-milk extrinsic sugars and refined carbohydrates in favour of unrefined NSP-rich carbohydrates, and fruits and vegetables. DRVs have been quoted as a guide, but as it is not practical in a domestic setting to weigh all food to be eaten, or to attempt calculation of the dietary constituents, translation of the guidelines into a working diet may, at first, seem impossible.

Pharmacists may be asked to explain why the changes are necessary and how, in practical terms, they may be effected. It should be borne in mind when recommending lifestyle adjustments of any sort that people are, by nature, resistant to change. Habits may be firmly entrenched, and it may seem that change requires a lot of hard work and effort. The idea that 'anything that is good for you is bound to be unpleasant' may remove the incentive to even attempt a change. All of these obstacles may be removed by careful and thoughtful counselling. The changes do not have to be made overnight, and for many, a gradual transition, dealing with one component at a time, may be preferable.

Pharmacists should also be aware that there is a limit to how much information a person can assimilate on one occasion. For many people, the ideas discussed by the media and the recommendations made are too numerous and, in some instances, extremely vague. It is all very well to state that consumption of an item should be increased or reduced, but by how much? Acceptance of change is more likely if the number of recommendations are kept to a minimum, and if specific messages are conveyed. It is also important not to suggest too many negative changes without qualifying them in some way. If a particular component of the diet is to be avoided, pharmacists should suggest alternatives, and thereby encourage a positive attitude with a greater chance of compliance.

Diet is largely based on habit, both in terms of the food eaten and when it is eaten. One of the causes of a bad diet is missed or irregular meals. The quickest way to satisfy hunger in busy lifestyles is to resort to ready-prepared snack foods, but unfortunately many of those that are widely available contain a high proportion of fats or sugars, or both, and low concentrations of vitamins and minerals. Additionally, such foods may be low in bulk and, although they may meet energy requirements, they do not necessarily satiate. When making dietary changes, it is essential to avoid long periods without food because growing hunger may reduce will-power and cause a regression into bad habits. The value of regular meals cannot be overemphasised, and perhaps the first stage in effecting dietary changes is to establish a good routine that fits in with an individual's lifestyle. There is a growing trend towards snack meals and away from the traditional idea of sitting down two or three times a day to a full meal. There is evidence that several small meals a day may be more beneficial than a smaller number of large meals, provided that the foods consumed are selected with care and that the total daily dietary energy requirements are not exceeded.

It may be necessary, initially, to allow more time to plan and shop for food, so that alternatives to items eaten formerly may be sought. However, it should be stressed that it is not necessary to shop exclusively at 'health food' or 'whole food' shops. In fact, some of the snack foods available in such stores may be just as high in sugars and fats as any other type of snack food. Supermarkets have been changing their policies to make available more healthy foods, with a wide variety of breads, fruits and vegetables. Careful selection of food is necessary, taking note of the product labels on processed foods and using fresh, unprocessed foods whenever possible. Pharmacists can be of great help in this field by explaining how to interpret the data and clarifying the various claims on labels. New recipes may be required to meet the adjustments or alternatively old ones could be adapted. Eventually, new ways will themselves become habits, and the time spent in planning and preparing meals should revert to what it was previously.

Foods should not be considered in isolation as being healthy or unhealthy: a diet consisting solely of oranges would be just as harmful as one made up entirely of chocolate. The most important factors in a healthy diet are variety and balance. In many instances, food is used as a reward or a comfort, and the types of food chosen for this function are generally high in fats and sugars. To abolish these items totally from the diet would be quite unacceptable to many, and unnecessary in most cases. As long as such foods do not form the major part of a diet, and are really only used as infrequent treats, they are not harmful.

The most important change to be made is reduction of total fat intake and alteration of the balance between polyunsaturated fatty acids and saturated fatty acids (*see* Fats and cholesterol *above*). The amount of non-milk extrinsic sugars ingested in the diet should also be reduced (*see* Carbohydrates *above*). Reducing the consumption of fats and sugars should automatically lead to the desired changes in other aspects of diet. The reduced energy intake will cause hunger, and the deficit should be made up with complex carbohydrates. Once fruits and vegetables are added to increase variety and interest, then most of the major adjustments will have been made; there is also an added advantage in that the intake of vitamins and minerals should increase.

It is recommended that the amount of NSP in the diet should be increased. However, NSP should not be thought of as a separate component in itself, but rather as a constituent of those foods of plant origin. The amount present in different sources varies widely, and more is found in cereals than fruits and vegetables. As the intake of complex carbohydrates increases with decreasing fat consumption, NSP intake will automatically increase if the carbohydrate sources are chosen carefully. The emphasis should be towards those foods that utilise whole grains and have undergone minimal processing. A variety of NSP-rich carbohydrates should be chosen; there is no nutritional advantage to be gained by merely sprinkling all food with wheat bran. An increase in NSP intake may result initially in reduced absorption of some minerals, but this is not considered a problem for those consuming a mixed diet. Fruits and vegetables also provide NSP, especially those in which the skins are eaten. Nuts are also a good source, but meat provides absolutely none.

Pharmacists should be aware of the nutritional needs of specific groups (*see* Dietary needs of specific groups *above*). In general, however, if the recommendations for the population as a whole are followed, these groups will receive an adequately balanced diet. The main differences are focused on energy requirements, which must either be increased during periods of active growth, or reduced in the overweight and obese. Pharmacists should take an active role in helping those having difficulty with any dietary adjustments, and encourage them to discuss their problems. Those on restricted diets (e.g. vegetarians) may need to pay particular attention to the food sources of some of the nutrients that may be lacking in their diets, particularly if they are raising young children, and advice from pharmacists may be welcome.

Pharmacists are often asked to counsel and advise the overweight, and this group, in particular, is faced with an overwhelming amount of information from the media. Being overweight can be extremely distressing, both psychologically and physically, and attempting weight-reduction requires a lot of support from family, friends and healthcare professionals. Pharmacists are in an ideal position to play an active role and should encourage such people in every possible way. Pharmacists should explain the principles of energy balance and draw attention to the dangers of obesity. Each person's lifestyle is individual and it is necessary to consider how changes may best be effected with minimal disruption. Greater compliance may be achieved if the individual is actively involved in decision-making and develops an interest in nutrition. Effective dieting is a long-term commitment, and once the novelty has worn off, it is essential that bad practices are not resumed.

Pharmacists should make it clear that they are always available for advice if necessary; compliance could be encouraged by arranging weekly 'weigh-ins' if there are suitable weighing scales in the pharmacy. This would provide an opportunity to offer praise if weight has been lost and thus give an incentive to carry on, or to re-evaluate a diet if there has been no loss or even a gain in weight.

Pharmacists may be consulted about the problems relating to contamination of food with residues of chemicals and drugs used in agriculture, or micro-organisms. Food additives used in commercial processing are also of great concern to many.

References

Department of Health (1991). Dietary reference values for food energy and nutrients for the United Kingdom. *Report on Health and Social Subjects No. 41*. London: HMSO.

Department of Health (1994). Weaning and the weaning diet. Report on Health and Social Subjects No. 45. London: HMSO.

Department of Health and Social Security (1987). The use of very low calorie diets in obesity. *Report on Health and Social Subjects No. 31*. London: HMSO.

Department of Health and Social Security (1988). Present day practice in infant feeding: Third report. *Report on Health and Social Subjects No. 32*. London: HMSO.

Harman R J (1989). Dietary products. In: *Patient Care in Community Practice: A Handbook of Non-medicinal Health-care*. London: Pharmaceutical Press, 107–138.

Harman R J, ed. (1990). Child health and immunisation. In: *Handbook of Pharmacy Health-care: Diseases and Patient Advice*. London: Pharmaceutical Press, 389–403.

Further reading

Department of Health (1989). Dietary sugars and human disease. *Report on Health and Social Subjects No. 37*. London: HMSO.

Department of Health (1990). *Clean Food: Food Handlers Guide*. London: HMSO.

Department of Health (1992). The nutrition of elderly people. *Report on Health and Social Subjects No 43*. London: HMSO.

Department of Health (1994). Nutritional aspects of cardiovascular disease. *Report on Health and Social Subjects No. 46*. London: HMSO.

Department of Health (1998). Nutrition and bone health. *Report on Health and Social Subjects No 49*. London: HMSO.

Department of Health (1998). Nutritional aspects of the development of cancer. *Report on Health and Social Subjects No 48*. London: HMSO.

Department of Health (2000). Folic acid and the prevention of disease. Report on Health and Social Subjects No. 50. London: HMSO.

Food and Agriculture Organization/World Health Organization (1998). Evaluation of certain veterinary drug residues in food: forty-seventh report of the joint FAO/WHO expert committee on food additives. *WHO Tech Rep Ser 876*.

Food and Agriculture Organization/World Health Organization (1999). Evaluation of certain food additives and contaminants: forty-ninth report of the joint FAO/WHO expert committee on food additives. *WHO Tech Rep Ser 884*.

Hobbs B C, Roberts D (1987). *Food Poisoning and Food Hygiene*, 5th edn. London: Edward Arnold.

Institute of Food Science & Technology (UK) (1989). Nutritional enhancement of food. (Benefits, hazards and technical problems.) *IFST Technical Monograph No. 5*.

Mason P (2000). *Nutrition and Dietary Advice in the Pharmacy*, 2nd edn. Oxford: Blackwell Scientific Publications.

Ministry of Agriculture, Fisheries and Food (1985). *Manual of Nutrition*, 9th edn. London: HMSO.

Useful addresses

Diabetes UK
10 Queen Anne Street
London W1G 9LH
Tel: 020 7323 1531

The British Dietetic Association
5th Floor, Elizabeth House
22 Suffolk Street
Queensway
Birmingham B1 1LS
Tel: 0121 616 4900

The British Nutrition Foundation
High Holborn House
52–54 High Holborn
London WCIV 6RQ
Tel: 020 7404 6504

The Food Commission
94 White Lion Street
London N1 9PF
Tel: 020 7837 2250

Henry Doubleday Research Association
Ryton Organic Gardens
Ryton-on-Dunsmore
Coventry CV8 3LG
Tel: 024 7630 3517

Hyperactive Children's Support Group
71 Whyke Lane
Chichester
West Sussex PO19 2LD
Tel: 01903 725182

The Institute of Food Science and Technology
5 Cambridge Court
210 Shepherd's Bush Road
London W6 7NJ
Tel: 020 7603 6316

Ministry of Agriculture, Fisheries and Food (MAFF)
Whitehall Place
London SW1A 2HH
Tel: 020 7270 8080

The Vegan Society
Donald Watson House
7 Battle Road
St Leonards-on-Sea
East Sussex TN37 7AA
Tel: 01424 427393

The Vegetarian Society (UK) Ltd
Parkdale
Dunham Road
Altrincham
Cheshire WA14 4QG
Tel: 0161 928 0793

Weight Watchers (UK) Ltd
Kidwells Park House
Kidwells Park Drive
Maidenhead
Berks SL6 8YT
Tel: 0345 123000

Women's Nutritional Advisory Service
incorporating
The Pre-Menstrual Tension Advisory Service
PO Box 268
Lewes
East Sussex BN7 1QN
Tel: 01273 487366

3

Dental healthcare

Derrick Garwood

It is now reasonable to expect a set of permanent teeth to last a lifetime. This contrasts starkly with the situation only a generation ago, when it was widely accepted that teeth would have to be extracted and replaced by dentures well before old age.

Loss of teeth, other than by accident, is caused by two different pathological processes: dental caries and periodontal disease. Today, these are very rarely life-threatening, although dental treatment may produce adverse effects in susceptible individuals. Certain pre-existing medical conditions dramatically increase the risks of treatment. For example, haemophiliacs are at risk of severe haemorrhage after dental procedures. Subacute bacterial endocarditis may occur in individuals with a history of rheumatic fever or valvular heart disease, as a result of a bacteraemia following extractions, calculus removal (scaling), or other invasive dental procedures. Dental healthcare in susceptible individuals is, therefore, extremely important. However, for most people, dental disease is more of a social embarrassment and inconvenience than a serious health risk; at worst, it may reduce the quality of life if many teeth are lost.

In terms of the effects of dental disease on the community, its treatment is costly and results in loss of time from school or work. Unfortunately, most expenditure is on the treatment of established disease rather than disease prevention. In the UK, millions of teeth are extracted every year. Some extractions are unavoidable (e.g. to reduce overcrowding), but the overwhelming majority are a direct result of dental disease. An even greater number of teeth undergo some form of restorative treatment. A dedicated commitment to prevention by the individual is of far greater benefit than treatment.

The link between dental caries and diet has long been recognised. The incidence of dental caries increased significantly after the seventeenth century with the greater consumption of refined carbohydrates, particularly sugars. The prevalence in developing countries has until recently been low compared with western nations, but is now increasing as western-style diets are adopted. Conversely, the high prevalence in western nations reached a peak in the 1960s, but is now declining as a result of improved dental health education and the use of fluoride, especially in fluoride-containing toothpastes (*see* Anatomy and morphology *below*).

Surveys were conducted in the UK in 1973, 1983 and 1993 to assess the dental health of children. The results show that over 20 years, the total decay experience of children has fallen dramatically (Downer, 1994):

- by 55% at five years of age
- by 82% at eight years of age
- by 75% at 12 years of age
- by 74% at 14 years of age.

In 1973, just 7% of children of 12 years of age had no experience of permanent tooth decay; by 1993 this figure had risen to 50%. However, marked regional inequalities remain, with much higher caries rates in Northern Ireland and Scotland than in England. It also appears that the rate of decline has levelled out in children of five years of age, so there is still room for improvement.

Periodontal disease is responsible for the loss of more teeth than dental caries. Although generally considered a disease of adults, it also occurs in children. Surveys of the dental health of adults in the UK have shown that the majority of people aged over 35 with some natural teeth exhibit evidence of periodontal disease. As the incidence of caries decreases, and the number of teeth that are retained consequently increases, periodontal disease will assume even more importance as a cause of tooth loss. In the past, periodontal disease was thought to be a normal process of ageing, but this is not the case; it is totally preventable.

Dental healthcare is not new; people have attempted to clean their teeth with various abrasive substances throughout history. Ancient Egyptians used mixtures of burnt egg shells, myrrh, ox hoof ashes and pumice; ancient Greeks used granulated alabaster stone, coral powder, emery, pumice, rust and talcum; and the Romans used bones, hooves, horns, shells and myrrh. Mouthwashes have also been used throughout history, and ancient Chinese writings advocate the use of urine to treat periodontal disease. Toothbrushes or toothpicks in a variety of forms have been employed for thousands of years.

Modern dental healthcare products have evolved as understanding of the mechanism and prevention of dental disease has increased. These products have traditionally been sold through community pharmacies, so the pharmacist can make a significant contribution to dental health education. However, a sound knowledge of the properties, actions and uses of the products is essential, together with a basic understanding of dental anatomy and the aetiology of dental disease and its prevention. These subjects and the pharmacist's role are discussed below.

This chapter is concerned only with diseases that affect the teeth and gums. For diseases of other tissues in the oral cavity, the reader is referred to Disorders of the ear, nose, and oropharynx in Harman (1990).

Dental anatomy and physiology

The oral cavity is the area between the cheeks, lips, hard and soft palates, and the pharynx; the floor of the oral cavity is formed by the tongue and its associated muscles. The structures surrounding the oral cavity have important roles in:

- masticating food
- initiating digestion by salivary enzymes
- swallowing food, fluid and saliva
- respiration
- speech.

Gingivae

The gingivae (gums) cover the alveolar ridges: bony horseshoe-shaped projections of the maxillae (upper jaw bone) and mandible (lower jaw bone). The gingival epithelium is continuous with the mucous membrane of the inner surface of the lips and cheeks, and with the epithelium of the hard palate and the floor of the oral cavity. Healthy gingivae are coral pink with a stippled surface, whereas the oral mucous membrane is red. Folds of soft tissue (called fraena) run between the alveolar ridges and the lips and cheeks. Gingival connective tissue forms a collar around each tooth, and is attached to the tooth surface by junctional epithelium. There is a shallow trough (the gingival crevice, Figure 3.1) between the crest of gingival tissue and the tooth, which in health is between 0.5 and 1 mm in depth.

Teeth

The teeth are supported on the upper and lower alveolar ridges, and are important structures required for mastication. They also profoundly affect speech, and facial appearance and expression.

Anatomy and morphology

Each tooth consists of the crown, which projects through the gingivae into the oral cavity, and one or more roots, which anchor the tooth in its socket (*see* Figure 3.1). The different types of teeth (Figure 3.2) reflect their varied functions:

- incisors are chisel-shaped and used for cutting into food
- canines have a pointed surface (the cusp) for tearing and shredding food

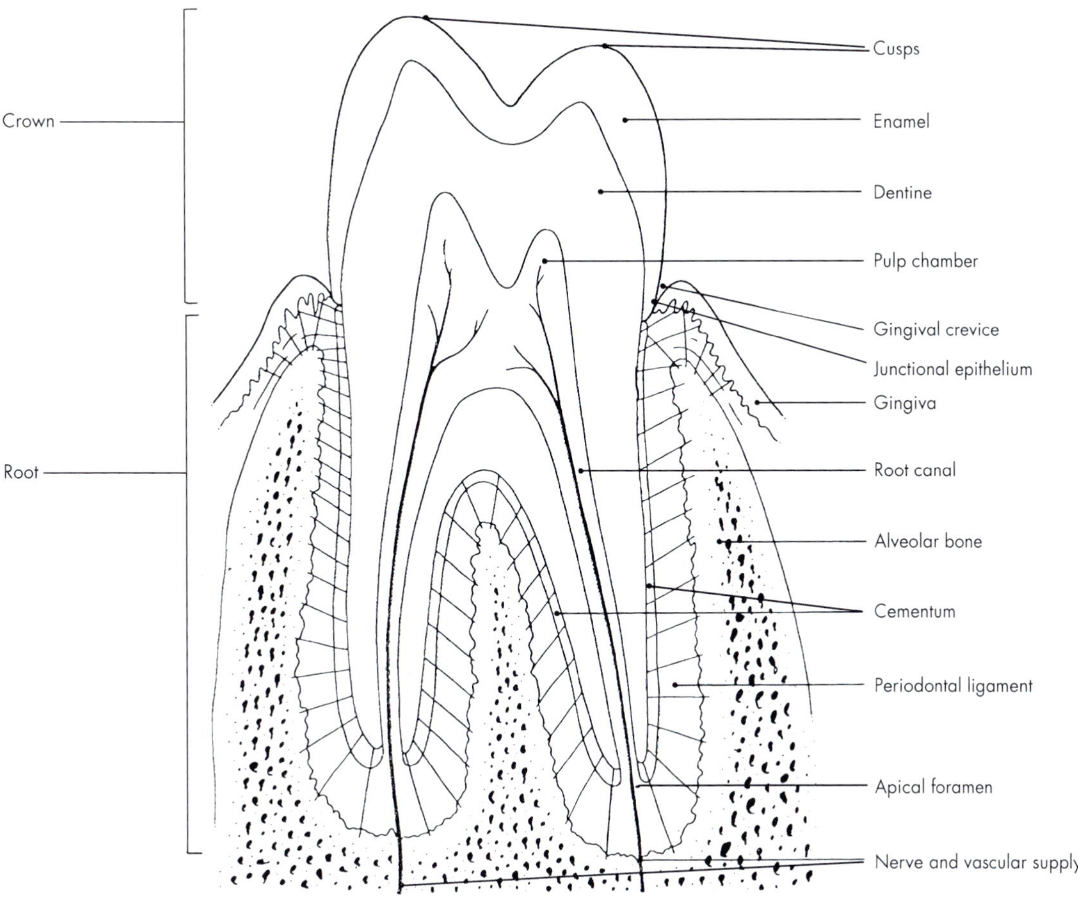

Figure 3.1 Section through a molar to show the anatomy of a typical tooth.

- premolars (bicuspids) have two cusps for chewing food
- molars have four cusps for crushing and grinding.

The cusps of premolars and molars are separated by fissures, and the whole biting surface of these teeth is called the occlusal surface. Other surfaces include:

- the palatal surface – the surface of upper teeth nearest the palate
- the lingual surface – the surface of lower teeth facing the tongue
- the labial surface – the surface of incisors and canines facing the lips
- the buccal surface – the surface of premolars and molars facing the cheeks.

The surfaces facing adjacent teeth are also important because of their association with dental caries and early periodontal disease (*see* Dental disease *below*). For effective mastication, each tooth should meet its opposing tooth in the other jaw; if one of the pair is missing, the remaining tooth is less effective because it has nothing to work against.

Incisors, canines and premolars have only one root, with the exception of the upper first premolar, which usually has two. Lower molars usually have two roots and the upper molars three, except the third molars, which may have one, two or three.

The principal component of a tooth is dentine. In the crown, this is covered with enamel; in the root, it is covered with cementum.

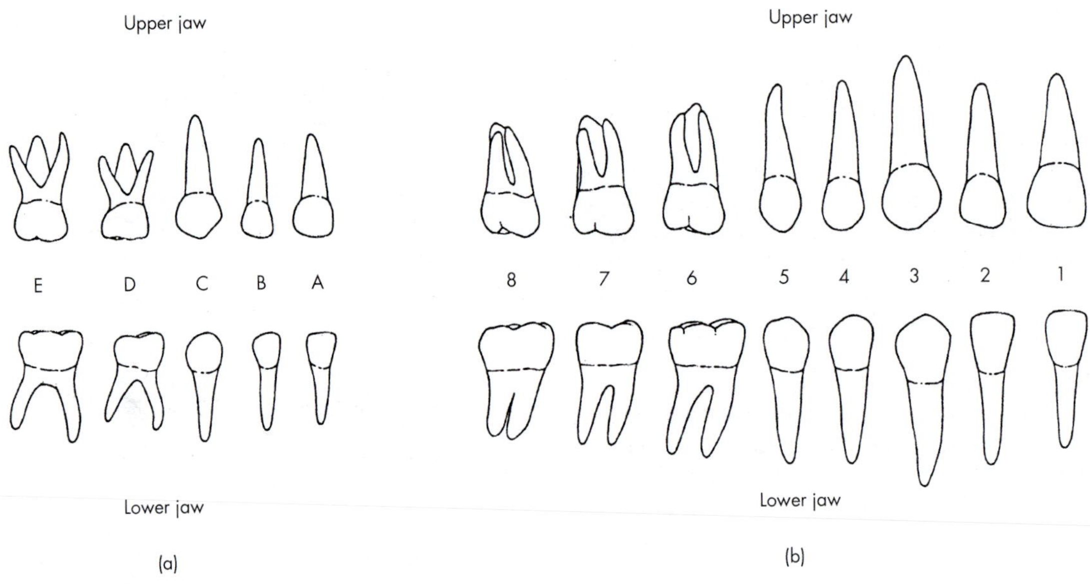

Figure 3.2 Morphology of teeth: (a) Primary dentition (b) Permanent dentition (*see* Table 3.1 for key to identification of teeth).

Dentine surrounds a cavity containing pulp; in the crown, the cavity is termed the pulp chamber; in the root, it becomes the root canal.

Dentine

Dentine is a hard yellowish substance consisting of calcium hydroxyapatite, water and an organic matrix of collagen and mucopolysaccharides. It is sensitive to touch and extremes of temperature, although the exact reason for this is not known. Dentine is deposited continuously throughout life, gradually reducing the size of the pulp cavity. This normal physiological process proceeds at a relatively slow rate compared with the secondary deposition of dentine following loss of tooth substance (e.g. as a result of dental caries, excessive wear or cavity preparation).

Enamel

Enamel is the hardest substance in the animal kingdom, and consists mainly of calcium hydroxyapatite; the remainder is water and an organic matrix similar to keratin. The primary function of enamel is to protect teeth from the forces of mastication, which would otherwise eventually wear them away. Enamel also insulates teeth from heat, cold and other pain-producing stimuli. However, it is brittle and requires the support of dentine; if this support is lost (e.g. as a result of caries) it readily fractures. Enamel is thinnest where it approaches the root, but at the cusps (or edges of incisors) it may be up to 2.5 mm thick. Its colour is governed by its thickness, and it appears lightest and almost translucent at the tooth tip. Where the enamel layer is thin, the tooth appears yellow because the dentine beneath shows through. Colour, however, does not indicate the strength of teeth, which tend to darken with age.

Cementum

Cementum is softer than dentine. It is a bone-like substance consisting of calcium hydroxyapatite and an organic matrix of collagen and mucopolysaccharides. It is laid down continuously, and the thickness may treble throughout life; some cementum is resorbed, but these areas are repaired by further deposition. Cementum attaches the tooth to the socket by means of the periodontal ligament (*see below*).

Pulp

Pulp is composed of loose areolar connective tissue richly supplied with blood vessels, lymphatic vessels and nerves, which reach it via the apical foramen. The nerve supply consists of sympathetic nerves and sensory nerves, but as the only sensory receptors are pain receptors, all stimuli are perceived as pain. Pulp becomes more fibrous and less vascular with age, and is reduced in overall size as dentine is laid down (*see above*). These changes reduce the sensitivity of teeth with age.

Periodontal ligament

A tooth is suspended firmly in its socket by the periodontal ligament, which connects the cementum to the underlying bone. Its function is to support the tooth, and protect both tooth and bone from excessive pressures during chewing and biting. The periodontal ligament is composed of collagenous fibrous connective tissue, with a rich vascular supply to provide essential nutrients to the cementum. Its nerve supply includes both touch and pain receptors, which are important in controlling mastication. Cementoblasts and osteoblasts are also present, and are responsible for laying down new cementum and bone, respectively, throughout life.

Dentition

The term dentition refers to the natural teeth and their position in the alveolar ridges. In humans, there are two dentitions: the primary dentition (deciduous teeth, baby teeth or milk teeth) and the permanent dentition. There are 20 primary and 32 permanent teeth (Table 3.1).

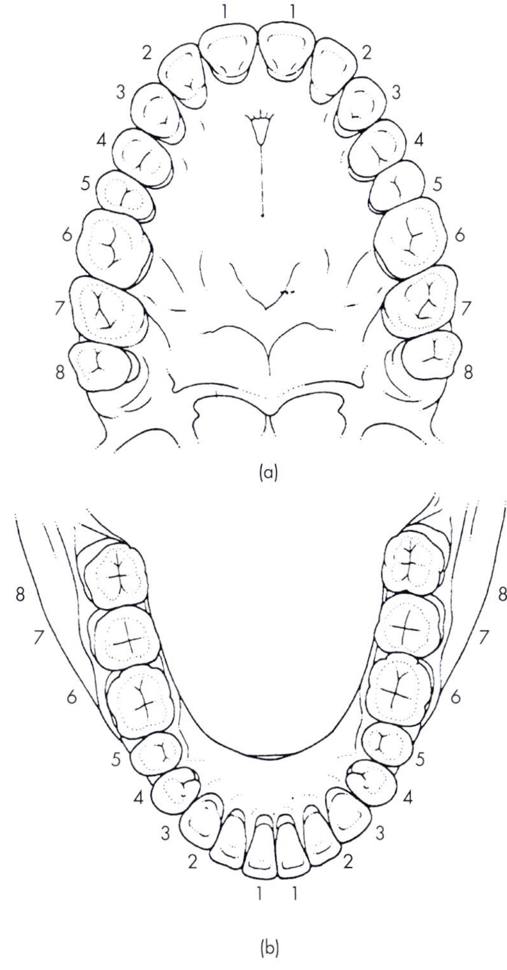

Figure 3.3 Permanent dentition: (a) Upper jaw (b) Lower jaw (*see* Table 3.1 for key to identification of teeth).

Table 3.1 The dentitions

(a) Primary dentition	(b) Permanent dentition
A (1) central incisor	1 central incisor
B (2) lateral incisor	2 lateral incisor
C (3) canine	3 canine
D (4) first molar	4 first premolar
E (5) second molar	5 second premolar
	6 first molar
	7 second molar
	8 third molar (wisdom tooth)

Dental notation

Two different systems are used to identify the teeth in their positions in the alveolar ridges. In both systems, the two dental arches are divided into four quadrants: the upper left and right, and the lower left and right (Figure 3.3).

Traditionally, a tooth has been identified by specifying the quadrant in which it is situated and the number or letter of the tooth itself; for example, the upper right six or the lower left D. Note, however, that it is always assumed that the observer is facing the patient, causing lateral inversion – as in a mirror. Thus the upper left six is written as |6 and the upper right C as C| (Figure 3.4).

Today, the International Tooth Numbering System is becoming accepted all over the world as the standard system of tooth identification. In this system, each quadrant is assigned a number (Table 3.2).

A tooth is denoted by specifying its quadrant number and then its individual number. In this system, the deciduous teeth are given the numbers 1 to 5, not the letters A to E. Thus, the upper left six now becomes 26, and the upper right C becomes 53 (Figure 3.5). In speech, these are referred to as 'two-six' and 'five-three', not 'twenty-six' and 'fifty-three'.

QUADRANT 5	QUADRANT 6
55 54 53 52 51	61 62 63 64 65
85 84 83 82 81	71 72 73 74 75
QUADRANT 8	QUADRANT 7

(a) Primary dentition

QUADRANT 1	QUADRANT 2
18 17 16 15 14 13 12 11	21 22 23 24 25 26 27 28
48 47 46 45 44 43 42 41	31 32 33 34 35 36 37 38
QUADRANT 4	QUADRANT 3

(b) Permanent dentition

Figure 3.5 The International Tooth Numbering System.

UPPER RIGHT QUADRANT	UPPER LEFT QUADRANT
E D C B A	A B C D E
E D C B A	A B C D E
LOWER RIGHT QUADRANT	LOWER LEFT QUADRANT

(a) Primary dentition

UPPER RIGHT QUADRANT	UPPER LEFT QUADRANT
8 7 6 5 4 3 2 1	1 2 3 4 5 6 7 8
8 7 6 5 4 3 2 1	1 2 3 4 5 6 7 8
LOWER RIGHT QUADRANT	LOWER LEFT QUADRANT

(b) Permanent dentition

Figure 3.4 Traditional notation system.

Table 3.2 Quadrants in the International Tooth Numbering System

1	upper right quadrant, permanent dentition
2	upper left quadrant, permanent dentition
3	lower left quadrant, permanent dentition
4	lower right quadrant, permanent dentition
5	upper right quadrant, deciduous dentition
6	upper left quadrant, deciduous dentition
7	lower left quadrant, deciduous dentition
8	lower right quadrant, deciduous dentition

Tooth development

Teeth usually start erupting at about six months of age with the emergence of the central incisors, followed at about eight months of age by the lateral incisors. The first molars appear at about 12 months of age, the canines at about 18 months of age, and the second molars at about 24 months of age, although there is wide individual variation. As a general rule, lower teeth tend to erupt before the corresponding upper teeth.

Contrary to popular belief, there is little evidence to suggest that the eruption of teeth in children causes systemic illness. As teeth begin to erupt, the shape of the jaw bone changes. Premature loss of primary teeth may adversely affect the subsequent spacing of the permanent teeth and the shape of the jaws.

Teeth are mineralised before eruption, so they are hard enough to withstand the rigours of mastication immediately. Secondary maturation takes place after eruption; this is an important process in increasing their resistance to dental caries (*see* Dental disease *below*). Fluoride is particularly important in this process (*see* Prevention of dental disease *below*).

Teeth may become stained during development as a result of:

- systemic administration of some drugs (e.g. tetracyclines)
- ingestion of high levels of fluoride (*see* Prevention of dental disease *below*)
- systemic illness (e.g. chickenpox or measles).

These are intrinsic stains and cannot be removed from the tooth substance. Pathological lesions (e.g. dental caries or pulp necrosis, *see* Dental disease *below*) may cause intrinsic stains in developed teeth.

The entire set of primary teeth is lost between six and 12 years of age, and replaced by the permanent dentition. This permanent set is not, however, completed until adulthood. The first permanent teeth to erupt are the first molars at about six years of age, followed by the central incisors at about seven years of age. The lateral incisors appear at about eight years of age, and the canines, first premolars and second premolars between nine and 11 years of age. The second molars erupt at about 12 years of age, and the third molars (wisdom teeth) between about 17 and 21 years of age. Human evolution has resulted in a jaw that may be too small to accommodate the full dentition. In many cases, the third molars do not erupt fully but remain impacted; if they cause pain and infection, they must be surgically removed. In some cases, third molars fail to develop at all.

Saliva

Approximately 0.5 to 1.5 litres of saliva is secreted each day. There are three pairs of salivary glands: the sublingual and submandibular glands in the floor of the oral cavity, and the parotid glands (the largest) below each external auditory meatus. Salivary flow is affected by various factors (e.g. age, sex, nutritional and emotional state, time of day and season of the year). Over 50% of unstimulated saliva (resting saliva) is secreted from the submandibular glands, whereas more than 50% of stimulated saliva comes from the parotid glands.

Saliva is formed from serum and composed of water (99.5%) containing dissolved proteins and inorganic ions. The proteins include glycoproteins (mucin), albumins, globulins and enzymes. One major protein component is the enzyme amylase, which initiates digestion of starch in the oral cavity. Antibacterial enzymes are also present. The watery and mucinous character of saliva is important in:

- lubricating the mucous membranes of the oral cavity
- facilitating chewing and swallowing
- assisting speech.

The inorganic component includes bicarbonate, calcium, chloride, magnesium, phosphate, potassium, sodium and sulphate.

The proportions of the different components vary with the source of the saliva and also with the flow rate. This has the effect of changing the pH of submandibular saliva from 6.47 (flow rate of 0.26 mL/minute) to 7.62 (flow rate of 3.0 mL/minute), and of parotid saliva from 5.8 (flow rate of 0.1 mL/minute) to 7.8 (flow rate of 3.0 mL/minute).

Saliva helps maintain oral hygiene and prevent dental disease in several ways:

- the bicarbonate and phosphate content acts as a buffer in acidic environments
- antibacterial enzymes (e.g. lysozyme and lactoperoxidase) control oral bacteria
- inorganic components help re-mineralise tooth enamel and prevent dental caries
- water and mucin assist the tongue in clearing food debris and bacteria from the gingivae and teeth.

Saliva is continuously secreted to keep the mucous membranes moist, but the flow increases dramatically in response to stimulation by food. Heavy secretion of saliva continues after food has been swallowed, to clean the mouth and buffer any acidic components.

Reduced secretion of saliva causes a dry mouth (xerostomia). This may result from certain medical conditions (e.g. anaemia or diabetes mellitus) or as a side-effect of some drugs (e.g. adrenergic neurone blocking drugs, antidepressants, antihistamines, antimuscarinics, anxiolytics, diuretics, hypnotics or lithium). Sympathetic stimulation in response to fear or anxiety causes the glands to stop secreting, giving a characteristic lack of saliva. Radiotherapy to the head and neck can also reduce salivary flow, although it usually returns to normal after a period of months.

Dry mouth may be relieved by administering Artificial Saliva DPF, an inert, slightly viscous, aqueous liquid containing sodium chloride, hypromellose '4500', benzalkonium chloride, saccharin sodium, thymol, peppermint oil, spearmint oil and amaranth solution. Alternative formulations may be used, and several commercial preparations are available. Frequent sips of cool drinks and sucking pieces of ice or sugar-free pastilles may also be of value.

Dental disease

Two distinct dental diseases may ultimately result in loss of teeth: dental caries and periodontal disease. Both diseases can occur at any age, but dental caries is generally more prevalent in children, and periodontal disease in adults. The aetiology of each disease is different, but the common factor is the presence of bacteria in dental plaque.

Plaque

Plaque is a film of soft material that forms on the teeth, gingivae, restorations and orthodontic appliances. It is composed predominantly of micro-organisms, but other constituents include:

- dietary carbohydrates
- organic acids formed by the bacterial metabolism of carbohydrates
- glucans (dextrans) resulting from the metabolism of dietary carbohydrates by streptococci
- proteins (including enzymes) from saliva
- leucocytes
- toxins from Gram-negative bacteria.

The first stage of plaque formation is the development of the salivary pellicle, a thin layer of mucoproteins derived from the glycoproteins of saliva. Mucoproteins are unstable in solution and adsorb to hydroxyapatite in tooth enamel. Pellicle formation begins immediately after cleaning the teeth, and the whole of the crown, except areas exposed to friction, becomes covered. The pellicle readily takes up extrinsic stains (*see below*). These are not necessarily harmful to the teeth, but are unattractive and generally considered socially unacceptable. The pellicle is very quickly colonised by commensal bacteria to form plaque.

Streptococcus spp. are usually the first bacteria to form colonies on the salivary pellicle, after about three to eight hours. *Streptococcus mutans* is of particular importance. *Actinomyces* spp. may also be found at this stage. After 24 hours, other species, including Gram-negative anaerobes, are attracted and start to multiply. The bacterial composition continues to become more complex, and the earlier species of colonising microorganisms assume less importance. Plaque reaches its mature state after about seven days. Micro-organisms make up about 70%, although the exact composition varies from one area of the oral cavity to another, depending upon the micro-environment and accessibility for cleaning. Mature plaque has a different role from new plaque in the aetiology of dental disease.

Food is not essential for plaque formation, but the presence of dietary sugars, especially sucrose, increases its rate of formation and thickness. Bacteria utilise sugars as an energy substrate, producing extracellular mucilaginous polysaccharides (glucans), which provide the plaque matrix and facilitate the firm adhesion of plaque to the tooth surface.

Plaque is highly tenacious and can only be removed from the teeth by mechanical means (*see* Prevention of dental disease *below*). It forms rapidly over all tooth surfaces after cleaning, and is virtually always present in areas that are difficult to clean. Plaque can only be detected during the initial stages of formation by using disclosing agents (*see* Prevention of dental disease *below*). However, if deposits are allowed to build up, it becomes clearly visible. In the early stages of development, plaque is thought to be cariogenic; mature plaque, however, is more likely to influence the development of periodontal disease.

Staining of the salivary pellicle or plaque may occur. Such extrinsic stains can be removed and should not be confused with permanent intrinsic stains that are part of the tooth substance (*see* Anatomy and morphology *above*). The commonest extrinsic stain is tar from tobacco, usually found on the lingual surfaces of the lower teeth and ranging in colour from light brown to black. The degree of staining generally reflects the standard of oral hygiene rather than the amount of tobacco smoked. Brown-black stains may occur following use of chlorhexidine mouthwashes, and plaque may become stained a dull yellow by food dyes. Children sometimes have black or green stains; these are thought to be derived from chromogenic bacteria.

Calculus

Dental calculus (tartar or scale) is mineralised plaque, which may occur in any area of the mouth. Prevalence is high in most populations and increases over 30 years of age. Calculus is composed of inorganic salts (70%) plus organic material and micro-organisms (30%). Composition varies with location and the age of the calculus. The organic constituents are similar to those of plaque, and the micro-organisms comparable to those in mature plaque.

Plaque acts as an organic matrix for calculus formation, although the exact mechanism is unknown; it is possible that a plaque component acts as a seeding agent. Calculus provides a hard, rough surface for the formation of more plaque, which is difficult to remove and may itself become calcified; in this way, incremental layers of calculus are built up. Calculus formation usually begins between two and 14 days after the start of plaque development, but may be as early as four to eight hours in some individuals, and does not appear to be dependent on diet.

Calculus above the gingival margin (supragingival calculus) is formed from the minerals in saliva. It is especially prevalent opposite the ducts of the principal salivary glands (i.e. on the lingual surface of lower front teeth and the buccal surface of upper molars). Supragingival calculus is moderately hard and usually white or pale yellow, although it may become stained by tar from tobacco or pigments from food.

Subgingival calculus occurs below the gingival crest. It contains fewer micro-organisms than supragingival calculus, is difficult to remove, very hard, and stained a dark colour by the breakdown products of blood. Previously thought to cause periodontal disease, subgingival calculus is now considered to be merely an indicator of its presence. However, calculus does influence the development of periodontal disease by virtue of the plaque deposits present on its surface.

Dental caries

Definition and aetiology Dental caries destroys the mineralised portion of the tooth, and is one of the most common diseases in western society; prevalence in the UK is particularly high. Once established, the disease process is irreversible; unless treated, it leads inexorably to destruction of the tooth.

Dental caries is a disease of the modern world. Numerous studies have demonstrated that a high sugar diet is implicated in its aetiology, although the exact mechanism remains unclear. However, it is known that sugars alone do not cause dental caries; it is the combination of sugars in the oral cavity and plaque on the teeth. Dietary sugars dissolved in saliva readily diffuse into plaque, where bacteria (particularly streptococci in early plaque) ferment them to produce organic acids (e.g. lactic acid). These acids demineralise tooth enamel and dentine. Bacteria then invade, causing infection and inflammation. The infection progressively destroys the dentine until the pulp is reached. If unchecked, this eventually results in pulp death. Infection then spreads through the apical foramen to the apical part of the periodontal ligament and an abscess may result.

The frequency of sugar consumption has a greater influence than the quantity consumed (National Dairy Council, 1995). However, the quantity consumed is important in increasing plaque thickness and the rate of formation (*see* Plaque *above*). The incidence of caries is higher in children and adolescents than in adults because secondary maturation of dental enamel gradually increases its resistance to acid attack. Fluoride also increases the resistance of enamel.

Several host factors may influence the initial development of caries or the rate of decay. The structure of teeth varies between individuals, and the presence of deep fissures and pits predisposes to caries formation. The chemical composition of enamel also varies, and some people have teeth that are more resistant to acid attack than others. Crowded or badly aligned teeth render good plaque control difficult; the resultant stagnation areas are more susceptible to caries.

Although dental caries may attack any surface of the tooth, more than 50% of lesions affect the occlusal surfaces of back teeth, with marginally more occurring in the upper arch than the lower. First molars appear to be more susceptible than other teeth, whilst the lowest prevalence is in lower incisors and canines. There are three types of caries:

- Pit and fissure caries
  Lesions that occur in pits and fissures are the most common type of caries. The initial break in the enamel is seen as a small black pit, which may extend into dentine. The underlying dentine is destroyed more quickly than enamel, and eventually a bluish-white area appears around the initial pit. The enamel collapses as more of the underlying dentine is destroyed, and the later stages are marked by an open cavity.
- Smooth surface caries
  Smooth surface caries is the least common. It can occur on any smooth surface, but particularly on the proximal surfaces between teeth. Lingual surfaces are affected less frequently than buccal or labial surfaces. The lesion initially appears chalky-white, becoming gradually rougher as the enamel starts to break down. The subsequent stages are the same as in pit and fissure caries.
- Cervical caries
  Cervical caries is more common in older people. It attacks exposed dentine at the neck of the tooth, where the crown meets the root. As there is no enamel at this point, an open cavity is formed from the beginning. The subsequent stages are as described above under pit and fissure caries.

On average, it takes about two years for a cavity to be clinically visible in permanent teeth, although there is wide individual variation. The time span may be as short as three months in primary teeth.

Rampant caries ('dummy' caries or 'bottle' caries) occurs in infants allowed to suck comforters (dummies) coated with sugary substances (e.g. honey, jam or undiluted fruit syrups). Drinking concentrated sweetened liquids from feeding bottles produces the same effect. Such practices allow prolonged contact between the teeth and sugar, resulting in severe and extensive caries affecting several teeth, particularly the upper incisors.

The properties of saliva (e.g. mineral composition, viscosity and rate of production) vary between individuals, affecting their susceptibility to caries. Saliva is the body's natural means of cleaning and buffering the oral cavity. It is also involved in the re-mineralisation of enamel, which can reverse early dental caries (*see below*). Xerostomia, caused by a reduction in salivary secretion (*see* Anatomy and morphology *above*), is associated with an increased incidence of caries.

Symptoms The initial stages of dental caries are asymptomatic. Pain is first felt when dentine is exposed during the open-cavity stage, although there is wide variation in the degree of pain experienced. Short-term pain on exposure to heat, cold or sweet substances during the early stages of decay indicates that prompt treatment may save the pulp from irreversible damage.

Inflammation of the pulp (pulpitis) produces swelling of the pulp tissue in an enclosed area. This sometimes results in a throbbing pain that is exacerbated by heat and relieved by cold. Pain lasting for some time (e.g. up to 20 minutes) indicates that damage to the pulp is irreversible. Severe pain that is unconnected with any stimuli or disturbs sleep signifies extensive decay. If untreated, the pain eventually subsides once pulp necrosis occurs, because of degeneration of the nerve supply. However, the infection may spread through the apex and cause inflammation of adjacent tissues. A periapical abscess may then occur, which can be extremely painful during the acute phase as pressure builds up in the enclosed space around the apical foramen. The pain is exacerbated by pressure on the tooth and subsides once the pus has discharged.

Treatment Early dental caries is reversible because minerals present in saliva allow re-mineralisation of the enamel to take place. The organic matrix is still intact at this stage, which allows the deposition of further crystals. Once the matrix collapses, this is impossible.

Re-mineralisation is more likely to be successful if further acid attack is kept to a minimum by strict plaque and dietary sugar control. Fluoride is highly beneficial in re-mineralisation (*see* Prevention of dental disease *below*), as it converts the inorganic hydroxyapatite in enamel to the more resistant fluorapatite.

Irreversible caries may require a variety of treatments, including:

- restorations (fillings)
- root canal treatment (endodontics)
- crowns or bridges
- extraction.

Analgesics may be given for pain relief until dental treatment is available, but controlling the pain does not in any way control the disease, and dental referral should not be delayed longer than necessary. For measures to prevent dental caries, *see* Prevention of dental disease *below*.

Periodontal disease

Definition and aetiology Periodontal disease encompasses several inflammatory disorders which affect the supporting structures of the teeth. It is one of the most common conditions in the world, affecting the vast majority of people at some stage in their lives. Chronic periodontal disease is slow, insidious and usually painless, but the eventual result may be destruction of the underlying bone. It causes the loss of more teeth than dental caries because the supporting structures cannot be repaired as effectively as teeth can be restored.

Like dental caries, periodontal disease is caused by plaque bacteria. However, diet is not thought to be an important factor in its development, and dental caries is not a cause; completely undecayed teeth can be affected. Plaque deposits around the gingival margin and within the gingival crevice are most important in the aetiology of periodontal disease.

Where inflammation is confined to the gingivae, the condition is called gingivitis. Spread of inflammation to the periodontal ligament and alveolar bone is termed periodontitis. Chronic gingivitis precedes chronic periodontitis, but does not always lead to it. The reason why some cases progress and others do not is not known. Prevention of chronic gingivitis therefore prevents chronic periodontitis. Gingivitis may also be an acute condition, but, unlike chronic gingivitis, this is always painful.

Chronic gingivitis

Definition and aetiology Chronic gingivitis is the result of inflammatory changes produced in the gingivae by endotoxins and enzymes from plaque bacteria. Undisturbed plaque deposits may cause the initial inflammatory reaction within two to four days.

Some medical conditions (e.g. diabetes mellitus, leukaemias and scurvy) may increase the risk of chronic gingivitis. The precise mechanism for this is unknown, but it may be a result of altered host response to bacterial products (e.g. toxins and enzymes). Administration of some drugs (e.g. cyclosporin, nifedipine, oral contraceptives or phenytoin) may also predispose to gingivitis. In some cases, these may cause severe gingival hyperplasia in which the gingivae cover most of the crown of the tooth. Any disorder or drug which reduces salivary secretion increases the susceptibility to chronic gingivitis (*see also* Dental caries *above*).

People who habitually keep their lips apart, particularly when asleep, show a greater incidence of inflammation of the anterior gingivae, most likely as a result of excessive drying of the tissues. Smokers are also more susceptible; it is not certain whether this is caused by tobacco smoke or poor oral hygiene, which has been shown to be greater in smokers than non-smokers.

Pregnant women are more susceptible to gingivitis ('pregnancy gingivitis') as a result of hormonal changes affecting connective tissues, including those of the gingivae. Some pregnant women may even complain of loose teeth. Scrupulous oral hygiene will prevent pregnancy gingivitis, and the tissues revert to normal after parturition. Puberty is also commonly associated with an increased incidence of gingivitis; again it is not clear whether this is associated with hormonal changes or poor standards of oral hygiene.

Symptoms Inflammation results in oedema, causing the gingival crevice to deepen and pockets to develop between the gingivae and the teeth. At this stage, these are called 'false pockets'; they should not be confused with the true periodontal pockets of chronic periodontitis (*see below*). The epithelium of the crevice becomes ulcerated. Subgingival plaque accumulates in the deepened crevices, and bacterial products produce further inflammation. A vicious cycle is set up, which causes the crevices to enlarge further.

In the presence of gingivitis, gingival crevicular fluid exudes through the junctional epithelium into the gingival crevice. This cannot be detected by the patient, but can be measured using crevicular strips (small filter paper strips), and is an indicator of the extent of inflammation. Crevicular fluid contains immunoglobulins (IgA, IgG and IgM) and neutrophils (polymorphonuclear leucocytes), which may exert a protective effect.

The outward symptoms of chronic gingivitis are mild, so many sufferers do not realise they have the condition. Established chronic gingivitis is marked by changes in appearance: the gingivae become reddened, glossy, soft and swollen. Halitosis may also be present. Pain is usually absent, although abrasive food or vigorous toothbrushing may produce discomfort. The main symptom, bleeding gums, is all too often attributed to toothbrushing trauma and ignored.

Treatment Mild chronic gingivitis can be treated by good plaque control (*see* Prevention of dental disease *below*). The only dental treatment required may be oral hygiene instruction, but it is wise to refer patients to their dentist. In many cases, scaling is necessary. This involves the removal of plaque and calculus from the crown and exposed root surfaces. The surfaces are then polished to remove any rough areas that may attract plaque accumulations. For measures to prevent chronic gingivitis, *see* Prevention of dental disease *below*.

Chronic periodontitis

Definition and aetiology Chronic periodontitis, which is always preceded by chronic gingivitis, results in irreversible damage to the periodontal ligament and alveolar bone. It is rare in children under 13 years of age, but becomes more common from the late teens onwards. It is the most common cause of loss of teeth in patients over 30 years of age.

Symptoms Inflammation spreads through the gingival crevice and eventually destroys the periodontal ligament, with the junctional epithelium moving downwards onto the root. A true periodontal pocket is formed and gingival recession may occur, exposing the coronal portion of the root. As periodontal pockets deepen, plaque and debris can collect within them, exacerbating the inflammatory process. The depth of the pockets may be measured using a dental probe and indicates the progression of the disease. Further spread of inflammation to the supporting bone causes resorption, which eventually loosens the teeth.

Many symptoms of chronic gingivitis are present. As the periodontal pockets deepen, however, the swelling and reddening of the gingivae may subside, leading to the mistaken belief by the patient that the gingivitis has resolved. In fact, inflammation is still present, but is now much deeper in the tissues. Chronic periodontitis eventually causes extensive damage that is largely irreversible, and patients should seek treatment at the earliest opportunity (Figure 3.6).

Treatment Treatment of chronic periodontitis is similar to that of chronic gingivitis (*see above*). It involves thorough scaling and polishing, usually over several appointments. Root planing to clean the roots and remove infected cementum is usually necessary. In severe cases, where periodontal pockets are very deep, surgery may

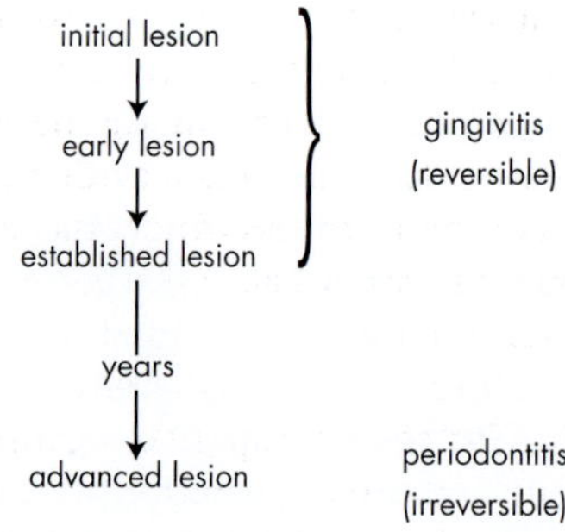

Figure 3.6 The chronological progression of gingivitis to periodontitis.

be required to reshape the gums and facilitate routine plaque removal by the patient. In the last few years, it has become possible to replace lost alveolar bone by sophisticated techniques (e.g. periodontal bone grafting and guided tissue regeneration), but these are highly specialised and not widely available.

Chlorhexidine mouthwash or gel may be useful to control plaque deposition, but is no substitute for toothbrushing. It is not recommended for long-term use, may stain the teeth, and should be restricted to the treatment phase.

Treatment of chronic periodontitis may be a long process, and is heavily dependent on improved home dental care by the patient. Oral hygiene measures alone will not arrest chronic periodontitis, but serve as a valuable adjunct to periodontal treatment and are essential to prevent further disease. Corrective measures (e.g. restorations or orthodontic procedures) in areas prone to plaque accumulation may also be beneficial. For measures to prevent chronic periodontitis, *see* Prevention of dental disease *below*.

Periodontal abscess

Definition and aetiology A periodontal abscess may develop from a periodontal pocket which becomes blocked with exudate or a foreign body (a lateral periodontal abscess). Alternatively, infection of the pulp may spread through the apical foramen (periapical periodontal abscess).

Symptoms Both types of periodontal abscess present with a throbbing pain, exacerbated by pressure on the tooth involved. Gingivae in the area of the abscess become red and swollen; this may spread to surrounding tissues (e.g. the cheeks or lips). Once pus has discharged, the acute phase subsides and, if untreated, often leads to a painless chronic abscess which may continue to exude pus. Abscesses cause further resorption of the surrounding bone.

Treatment Treatment of periodontal abscesses may involve drainage, mouthwashes and administration of antibiotics. Root canal therapy, extraction or periodontal surgery may subsequently be required.

Juvenile periodontitis

Definition and aetiology Juvenile periodontitis (periodontosis) is a chronic periodontal disease occurring in adolescents and young adults. Its development appears to be independent of the level of oral hygiene. The cause of this severe chronic periodontal disease is not known, although it has been suggested that the bacterial flora in the mouths of sufferers may be excessively virulent.

Symptoms The features of juvenile periodontitis appear similar to chronic periodontitis, but its early onset and associated bone loss make it a more serious condition. Pain is usually absent unless a lateral periodontal abscess develops. The most common presenting features are drifting of teeth and localised periodontal pockets. These are usually only apparent during dental examination; radiographs may also show severe bone loss. The disease often progresses relentlessly despite dental intervention, and the prognosis for affected teeth is not good.

Treatment Treatment is similar to that for chronic periodontitis, but more follow-up examinations are required to monitor progress of the disease. Periodontal surgery is not always successful. Treatment may have to rely on strict plaque control measures plus frequent scaling, root planing and polishing. Chlorhexidine solution is only of value if it can penetrate the periodontal pockets, which in juvenile periodontitis are very deep; use of a syringe with a suitable nozzle may be required.

Primary herpetic gingivostomatitis

Definition and aetiology Primary herpetic gingivostomatitis is an acute gingivitis occurring mainly in children between six months and five years of age. It is caused by a primary infection with herpes simplex virus type 1 (HSV 1). On recovery, the virus lies dormant in the ganglia of the trigeminal nerve and produces latent herpes labialis (cold sores) in response to various stimuli (e.g. emotional disturbance, fever, menstruation, sunlight or local trauma).

Symptoms Symptoms include fever, malaise, gingivitis, pharyngitis and generalised adenopathy. Vesicles appear all over the oral cavity and on the lips, rupturing to form excessively painful ulcers. Accompanying symptoms may include profuse salivation and halitosis. The child appears unwell, irritable, unable to eat, and has a high temperature.

Treatment The condition is self-limiting, and untreated ulcers heal without scarring within 14 to 21 days. Treatment is not generally given for primary HSV 1 infection, but measures that may be taken to relieve the discomfort include paracetamol for pain, bland mouthwashes and soft food. Chlorhexidine mouthwash or gel may be of value as an alternative to toothbrushing until the pain subsides. Where secondary infection occurs, systemic antibiotics may be necessary.

Acute ulcerative gingivitis

Definition and aetiology Acute ulcerative gingivitis (acute necrotising ulcerative gingivitis, trench mouth or Vincent's disease) is an acute, destructive, ulcerative condition affecting the gingivae. It occurs most commonly between 14 and 30 years of age. The micro-organisms most often present are fusiform bacilli and spirochaetes, but the evidence suggests that these are not the causative agents. Predisposing factors are stress, worry, and fatigue. After an initial attack there is a strong tendency for recurrence.

Symptoms Acute ulcerative gingivitis is of sudden onset, usually begins in the gingival papillae, and may extend throughout the gingivae. It is characterised by general malaise, marked gingival bleeding, inflammation and swelling. Fever is generally absent, but the pain may be so severe as to render eating and talking impossible. Halitosis and excessive salivation are also common. Characteristic 'punched-out' grey ulcers, which bleed readily, often develop at the crest of the gingival papillae. These ulcers develop a pseudomembrane composed of a necrotic grey slough.

Treatment Treatment comprises the administration of metronidazole or nimorazole in conjunction with local debridement of necrotic and infected tissue. Hydrogen peroxide mouthwashes may be used between dental appointments, and the patient should be fully instructed in good oral hygiene procedures. All patients should be followed up regularly as tissue destruction may make subsequent plaque removal difficult in some areas.

Tooth wear

Definition and aetiology Recent evidence suggests that tooth wear is now a significant problem in both children and adults (Smith, Bartlett and Robb, 1997). It is rarely possible to differentiate between the different aetiological factors, but the dental profession is particularly concerned about dental erosion. This may be defined as the progressive loss of hard dental tissues caused by the action of acids on the teeth, without the involvement of bacteria.

Erosion may result from occupational exposure to acid fumes or chronic contact with gastric acid as a result of frequent vomiting or oesophageal reflux. However, the frequent ingestion of dietary acids, in the form of carbonated drinks and fruit juices, is now considered to be of major importance, particularly in children. The extent of the problem was measured by the 1993 Child Dental Health Survey. 52% of children of five and six years of age had erosion of the deciduous incisors, and the permanent teeth of more than 30% of those of 14 years of age were affected (Office of Population Censuses and Surveys, 1994).

Prevention and treatment Prevention consists of reducing the frequency of contact with the causative agent, where this can be identified. Teeth that are severely worn may require extensive restoration work.

Gingival recession

Definition and aetiology Gingival recession may occur in healthy mouths, even in the young. Recession can take place around teeth that have a thin bone covering, teeth that are subject to excessive biting forces or where there are bony defects. Trauma produced by over-zealous toothbrushing may exacerbate this process.

Symptoms The gingivae are pushed back and the underlying cementum is worn away to expose dentine. This may cause increased sensitivity and pain, particularly on exposure to heat, cold or sweet substances. Gingival recession can increase the risk of developing root caries.

Treatment The primary cause of recession should be eliminated where possible. For example, selective grinding by the dentist is an effective way of equalising biting forces and reducing excessive loading on an individual tooth. Desensitising toothpastes (*see* Prevention of dental disease *below*) may be used to reduce the sensitivity of the dentine. Topical application of such a toothpaste directly to the sensitive area may also be beneficial. Fluoride varnishes may be applied by the dental surgeon to promote remineralisation of the exposed dentine. The patient should be encouraged to adopt a less vigorous toothbrushing technique to prevent further recession.

Halitosis

Definition and aetiology Halitosis (bad breath) is characterised by an offensive breath odour. It is highly prevalent and is a source of social embarrassment to many.

Halitosis is often a symptom of periodontal disease. However, abnormal breath odours are produced by elimination of certain substances via the lungs, and may be a symptom of systemic disease (e.g. ketones in uncontrolled diabetes mellitus or ammoniacal compounds in uraemia). However, in the majority of cases, halitosis results from anaerobic bacterial putrefaction in the oral cavity and is not caused by systemic disease. Malodorous breath may also arise following smoking, alcohol consumption or ingestion of certain foods (e.g. garlic).

Treatment Halitosis may be controlled by minimising the oral bacterial population. All measures advocated to reduce the level of gum disease and hence bleeding (*see* Prevention of dental disease *below*) will also improve breath odour.

Mouthwashes (*see* Prevention of dental disease *below*) are often used to freshen the breath, although their value in treating halitosis is questionable.

Prevention of dental disease

Dental disease may not be life-threatening, but it can severely affect the quality of life. Loss of many or all the permanent teeth necessitates the use of dentures, which can create a different set of problems. For the young, the social stigma of wearing dentures is now much greater than in the past, when the wholesale loss of teeth was common.

Lost teeth which are not replaced by dentures create problems for the remaining teeth, and may even alter the shape of the jaw. Adjacent teeth tend to tilt or drift into the gaps, which may alter the biting pattern. Loss of one tooth from a complementary pair may limit chewing movements because the remaining tooth has nothing to bite against, and it often over-erupts. There is also the psychological aspect of altered appearance, because gaps in the permanent dentition are not generally considered attractive. Premature loss of primary teeth may affect the spacing of the subsequent permanent teeth and influence jaw development.

Decayed teeth may be restored if treated in time, but scrupulous dental healthcare is essential to save them from further damage. Secondary caries may form around the margins or underneath a filling if bacteria and sugar can gain access. Should this occur, the tooth must be refilled. Subsequent fillings are larger, and eventually the tooth may need to be crowned or even extracted.

It is absolutely essential that the gingivae are in peak condition before advanced dentistry is carried out, because the position of the gingival margins is used as a reference point. Inflamed gingivae may be swollen and cover more of the crowns of the teeth than normal. If the inflammation subsequently subsides following improvements in dental healthcare, the margins may recede to a more normal position and, for example, expose the edges of crowns and bridges.

Almost all dental disease is completely preventable, but this requires a high degree of motivation on the part of the individual. The only passive measure available is water fluoridation, which reduces the incidence of dental caries but not periodontal disease. Both caries and chronic periodontal disease are painless conditions until the later stages, by which time irreversible damage has already occurred. Many people are unable to appreciate that a problem exists if there are no outward signs and symptoms. Consequently, they cannot easily be convinced of the need to take preventive measures. This represents one of the greatest barriers to be overcome in dental health education.

Plaque control

Plaque control is the basis of prevention of dental disease. Plaque bacteria, particularly those of mature plaque, are responsible for the vast majority of periodontal disease; therefore, prevention is aimed at keeping the level of plaque to an absolute minimum. The role of plaque in dental caries is more complex because it is the combination of sugar and plaque that results in tooth decay (*see* Dental disease *above*). Theoretically, if plaque were removed from the teeth immediately before consuming sugar, dental caries would not develop. However, for most people this is totally impractical. It is also unlikely that the teeth are ever completely plaque-free, because plaque forms extremely rapidly after cleaning, and some areas are inaccessible. Prevention of caries must, therefore, combine both good plaque control and sugar control.

The most effective means of removing plaque from teeth is with a toothbrush; invariably, toothpaste is used as well. Regular toothbrushing is begun by many people when young and continued throughout life. However, in many cases, the brushing regimen is inadequate for complete plaque control. Some areas of the dentition cannot be reached by a toothbrush, and additional methods (e.g. dental floss or interproximal brushes) must also be employed.

Disclosing agents

Plaque cannot readily be seen on teeth, making it difficult to convince an unwilling or sceptical person of its presence. A disclosing agent that stains plaque should be recommended. Various proprietary disclosing tablets and fluids are available. Some can distinguish between new and mature plaque, staining each a different colour. Re-application after brushing serves to illustrate the effectiveness of brushing technique and highlight areas where improvements may be required. Patients should be advised to smear white soft paraffin on their lips, to prevent discoloration by the dye contained in the disclosing agent.

Toothbrushing

Toothbrush design

Selecting a toothbrush can be daunting when faced with the vast array of designs available, backed up by impressive claims from manufacturers. In reality, there is no general consensus of opinion on the best design for a toothbrush, and the ultimate selection is based on personal preference. However, certain factors may help when making a choice.

Nylon bristles are preferable to natural bristles because they do not absorb fluids or harbour micro-organisms as readily, and the control of bristle quality during manufacture is easier. Natural bristle toothbrushes also have the disadvantage that they become soft (and therefore less effective) when wet. Multi-tufted, small bristles are better than fewer, larger bristles. Rounded ends to the filaments generally offer no major advantage over cut ends, although they may prevent soft tissue injury by over-enthusiastic toothbrushers.

Soft-texture brushes are less efficient in removing plaque than medium brushes, but may be of value for those with sensitive teeth, painful gum dis-orders or gingival recession. Hard brushes should be avoided because they may cause gingival trauma or recession. The brush-head should be small enough to reach awkward areas, but not so small that effective plaque removal requires prolonged brushing. A medium-sized brush-head with multi-tufted nylon bristles of medium texture is probably the best choice for most adults.

Interproximal brushes or brushes shaped like miniature bottle brushes may be required for extremely awkward areas (e.g. badly aligned teeth or bridges) or large interdental spaces.

Electric brushes can be particularly valuable for people with mental or physical disabilities. When used by the able-bodied, there is no evidence that they are intrinsically superior to manual toothbrushes, but they can achieve effective plaque removal much more quickly. Many people, especially children, find them pleasant to use, and are therefore more likely to maintain a satisfactory oral hygiene regime. Rechargeable electric toothbrushes are considered preferable to battery-operated brushes, which lose torque quickly.

Toothbrushes should be renewed relatively frequently. A worn toothbrush cannot effectively remove plaque, but there is no simple means of detecting when a toothbrush is past its prime. It has been estimated that the lifespan of a toothbrush being used correctly is probably only a few weeks.

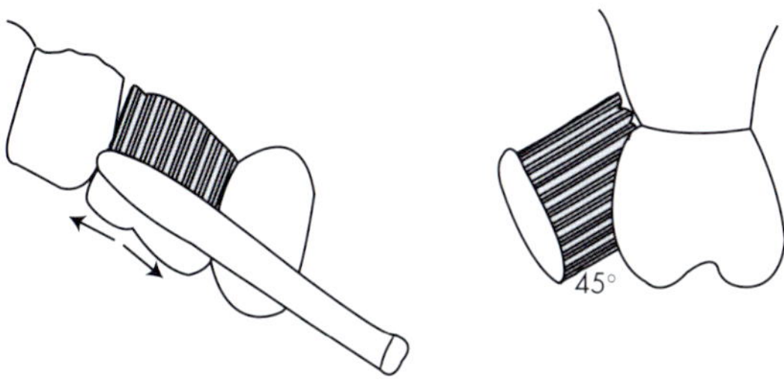

Figure 3.7 The Bass method.

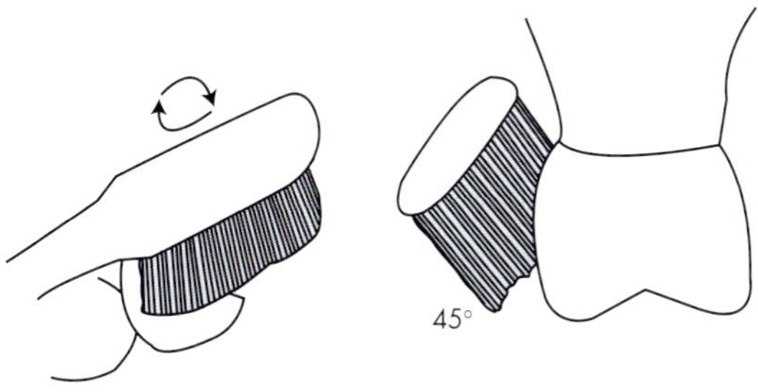

Figure 3.8 The Charters method.

Toothbrushing technique

The aim of toothbrushing is to remove plaque and food debris; it can also deliver the topical fluoride in toothpastes to the teeth. Toothbrushing technique has been the subject of much argument and many suggestions have been put forward. However, different dentitions may require different techniques; any technique that results in good plaque control without causing damage to the teeth or soft tissues can be regarded as satisfactory.

Two of the most frequently recommended techniques are the Bass and Charters methods. In the Bass method, the head of the brush is applied at an angle of 45° to the long axis of the teeth and pressed in an apical direction against the gingival margin (Figure 3.7). It is then moved anteroposteriorly with short vibratory strokes. In order to gain adequate access to the lingual surfaces of the anterior teeth, the brush must be turned into a vertical position. This method effectively removes soft deposits located above and below the gingival margin.

In the Charters method, the head of the brush is applied to the teeth at an angle of 45° to the occlusal plane (Figure 3.8), and jiggled back and forth in a circular motion. It is particularly useful if the interdental papillae have receded, leaving the proximal surfaces of the teeth accessible to the toothbrush.

Whichever technique is used, the most important factor in toothbrushing is that every accessible surface of every tooth should be thoroughly cleaned during each session. Many people concentrate on the buccal and labial surfaces, but forget the lingual and occlusal surfaces. It is helpful to divide the dentition into sections and concentrate on one section at a time. Patients who are concerned about their toothbrushing technique should be referred to their dental surgeon for evaluation.

Toothbrushing frequency

The most widely accepted routine is once in the morning and once at bedtime. Some authorities also advocate brushing the teeth after lunch, but this is probably not practical for many people. The thoroughness of plaque removal is more important than the frequency; nothing is gained by several cursory attempts at toothbrushing throughout the day.

Toothbrushing before bed is important to

prevent the reduced salivary flow during sleep allowing the build-up of thick plaque deposits. Therefore, removing as much plaque and debris as possible before sleeping considerably reduces overnight plaque levels. Theoretically, the best time to brush teeth would be before eating, because sugar is only cariogenic in the presence of plaque. In practice, plaque is unlikely to be completely removed, so it is probably best to recommend toothbrushing after meals, to remove plaque and sugars together.

However, toothbrushing should be avoided immediately after consuming acidic foods or drinks, and after vomiting. This is because at this point the enamel is particularly delicate, being in the first stages of acid attack. After approximately 30 minutes, the enamel is stabilised as a result of re-mineralisation.

Toothpaste

A toothpaste (dentifrice) is applied with a toothbrush to clean the teeth, but the action of the toothbrush is far more important than the toothpaste. It has even been suggested that toothpaste is not necessary for plaque removal. However, toothbrushing with water alone is of little benefit in stain removal. Toothpastes also polish the tooth surfaces, and plaque forms less readily on smooth surfaces than rough surfaces. Many people like the freshening effect toothpaste has in the mouth, particularly first thing in the morning.

Toothpastes are composed of the following ingredients:

- humectants, which prevent the toothpaste drying out, control microbial growth and provide a vehicle for the other ingredients
- abrasives, which polish the tooth surface and remove debris, plaque and stains
- surface-active agents, which loosen debris and facilitate its removal
- binders and thickeners, which prevent separation of the aqueous and non-aqueous constituents and thicken the formulation
- flavourings, which improve consumer acceptability, thereby increasing the likelihood of patients maintaining good plaque control
- colourings, used to improve appearance and consumer acceptability.

Toothpastes may act as vehicles for active ingredients. About 95% of all toothpastes sold in the UK contain fluoride (*see below*) in the form of sodium fluoride or sodium monofluorophosphate (MFP). The fluoride content of toothpaste is usually about 0.1%. Fluoride-containing toothpastes deliver fluoride to the enamel surface, which is extremely important in preventing dental decay. Desensitising toothpastes contain various compounds to block the perception of painful stimuli by dentine. Chlorhexidine (*see below*) inhibits plaque formation on the teeth and is included in toothpaste indicated for the control of gingivitis.

Most people cover the entire brush head with toothpaste, which is far in excess of the quantity needed. All that is required is an amount the size of a pea. Too much toothpaste generates a lot of foam and induces a premature desire to spit and rinse. For many people, this signals the end of toothbrushing. Ingestion of too much fluoride toothpaste by children, who swallow much more than adults, could possibly result in fluorosis, particularly if fluoride supplements are also being administered.

Dental floss and interdental woodsticks

Dental floss and interdental woodsticks are used to remove plaque from the areas between the teeth (embrasures) where a toothbrush cannot reach. These areas should be cleaned regularly, but not every time the teeth are brushed; once a day should be sufficient.

Dental floss

Dental floss is available in waxed or unwaxed forms; the choice is one of personal preference. Unwaxed floss splays out in contact with the tooth surface and may be more efficient at removing plaque. It may also be easier to pass through tight interdental spaces. However, the loose threads may tear against the margins of fillings, in which case waxed floss may be preferable. Dental tape, which is wider than dental floss, is also available, and special types of floss are manufactured for cleaning bridges. Correct use of floss may remove some subgingival plaque.

A long piece of floss (approximately 30 cm) should be wound around the first two fingers of each hand, leaving approximately 10 cm in between. The floss is held taut and carefully inserted into the space between two teeth. It is then held firmly against one of the teeth and carefully moved vertically up and down to remove the plaque. This is repeated for the tooth on the other side of the space. On no account should the floss be moved horizontally between the teeth; this can severely damage the gingivae. The procedure is repeated until all the teeth have been thoroughly cleaned.

An alternative method of using dental floss involves tying a length of floss (approximately 15 cm) into a loop. The lower teeth are cleaned by holding the floss between both index fingers. The left thumb and right index finger are used to clean the upper left quadrant, and the right thumb and left index finger to clean the upper right quadrant.

Interdental woodsticks

Interdental woodsticks should not be used without proper instruction from a dentist as they can cause tissue damage. They are less effective than floss and do not remove subgingival plaque; they should not be used where teeth are closely positioned.

Interdental spaces can be cleaned by inserting and manipulating the woodstick, taking care to follow the normal contour of the interdental papillae (Figure 3.9). The mouth must be clean and the gingivae healthy; rubbing inflamed gingivae over subgingival calculus will exacerbate periodontal disease. Regular use of woodsticks can improve the shape of the interdental papillae and reduce food stagnation.

Water irrigation

Water irrigation units direct jets of water at and between the teeth, and are promoted for plaque removal. However, plaque is an extremely sticky, tenacious substance and is unlikely to be removed by water alone. Water irrigation units are ineffective in removing stains from tooth surfaces. It is also possible that the water jet could force bacteria into the crevicular epithelium and the underlying connective tissue. Any resultant bacteraemia would pose a serious risk for patients susceptible to bacterial endocarditis (e.g. those with a history of rheumatic fever).

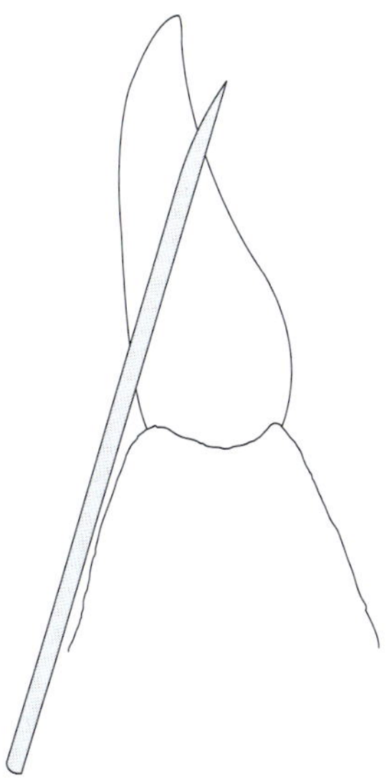

Figure 3.9 The woodstick should follow the gingival contour.

Mouthwashes

Mouthwashes are liquid preparations containing many of the same constituents as toothpastes (*see above*). Essential differences are the exclusion of abrasives and thickening agents. They may, in addition, contain antibacterial agents, astringents, demulcents or ethanol. Antibacterial mouthwashes may help control gingivitis, but not periodontitis; however, the evidence is not conclusive, except for chlorhexidine. Mouthwashes do assist in the removal of debris, tenacious mucus and purulent secretions, and in the cleansing of traumatised areas (e.g. aphthous ulcers).

Patients using mouthwashes to treat oral lesions should be referred to their doctor or dental surgeon if the condition persists for more than seven days; severe cases should be referred immediately. Anti-plaque mouthwashes intended to loosen plaque before toothbrushing have been developed, although the evidence for their effectiveness is inconclusive.

Chlorhexidine

Chlorhexidine is a cationic antibacterial agent available in a mouthwash or dental gel. Chlorhexidine gluconate has proven activity against plaque bacteria and prevents the build up of plaque deposits. However, it is not an effective substitute for toothbrushing, except for short-term use in painful oral conditions (*see* Dental disease *above*). In some cases, chlorhexidine stains the teeth a blackish colour along the gingival margins.

Hydrogen peroxide

The antimicrobial action of hydrogen peroxide is negligible.

Sodium chloride

A sodium chloride mouthwash can be prepared by dissolving half a teaspoon of salt in a tumblerful of warm water, or by diluting Compound Sodium Chloride Mouthwash BP in an equal volume of warm water. It is particularly useful in promoting healing (e.g. of extraction sockets and aphthous ulcers) and establishing the drainage of pus.

Sodium bicarbonate

Sodium bicarbonate may be used as a 2% solution to rinse the mouth. Its alkalinity makes it an effective mucolytic agent, but it does not have any antibacterial action.

Prevention of dental caries

Dietary management

Dental caries is unlikely to be prevented by plaque control alone; a reduction in sugar consumption is also important. Soft, sticky foods release sugars over a long period of time by clinging to tooth surfaces. Also, different sugars affect pH to varying degrees: lactose and galactose cause a smaller fall in pH than glucose, maltose, sucrose or fructose. There is no difference in cariogenic potential between refined and unrefined sugars, or some 'natural' (e.g. honey) and processed products. All should be avoided as far as possible. Fruits and vegetables are a preferred alternative to cakes, biscuits, puddings, confectionery and any other foods with a high sugar content.

Animal studies suggest that complex carbohydrates may be cariogenic, although to what extent is not known. However, suggesting that these should also be avoided would contradict the advice given to prevent other disorders. A compromise must be made so that the health of the body as a whole is considered. Thus, it is recommended that the frequency of carbohydrate consumption, rather than the amount, should be reduced. If snacks are eaten between meals, they should consist of non-sticky savoury rather than sticky sweet foods, but it must be borne in mind that sugar is also present in many processed savoury foods.

Non-cariogenic sugar substitutes may be used, although it is probably wiser to attempt to do without sweet foods and drinks. Sugar alcohols (e.g. sorbitol, mannitol and xylitol) are available; they are not as cariogenic as sugars because plaque bacteria are less able to utilise them as substrates to produce energy. However, large quantities cause osmotic diarrhoea, and the daily intake should not exceed 50 to 80 g. Hydrogenated glucose syrups are licensed for use in the UK, and available evidence suggests that they are less cariogenic than sucrose.

Fluoride

In the early 1900s, it was noted that the inhabitants of certain areas of America had mottled teeth. This was eventually found to be caused by increased levels of fluoride in the local drinking water; the condition was therefore called fluorosis. These people had a lower prevalence of dental caries than the population as a whole. Similar observations were made in the UK and elsewhere; children living in areas supplied with water containing a high level of natural fluoride had healthier teeth than those in areas whose water had a low fluoride content. The role of fluoride in the prevention of dental caries was investigated; worldwide epidemiological studies confirmed that caries is reduced in areas where the water supply contains at least 1 mg/L (1 ppm) of fluoride. However, concentrations of fluoride above 1 mg/L may cause fluorosis. Fluoride is also present in many foodstuffs, but significant amounts are found only in tea and the bones of sea-fish.

There is a strong anti-fluoridation lobby in the UK, which objects to fluoridation of water supplies on the grounds that it is dangerous, unnecessary, uneconomic and of negligible benefit. Careful and controlled studies have refuted all these claims, and fluoridated water has been shown to be safe and effective. However, most of the UK population does not benefit from fluoridated water supplies. This contrasts starkly with other nations (e.g. Russia and the USA) where fluoridation is widespread; it is mandatory in the Republic of Ireland.

Fluoride is effective both topically and systemically (Duckworth, 1993). The topical effect is now considered more important as the greatest concentrations of fluoride are found at the tooth surface. There are several theories to explain the mode of action of fluoride. The most popular is that the calcium hydroxyapatite in enamel is replaced by calcium fluorapatite. This has a lower critical pH and therefore increases the resistance of enamel to acid attack. Fluoride is also important in re-mineralisation and the reversal of early caries, especially smooth surface caries. Fluoride can block the enzymes of plaque bacteria and may inhibit the metabolic conversion of sugars to acids. Application of topical fluoride can re-mineralise enamel and completely reverse the development of early carious lesions; it may also arrest, or slow down, the progress of later lesions. There is some evidence that the presence of systemic fluoride during tooth development results in a smoother, less fissured morphology that is less susceptible to caries.

Oral fluoride supplements containing sodium fluoride may be given to children living in areas where the level of fluoride in the water is less than 1 ppm. Pharmacists should check the level with the water authority, and issue the following guidelines when selling fluoride supplements. Doses are expressed as the amount of fluoride ion to be taken daily. These guidelines are for temperate climates; the dose may be less in tropical climates where more water is consumed.

- Fluoride level less than 300 μg/L (0.3 ppm)
  six months to two years of age – 250 μg
  two to four years of age – 500 μg
  more than four years of age – 1000 μg
- Fluoride level of 300 to 700 μg/L (0.3 to 0.7 ppm)
  less than two years of age – no supplementation required
  two to four years of age – 250 μg
  more than four years of age – 500 μg
- Fluoride level above 700 μg/L (0.7 ppm)
  no supplementation required.

These doses take into account the small amount of fluoride ingested during toothbrushing. Two divided doses should be administered each day to avoid the plasma concentration peaking at a value that could cause fluorosis. However, this requires a high degree of motivation, and once daily administration (preferably in the evening) is an effective compromise; forgotten doses should not be doubled the following day. Fluoride tablets should be sucked or dissolved in the mouth rather than swallowed whole, to allow a topical as well as a systemic effect. In the UK, fluoride supplementation is now considered unnecessary for infants under six months of age, irrespective of local water concentrations.

Additional protection may be provided for those at increased risk of caries by the use of fluoride rinses or the application of fluoride gels. Rinses may be used daily or weekly. A concentration of 0.05% sodium fluoride may be used for daily rinsing, and of 0.2% for weekly or fortnightly rinsing. The mouth should be rinsed for one minute; the rinse should not be swallowed, and eating and drinking should be avoided for 15 minutes after use. Gels must be applied by a dental surgeon, usually twice a year; extreme caution is necessary to prevent any excess from being swallowed. Less concentrated gels have recently become available for home use. Fluoride varnishes may also be applied by the dental surgeon; they are particularly valuable for young or disabled children as the varnish adheres to the teeth and sets in the presence of moisture.

It should be borne in mind that fluoride does not confer complete protection, and minimal sugar consumption, together with good plaque control, is still essential to prevent dental decay.

Dental intervention

It cannot be emphasised too strongly that the most important preventive measures are those routinely undertaken by the individual at home. However, regular visits to the dental surgeon are necessary to identify early caries, some of which may be reversed. For lesions that cannot be reversed, restorative treatment limits the amount of tooth tissue lost. X-ray examination is essential to detect some cavities, especially those between teeth, and will also show early periodontal bone destruction.

Some individuals are more susceptible to caries than others. Some of the factors responsible may be outside their control (e.g. those that are genetically inherited or occur during tooth development, *see* Dental disease *above*). The risks may be minimised by strict attention to oral hygiene and use of fluoride products. However, dental intervention may be necessary to ensure effective plaque control (e.g. orthodontic procedures, which involve moving teeth into more favourable positions under mild pressure, or extractions to reduce overcrowding). Orthodontic appliances provide a surface for plaque build-up and can irritate the gingivae. They may increase susceptibility to dental disease, and must be kept scrupulously clean.

Fissures on the occlusal surfaces of molars and premolars are most prone to dental caries. Here, fluoride is less effective in preventing caries than in other areas of the tooth (*see above*). Deep fissures may be treated with proprietary sealants. This involves filling the fissures and pits with a plastic substance. If applied properly, no decay should occur as long as the sealant remains in place. Sealants should be applied as soon as possible after eruption. The method is painless but time-consuming, and may be difficult if a child is unco-operative.

Regular dental check-ups are also important for adults. The dental surgeon is able to offer advice and training in good plaque control techniques. It is generally recommended that routine check-ups should take place every six months, although some young children may benefit from visits every four months. Adults with good plaque control may only need an annual check-up. It must be stressed that regular dental check-ups are not a substitute for good oral hygiene.

Prevention of dental disease in children

In children, caries is more of a problem than periodontal disease, so dental healthcare measures should be directed towards reducing tooth decay. However, the practices and habits adopted during childhood will also combat periodontal disease if continued into adulthood.

Instilling good dietary habits (*see above*) is absolutely essential in the early years, together with fluoride supplementation (*see above*), if necessary. Parents should not add sugar to feeding bottles or coat dummies with sweet substances. Children should be discouraged from adding sugar to foods or drinks (e.g. cereals, fruit, tea or coffee). A taste for savoury foods should be encouraged because, once attained, a 'sweet tooth' is very difficult to eliminate.

Toothbrushing should be started as soon as the first tooth erupts, and the child encouraged to take an active part as soon as possible. Reasons for cleaning the teeth should be explained, and the presence of plaque demonstrated using a disclosing agent. Children's toothbrushes with small heads and short handles should be employed. Use of dental floss is not usually necessary in children, and would be difficult because of lack of manual dexterity. However, flossing should be started as soon as possible in adolescence. Thumbsucking should be actively discouraged, because it may alter the alignment and spacing of the front teeth.

Children should be introduced to the dental surgeon at an early age, certainly by the time all the primary teeth have erupted. Good oral hygiene practices reduce the necessity for treatment and ensure that a child builds a good relationship with the dental surgeon right from the start.

Care of dentures

Anyone who wears a complete set of dentures may assume that it is too late to worry about dental healthcare. However, plaque accumulates on dentures in exactly the same way as on natural teeth, and must be removed regularly to avoid mucosal inflammation. Removal of plaque and food debris also reduces the likelihood of bacterial putrefaction and the resultant offensive mouth odours. Plaque on dentures is subject to the same risks of staining (e.g. from coffee, tea, tobacco or red wine) as natural teeth. Regular cleaning will maintain an attractive appearance. Partial dentures must be kept scrupulously clean in order to preserve the remaining natural teeth. Dentures should always be cleaned out of the mouth, once or twice a day. They are not usually worn at night, when they should be placed in water to prevent them drying out and distorting.

Dentures are generally made of acrylic materials that are softer than enamel, so equipment and products designed for natural teeth should never be used. Some partial dentures are metal: chrome-cobalt alloy is most commonly used. Denture brushes resemble nail brushes on long handles. There is very often a thick tuft of bristles on the opposite side of the head, which can be used to clean awkward areas. Toothpastes specifically designed for dentures should be used and highly abrasive cleansers avoided, because of the risks of scratching; household bleach, disinfectants or antiseptics should never be used. Alternatively, brushing with soap and water can be just as effective. Disclosing solutions may be used to detect plaque on dentures and assess the thoroughness of cleansing routines in exactly the same way as for natural teeth.

Tablets or powders that release oxygen when dissolved in water may be used to soak the dentures to remove plaque; a stronger acidic cleanser may be required for stubborn stains. Soaking, however, is no substitute for brushing and can lead to 'crazing' of the acrylic surface; minute cracks develop which make the denture appear dull and render it much more susceptible to staining. Metal components may corrode in certain solutions, and the manufacturer's instructions should always be consulted before soaking. Some dentures have soft linings; the dental surgeon should be consulted about the safest way to clean these.

Dentures must be handled with great care; they should be cleaned over a bowl of water or a soft surface in case they are dropped. Denture repair kits are available to carry out emergency repairs, but should only be used as a very last resort; the slightest misalignment or excess of repair material can make a denture unwearable. Household adhesives should never be used; the dentures should be taken to a dental surgeon or dental technician for professional repair as soon as possible.

Once a tooth has been lost, the surrounding alveolar bone gradually resorbs, the rate varying dramatically between individuals. Dentures rest on the alveolar ridge and extensive bone loss results in a poor fit. Loose dentures affect eating and speaking; the effects may be severe enough to make the wearer withdraw socially. Eating may also be painful, because uneven contact means that the soft gingivae are excessively loaded in some areas. The hard palate provides a wide surface over which biting forces are distributed, whereas lower dentures can only cover the alveolar ridge, because the floor of the oral cavity is taken up by the tongue and its associated muscles. Consequently, lower dentures tend to be more difficult to wear than upper dentures. Denture fixatives, usually containing karaya gum or tragacanth, are used by many people to increase retention. However, anyone having problems should be referred to their dental surgeon.

The risk of developing oral lesions is increased in some systemic disorders. Pharmacists should always enquire about any underlying condition when a patient presents with denture problems (e.g. there is an increased incidence of oral candidiasis in diabetics). A dry mouth may also make wearing dentures difficult and uncomfortable, so pharmacists should be aware of the conditions and drugs that reduce salivary secretion (*see* Dental diseases *above*). Patients may need to be referred to their doctor as well as their dental surgeon.

New dentures may take getting used to, especially if the patient has not worn dentures before. They may produce gum discomfort and even sores or ulcers. Unless the symptoms are extremely mild, patients should be referred to their dental surgeon as the dentures may require adjustment. In the meantime, an oral preparation containing a local anaesthetic may be applied to the affected area.

The fit of dentures is rarely satisfactory for more than five years, and they must be renewed periodically. Denture wearers should visit their dental surgeon every one to three years (every six months if they have partial dentures) to have their dentures checked and the fit re-evaluated.

The role of the pharmacist

Pharmacists have traditionally been involved in selling dental products to the public, and are therefore ideally positioned to reinforce health education messages from the dental profession and other dental healthcare authorities. In addition, pharmacists can recognise disorders of the oral cavity and refer patients to general practitioners or dental surgeons as appropriate. Dental healthcare is essential for a healthy lifestyle, and should be placed equally among other forms of lifestyle modification. Pharmacists should not take over the role of dental health education from dental surgeons, but rather augment it. Much can be achieved by dental surgeons and pharmacists liaising. This also ensures that pharmacists endorse the dental healthcare advice given by the dental profession.

In most cases, the sale of dental healthcare products is a passive process. It would not be practical to become actively involved in every sale, but pharmacists may perceive that a problem exists (e.g. by noticing repeat purchases of mouthwashes or a customer's difficulty in selecting a toothbrush or toothpaste). Dental healthcare products should be positioned so that pharmacists can observe customers, and therefore offer help when necessary. In large pharmacies, locating the dental healthcare section close to the dispensary serves to raise the status of dental products in the eyes of the public from mere toiletries to essential healthcare items.

Pharmacists should be aware of the importance of sugar control in the prevention of dental caries, and therefore only counter-prescribe non-cariogenic liquid medicines, particularly for children. Mouth and throat lozenges may contain cariogenic sugars, and this should be pointed out to patients. Pharmacists have little control over medicines supplied on prescription unless generic items are requested. However, a discussion with local doctors to make them aware of any sugar-free alternatives may be valuable. Pharmacists should also check the manufacturer's information to see if alternative diluents to syrup may be used when dispensing reduced-strength preparations.

Whenever the opportunity arises, pharmacists should stress:

- the insidious and painless nature of dental disease
- prevention is better than cure
- complete prevention is totally feasible
- regular dental check-ups are essential at any age.

It should also be emphasised that periodontal disease is not a normal ageing process, but a pathological disease that can be prevented by good oral hygiene. Children should be encouraged to adopt good habits from as early an age as possible.

Pharmacists should be familiar with diseases and drugs that may increase the susceptibility to dental caries or periodontal disease (*see* Dental diseases *above*), and offer counselling on preventive measures where appropriate. It is imperative, however, that pharmacists do not compromise patients' confidence in prescribed medicines, or increase their anxiety over a disease state. The discussion needs to be handled with tact and sensitivity, maintaining a positive attitude throughout and emphasising there is nothing difficult about good dental heathcare. Sometimes, there is no alternative to a prescribed medicine, and the patient's medical health may seem more important than their dental health. Neither should be compromised at the expense of the other and, in most cases, dental health can be maintained with good plaque and sugar control. If a patient is over-anxious, pharmacists should discuss the matter with the patient's doctor and dental surgeon in an attempt to resolve the difficulty. Pregnant women are prone to gingivitis and should be counselled that good plaque control will minimise problems. It is also essential that pregnant women and children do not take tetracyclines, as these may cause intrinsic discoloration of children's permanent teeth during the developmental stages.

There may be occasions when patients consult pharmacists about dental problems. Anyone with dental pain should always be referred to a dentist, because it may be difficult to establish the cause, and usually only a dentist will be able to carry out the treatment necessary to alleviate the patient's discomfort. If patients are unable to obtain emergency treatment from their own dental surgeon, pharmacists should supply the address and telephone number of the nearest emergency dental service. Analgesics may be administered in the meantime, but it must be stressed that the problem does not disappear with the pain, and dental treatment must be sought at the earliest available opportunity. The belief that placing an aspirin tablet against the offending tooth will relieve toothache should be firmly discouraged, because of the risk of extensive mucosal ulceration; aspirin is of greater benefit in pain relief if taken systemically.

Some patients may have been given the all-clear by their dentist, or told that their problem is due to gingival recession and exposure of the root surface. In this case, pharmacists can recommend one of the proprietary brands of desensitising toothpaste, preferably one containing fluoride. It should be explained that two or three weeks' conscientious brushing is required before these toothpastes exert their maximum effect.

Most people have mouth ulcers occasionally. Aphthous ulcers are the ordinary mouth ulcers that appear singly or in small numbers, often at times of stress. Various proprietary remedies are on the market, some of which contain a local anaesthetic to render the ulcers less painful. Pharmacists should recommend an appropriate product, as well frequent hot salty mouthwashes, which often have a beneficial effect.

A patient with mouth ulcers need only be referred to a dental surgeon if the ulcers are:

- particularly large
- last more than ten days or so
- repeatedly occur in the same place, which implies that they could be traumatic in origin (e.g. caused by a sharp tooth or rough filling)
- widespread or in large clusters, especially in young children, which could indicate infection with herpes simplex virus
- associated with an objectionable taste or halitosis
- caused by dentures.

A number of emergency kits are available for patients to insert their own temporary fillings and temporarily cement crowns that have become detached. These are a good interim measure, but often require a high degree of manual dexterity on the part of the patient. At all costs, patients should be dissuaded from using household glues to re-cement a crown. The result can be painful and cause difficult and expensive dental problems.

Teeth which have been knocked out in an accident may be successfully re-implanted; however, they may not survive a lifetime, or may discolour and require crowning. Such teeth should be placed in a clean container of milk and immediately taken by the patient to the dental surgeon. On no account should the teeth be washed, rinsed or cleaned in any way. It is vital that there is the minimum delay possible in seeking treatment. If the tooth has fallen onto a dirty surface, the patient may require immunisation against tetanus.

People who visit a dental surgeon have been sufficiently motivated to make an appointment. However, many people never see a dental surgeon, but buy dental healthcare products. Others may not follow any sort of oral hygiene regimen, but still visit a pharmacy for other reasons. Pharmacists, therefore, can interact with significantly more people than dental surgeons, and should take advantage of this situation whenever possible. The impact of any educational material (e.g. books, leaflets or posters) in a pharmacy is potentially greater than in a dental surgery, and pharmacists would do well to include dental health information among their displays.

References

Downer M C (1994). The 1993 national survey of children's dental health: a commentary on the preliminary report. *Br Dent J* 176: 209–214.

Duckworth R M (1993). The science behind caries prevention. *Int Dent J* 43: 529–539.

Harman R J, ed. (1990). Disorders of the ear, nose, and oropharynx. In: *Handbook of Pharmacy Health-care: Diseases and Patient Advice*. London: Pharmaceutical Press, 239–248.

National Dairy Council (1995). *Diet and Dental Health*. London: NDC.

Office of Population Censuses and Surveys (1994).

Dental disease among children in the United Kingdom. *OPCS Monitor*. London: OPCS.

Smith B G N, Bartlett D W, Robb N D (1997). The prevalence, aetiology and management of tooth wear in the United Kingdom. *J Prosthet Dent* 78: 367–372.

Further reading

Centre for Pharmacy Postgraduate Education (1995). A distance learning course for community pharmacists. *Oral Health,* Volumes I & II. London: HMSO.

Ekstrand J, Fejerskov O, Silverstone L M, eds (1988). *Fluoride in Dentistry*. Copenhagen: Munksgaard.

Embery G, Rolla G, eds (1992). *Clinical and Biological Aspects of Dentifrices*. Oxford: Oxford University Press.

Levine R, ed. (1996). *The Scientific Basis of Dental Health Education*. London: Health Education Authority.

Löe H, Kleinman D V, eds (1986). *Dental Plaque Control Measures and Oral Hygiene Practices*. Oxford: IRL Press.

Mehta D, ed. (1998). *Dental Practitioner's Formulary 1998–2000*. London: British Medical Association and Royal Pharmaceutical Society of Great Britain.

O'Brien M (1993). *Children's Dental Health in the United Kingdom*. London: HMSO.

Rugg-Gunn A J (1993). *Nutrition and Dental Health*. Oxford: Oxford University Press.

Tay W M, ed. (1990). *General Dental Treatment*. Edinburgh: Churchill Livingstone.

WHO (1985). Prevention methods and programmes for oral diseases: report of a WHO expert committee. *WHO Tech Rep Ser 713*.

Useful addresses

British Dental Association (BDA)
64 Wimpole Street
London W1M 8AL
Tel: 020 7935 0875

British Fluoridation Society
Sandlebrook
Mill Lane
Alderley Edge
Cheshire SK9 7TY
Tel: 01565 873936

British Society for Disability and Oral Health
Department of Sedation and Special Care Dentistry
Floor 26, Guy's Tower
London SE1 9RT
Tel: 020 7955 5000 Ext. 3047

General Dental Council
37 Wimpole Street
London W1M 8DQ
Tel: 020 7887 3800

The Oral and Dental Research Trust
Keats' House
36 St. Thomas Street
London SE1 9RN
Tel: 020 7955 4699

FDI World Dental Federation
7 Carlisle Street
London W1V 5RG
Tel: 020 7935 7852

4

Contraception

Susan Shankie

Fertility and contraception

Fertility and fertilisation

Men produce sperm at the prodigious rate of about 1000 per second from each testicle, and in the normal ejaculate volume of 3 to 5 mL, there are up to 300 million sperm. Only one of these is necessary to fertilise an ovum but, in practice, the presence of 3 million highly motile and active sperm is necessary to ensure a possibility of fertilisation. Sperm can normally survive for up to six hours in the vagina, although this durability is subject to wide variation. Survival times in the fluids of the cervix, uterus, and Fallopian tubes have been variously estimated as between three and five days, but can be as long as nine days.

Women produce, on average, only one ovum in each monthly cycle (*see below*) that, under normal circumstances, is only capable of being fertilised for about 12 hours (maximum 24 hours) after it is released into the Fallopian tube. Ovulation occurs 12 to 16 days before the next period. The menstrual cycle is generally considered to last about 28 days, although it may vary from as short as 21 days to as long as 40 days or more. The average is 25 to 35 days. However, women may not have regular menstrual cycles and the time of ovulation may be difficult to predict.

The menstrual and ovarian cycles

The stages of a theoretical 28-day regular menstrual cycle, in the absence of fertilisation, are represented in Figure 4.1. These changes generally occur on a cyclical basis throughout a woman's life, from puberty until the menopause. An ovum is produced within the ovary from a primary oocyte by meiosis (oogenesis). The ovum is formed within the fluid-filled Graafian follicle and, at ovulation, is released from the follicle into the pelvic cavity. The ovum is guided into the funnel-shaped infundibulum of the Fallopian tube by finger-like ciliary projections (the fimbriae). The remaining cells of the Graafian follicle in the ovary multiply rapidly and form the yellow, highly vascularised corpus luteum. The corpus luteum secretes oestrogens and progesterone, which act on the endometrium to increase its blood supply and thickness in preparation for the receipt of a fertilised ovum.

In normal menstrual cycles, variations occur in the plasma concentrations of the gonadotrophins, follicle-stimulating hormone (FSH) and luteinising hormone (LH), and of the female sex hormones, the oestrogens and progesterone. FSH and LH are secreted by the anterior lobe of the pituitary gland in response to gonadorelin (gonadotrophin-releasing hormone or GnRH) produced by the hypothalamus.

At the start of a cycle, FSH stimulates the development of 20 to 25 ovarian follicles that will ultimately produce one ovum. FSH also stimulates the secretion of oestrogens from the follicular cells. Rising oestrogen concentrations inhibit gonadorelin (and consequently secretion of FSH), but stimulate the secretion of LH (the LH surge). LH stimulates further development of the follicles and, together with oestrogens, stimulates the release of the ovum from the ovary. LH also stimulates the formation of the corpus luteum.

If fertilisation does not occur, the continued secretion of oestrogens and progesterone inhibits the release of gonadorelin and, therefore, the secretion of LH. The corpus luteum remains for about 14 days before it degenerates and

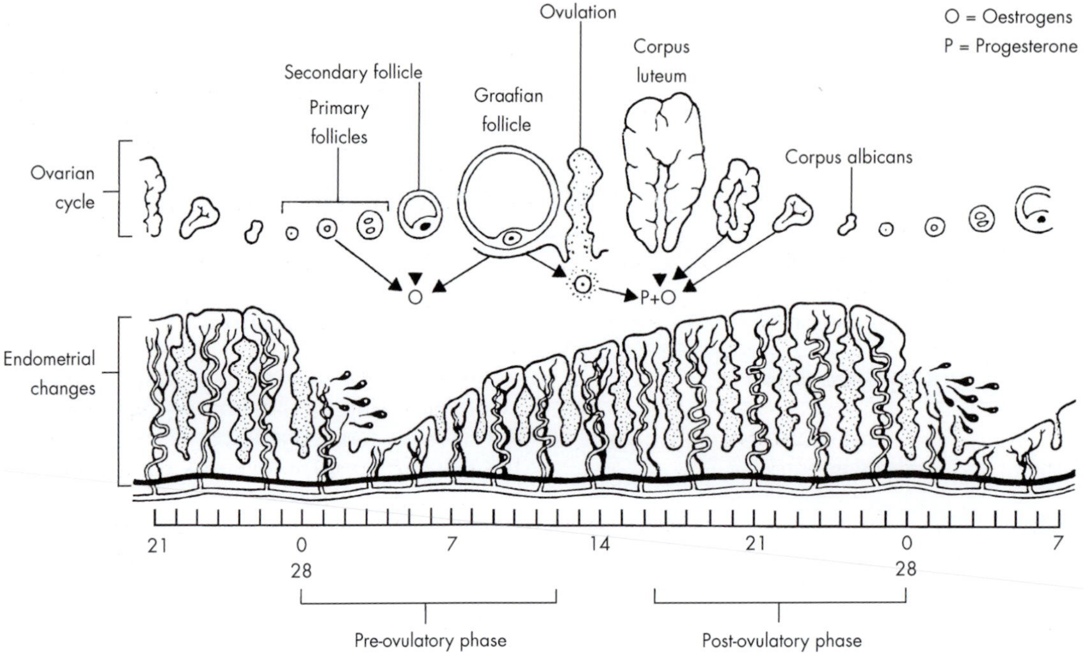

Figure 4.1 Menstrual cycle in the absence of fertilisation (*see also* Table 4.1).

consequently concentrations of oestrogens and progesterone decline, and menstruation occurs. Falling concentrations of oestrogens and progesterone cause gonadorelin to be secreted, which in turn stimulates the release of FSH and the start of a new cycle. The main events during the menstrual and ovarian cycles are summarised in Table 4.1.

Fertile and infertile phases

Combining a knowledge of the survival time of the ovum after ovulation with the survival time of sperm in the female genital tract (*see above*) permits the different stages of the monthly cycle to be considered as infertile or fertile. The first infertile phase of each menstrual cycle begins on the day that menstruation starts. This phase is terminated on the day when sperm can enter the reproductive tract and possibly lead to a pregnancy. The length of this period is determined by the speed at which the ovum is produced by maturation of the primary follicle. The fertile phase includes the one day that the ovum can be fertilised, plus the preceding seven days that sperm may survive in the reproductive tract. A safety margin of an extra day should be allowed. Fertilisation of an ovum can occur if sexual intercourse takes place at any time between days 9 and 17 of a 28-day cycle, but the variability of the time of ovulation produces a much wider range for the possible days on which fertilisation can occur. The presence of sperm already in the Fallopian tubes as an ovum is released from the Graafian follicle produces the greatest likelihood of fertilisation.

The second infertile phase lasts from the day after ovulation until the start of the next menses.

The likelihood of pregnancy resulting from intercourse has been estimated by Drife (1983). If 100 couples have frequent intercourse timed to take place during the most fertile period of the month, 85 of the women will have a fertilised ovum within one month. Of these, 15 will fail to implant in the uterus; and of the 70 that do become implanted, about half will be lost. Chorionic gonadotrophin will be detectable in 36 women, of whom only 24 will fail to menstruate the following month. Of the remaining 24, 3 or 4

Table 4.1 The stages of the menstrual and ovarian cycles (*see also* Figure 4.1)

Days	Events occurring
1 to 3	FSH stimulates production of approximately 20 to 25 primary ovarian follicles, that start to secrete oestrogen
4 to 5	Approximately 20 of the primary follicles develop into secondary follicles, that continue to secrete oestrogen
6 to13	FSH and LH stimulate further secretion of oestrogen from follicles; oestrogens stimulate repair of the endometrium
	One of the secondary follicles matures into a Graafian follicle, and oestrogen production continues to increase
	Small amounts of progesterone start to be secreted at the end of this phase
	High oestrogen levels inhibit GnRH, which decreases secretion of FSH, but the high oestrogen level increases secretion of LH (the LH surge)
14	LH surge causes release of an ovum into the pelvic cavity, from where it is guided into the Fallopian tube
15 to 28	LH secretion stimulates the development of the corpus luteum from the remaining follicular cells of the Graafian follicle; the corpus luteum secretes oestrogen and progesterone; and progesterone prepares the endometrium to receive a fertilised ovum
	In the absence of fertilisation, LH secretion decreases as a result of the negative feedback effect of rising oestrogen and progesterone levels (from the corpus luteum) on GnRH. As the secretion of LH falls, the corpus luteum degenerates, therefore the secretion of oestrogen and progesterone decreases, and the endometrium is shed (menstruation)
	Falling levels of oestrogen and progesterone cause the release of GnRH, which in turn stimulates the release of FSH, which stimulates the development of ovarian follicles, and a new cycle commences

will miscarry, leaving an approximate fertility rate of about 20%. The major cause of the high wastage rate is foetal chromosomal abnormalities.

Fertility at puberty

The menarche commonly occurs in healthy young girls between 11 and 12 years of age, although there is wide individual variation. However, the onset of the first period does not necessarily infer that ovulation will regularly occur; indeed, for up to two years after the menarche, ovulation may be infrequent and irregular. More importantly, the occurrence of menarche does not necessarily indicate the onset of fertility, although pregnancies have been reported in girls as young as 11 and 12 years of age.

Amenorrhoea and other menstrual disturbances may arise with the onset of further growth and development during the middle and late teens, particularly if associated with psychological upheavals (e.g. moving away from home). From the point of view of the need for contraception, however, the absence of periods does not preclude ovulation, and pregnancy can still occur.

Contraception

The desire to interrupt the normal physiological events that regulate conception has led to the development of a wide range of contraceptive methods. Each of the methods has associated adverse effects and benefits, and the usefulness and appropriateness of each of the available methods varies with the circumstances of the woman and her partner. Various factors relating to the contraceptive method will influence choice, including failure rate, reversibility, ease of use, mechanism of action, adverse effects and non-contraceptive benefits. Factors relating to the woman that influence the choice of contraceptive method include age (and therefore fertility), parity, medical disorders, smoking status and risk of sexually-transmitted diseases. Religious and cultural considerations may also influence choice. The contraceptive method of choice will thus probably vary during the course of a woman's life. The range of methods available will also change over time, as research is always underway into new methods of contraception and modifications of existing methods.

Failure rates, or effectiveness rates, are often given for the different contraceptive methods. Rates obtained from clinical trials generally refer to the failure rate that occurs with correct use of the contraceptive method. Some contraceptive methods (e.g. condoms, diaphragms, caps or oral contraceptives) require correct use for them to be effective (i.e. they are subject to 'user' failure). When these methods are used in practice, rather than in a clinical trial situation, the failure rates will be higher than those experienced during the trials. Other methods, such as injectable contraceptives and intra-uterine devices, have no 'user' failure associated with them, and the failure rates cited in clinical trials provide an accurate picture of the failure rates that may be expected in practice. Failure rates are often given as a number of pregnancies per 100 woman years. One hundred woman years is equivalent to 100 women using the method for one year.

Hormonal contraception

The introduction of hormonal contraception in the USA in 1960 and in the UK in 1961 revolutionised the techniques of contraception and led to the involvement of medical practitioners in a contraceptive advisory role that they had previously shunned.

There are two main types of oral hormonal contraceptive (known as 'the pill'): the combined oral contraceptive, which contains an oestrogen and a progestogen in varying strengths, and the progestogen-only oral contraceptive. Other forms of hormonal contraceptive available are progestogen-only injectable contraceptives and a progestogen-only intra-uterine contraceptive. Progestogen-containing subdermal implants were formerly available in the UK.

The oestrogens and progestogens used in oral contraceptive preparations available in the UK are listed in Table 4.2. The use of hormonal oral contraceptives in emergency contraception is discussed in Emergency contraception *below*.

Table 4.2 Oestrogens and progestogens contained in oral contraceptive preparations available in the UK

Oestrogens	Progestogens
Ethinlyoestradiol	Desogestrel
Mestranol	Ethynodiol diacetate
	Gestodene
	Levonorgestrel
	Norethisterone
	Norethisterone acetate
	Norgestimate
	Norgestrel

Combined oral contraceptives

Combined oral contraceptives provide very effective contraception. The failure rate of combined oral contraceptives with correct usage is less than one pregnancy per 100 woman years, although in practice failure rates of up to seven pregnancies per 100 woman years may be found. They are suitable for healthy, non-smoking women; smokers are advised to use alternative methods once they are over 35 years of age, and more suitable alternatives are available for women older than 50 years of age. However, they provide no protection against sexually-transmitted diseases, including human immunodeficiency virus (HIV).

Mode of action

Combined oral contraceptives act by disturbing the normal release of endogenous hormones and the regulatory feedback mechanisms. The method, therefore, imitates those changes in hormone concentrations that occur at the onset of pregnancy. Combined preparations inhibit ovulation and render the endometrium less favourable to implantation should ovulation occur. These preparations also increase the viscosity of cervical mucus, reducing the ability of sperm to reach the ovum.

Types of combined oral contraceptives

A complete list of the combined oral contraceptive preparations available in the UK is given in BNF 7.3.1. A number of factors should be considered when selecting a product, and these include:

- The strength of the oestrogen component
  Since the introduction of the combined oral contraceptive in the early 1960s, the dose of both the oestrogen and progestogen components has been reduced considerably. Combined oral contraceptives are classed as low-dose, standard-dose or high-dose oestrogen. Low-dose oestrogen preparations contain 20 µg of oestrogen (ethinyloestradiol) and are suitable for obese or older women if there are no other contra-indications. Standard-dose preparations contain 30 or 35 µg of oestrogen (ethinyloestradiol) in monophasic preparations or 30/40 µg in phased preparations and are suitable for most women (but *see* advice on progestogen content *below*). High-dose preparations contain 50 µg of oestrogen (either ethinyloestradiol or mestranol) and are generally reserved for circumstances where bioavailability is reduced (e.g. in concomitant use of enzyme-inducing drugs). Preparations with as low a dose of oestrogen consistent with effective contraceptive cover are recommended to minimise the incidence of adverse effects (*see below*).
- The strength of the progestogen component
  It is recommended that the lowest effective dose of progestogen with the most appropriate strength of oestrogen should be used.
- The selection of progestogen
  Gestodene, desogestrel and norgestimate have been reported to produce fewer adverse effects in combination with ethinyloestradiol than some other progestogens. However, recent evidence has indicated that combined oral contraceptives containing gestodene and desogestrel (so-called 'third-generation' combined oral contraceptives) are associated with a slightly higher risk of thromboembolism than those containing other progestogens (all combined oral contraceptives carry a small increased risk) (WHO Collaborative Study Group, 1995; WHO, 1997). There is insufficient evidence to know whether norgestimate also carries an increased risk. The UK Committee on Safety of Medicines (CSM) initially recommended that gestodene and desogestrel should therefore be reserved for women intolerant of other combined oral contraceptives. However, its current recommendation is that, provided women are informed of the risks and do not have contra-indications, the selection of a particular type of combined oral contraceptive should rest on clinical judgement (Committee on Safety of Medicines/Medicines Control Agency, 1999).
- Varying the hormone content during the month
  Combined oral contraceptives are available in monophasic, biphasic, and triphasic forms. Monophasic tablets contain a fixed dose of oestrogen and progestogen and are the most widely used. Biphasic and triphasic preparations contain two and three different hormone combinations respectively in the 21-day dosage schedule. They aim to provide a lower total dose of hormone over each cycle and to mimic more closely the pattern of endogenous secretion.
- Tablets to be taken for 21 or 28 days
  Regular compliance may be enhanced if one tablet is taken each day throughout the month, rather than discontinuing administration for seven days to provoke withdrawal bleeding. Some preparations (known as 'every day' tablets) include seven inert (or placebo) tablets to achieve continuous pill taking while still provoking withdrawal bleeding.

Dosage and administration

Combined oral contraceptives are generally taken at approximately the same time each day for 21 days and then stopped for seven days (but *see above*). If a dose is delayed by more than 12 hours, contraceptive protection may be lost. 'Every day' tablets are taken continuously. Withdrawal bleeding occurs during the pill-free (or inert tablet) week, usually 48 to 72 hours after discontinuing the last active pill, and is usually lighter and shorter than a normal menstruation. Withdrawal bleeding is not synonymous with the blood loss at menstruation since there is no unfertilised ovum that needs to be discarded and the endometrium does not break down. In theory, there is no need for withdrawal bleeding to take place. Continuous daily administration of combined oral contraceptives can be maintained in the short term, but the safety profile of long-term, continuous administration is not proven. In practice, however, many women are reassured by the regular monthly loss of blood as it confirms the absence of pregnancy.

During the pill-free week, there may be an increase in endogenous oestrogen concentrations. There is wide individual variation and some women may not exhibit any increase, whereas in others this increase may approach concentrations that could result in an LH surge and, subsequently, ovulation if a follicle is mature at that time (*see* Fertility and contraception *above*). In these cases, conception is a possibility and could account for rare pill-failures in the presence of perfect compliance. This effect is equally important in the event of any missed doses. If any pill is missed at the beginning or end of the monthly packet, the pill-free week will be increased beyond seven days. Consequently, there is a risk of endogenous oestrogen concentrations rising to levels that could result in an LH surge.

The general procedure for starting the first dose of the first course and the action to be taken in the event of a missed dose are outlined in Boxes 4.1a and 4.1b. Following childbirth, a combined oral contraceptive may be started at three weeks postpartum if the woman is not breast-feeding. A progestogen-only oral contraceptive (*see below*) is preferred in women wishing to use oral contraceptives who are breast-feeding. If combined oral contraceptives are started later than three weeks postpartum, additional contraceptive measures must be used for the first seven days. Following termination of pregnancy or miscarriage, combined oral contraceptives can be started on the same day. In women with secondary amenorrhoea, tablets may be started on any day once pregnancy has been excluded; additional contraceptive precautions are necessary for the first seven days. Special precautions are necessary in women undergoing surgery: oestrogen-containing oral contraceptives should be discontinued four weeks before major elective surgery and all surgery to the legs. They should normally be recommenced at the first menses that occurs at least two weeks after full mobilisation. When discontinuation is not possible (e.g. after trauma) or if, by oversight, a patient admitted for an elective procedure is still on an oestrogen-containing oral contraceptive, some consideration should be given to subcutaneous heparin prophylaxis. These recommendations do not apply to minor surgery with short duration of anaesthesia (e.g. laparoscopic sterilisation or tooth extraction) or to women taking oestrogen-free hormonal contraceptives.

Beneficial effects

The primary advantage of combined oral contraceptives, and the main reason why their use has become so widespread, is that they provide an extremely effective form of contraception for women, allied to minimal disruption to lifestyle. Other subsidiary benefits, which may themselves be primary indications for their administration, are the many improvements in gynaecological conditions produced by combined oral contraceptives.

Effects on menstruation

If a woman's periods are heavy, painful or irregular, administration of combined oral contraceptives will normally result in lighter, pain-free and regular withdrawal bleeding. Symptoms of premenstrual syndrome may also be improved.

Benign mammary dysplasias

Long-term administration of combined oral contraceptives can also protect against the development of benign, and particularly cystic, breast disease; this is in direct contrast to the postulated link between combined oral contraceptive use and malignant breast disease (*see below*).

Functional ovarian cysts

Administration of combined oral contraceptives has also been reported to reduce the incidence of functional ovarian cysts, primarily as a result of inhibition of ovulation.

Endometriosis

Combined oral contraceptives may help to suppress endometriosis and prevent the development

Box 4.1a Dosage regimen and missed-pill guidance for combined oral contraceptives

Dosage regimen

The dosage regimen for combined oral contraceptives is usually one tablet daily (at approximately the same time each day) for 21 days followed by a seven-day interval during which withdrawal bleeding occurs. It is usually recommended that tablets are started on the first day of the cycle (i.e. the first day of bleeding), in which case no additional contraceptive precautions are necessary. If the first course is started on the fourth day or later of the cycle, ovulation may not be inhibited during that cycle and additional contraceptive precautions should therefore be taken during the first seven days. Additional contraceptive precautions should also be used when changing from a high to a low oestrogen preparation.

Phased formulations more closely mimic normal endogenous cyclical activity. They are generally recommended for a day one start. If they are started on any other day, additional contraceptive precautions must be used for the first seven days. The tablets must be taken in the correct order.

'Every day' tablets should also be started on the first day of the cycle (beginning with active tablets). If the tablets are started on the fourth day of the cycle or later, additional contraceptive precautions must be used for the first 14 days (in case inactive tablets have been taken inadvertently). The tablets must be taken in the correct order.

When changing to a combined oral contraceptive containing a different progestogen, the new pack should be started without a seven-day break (or inert tablets). If there is a break between packs, additional contraceptive measures must be used for the first seven days (or 14 days for 'every day' tablets) of the new brand.

When changing to a combined oral contraceptive from a progestogen-only oral tablet, start the new tablets on the first day of the cycle, or, if amenorrhoea is present, start on any day once pregnancy is excluded.

Missed-pill guidance

If you forget to take a pill, take it as soon as you remember, and take the next one at your normal time. This may mean taking two tablets in one day. Provided that you are no more than 12 hours late in taking the forgotten tablet, contraceptive protection is not reduced.

If you are more than 12 hours late in taking one or more pills, you may not be protected. As soon as you remember take the missed pill, or, if more than one pill is missed, take the last missed pill and take the remainder of that month's course as usual. Either avoid sexual intercourse or use an extra contraceptive method for the next seven days. If these seven days run beyond the end of your pack, start the next pack as soon as you have finished the present one. In other words, do not leave a gap between packs. With 'every day' tablets, discard the inert tablets. This will mean you may not have a period until the end of two packs, but this will not harm you. Nor does it matter if you have some bleeding on days when you take the pill.

Extra contraceptive measures are also advised during, and for seven days after, vomiting or diarrhoea. If these seven days run beyond the end of your pack, omit the pill-free days (or the inert tablets in the case of 'every day' tablets) and start the next pack immediately.

If you are in doubt about these instructions contact your doctor or family planning clinic.

of endometrial and ovarian cancer. These beneficial effects can persist for many years after administration of combined oral contraceptives has stopped.

Other beneficial effects produced by administration of combined oral contraceptives are listed in Table 4.3.

Box 4.1b Dosage regimen and missed-pill guidance for progestogen-only oral contraceptives

Dosage regimen

Oral progestogen-only contraceptives are started on the first day of the cycle and taken every day at the same time (preferably in early evening) without a break. Additional contraceptive precautions are unnecessary when initiating treatment. When changing from a combined oral contraceptive to a progestogen-only preparation, treatment should start on the day following completion of the combined oral contraceptive course, so that there is no break in tablet taking (in the case of 'every day' tablets, the inert tablets must be omitted).

Missed-pill guidance

If you forget a pill, take it as soon as you remember and take the next one at your normal time. If you are more than three hours overdue in taking a pill, you are not protected. Continue normal pill taking but you must also use another method of contraception for the next seven days. If you have vomiting or very severe diarrhoea, the pill may not work. Continue to take it, but you may not be protected from the first day of vomiting or diarrhoea. Use another method of contraception for any intercourse during the stomach upset and for the next seven days.

Table 4.3 Beneficial effects of administration of combined oral contraceptives

System	Beneficial effect
Breast	Reduced incidence of benign breast disease
Endocrine system	Protection against thyroid disease
Gastro-intestinal tract	Protection against peptic ulceration
Genital system	Dysmenorrhoea reduced Endometriosis controlled Functional ovarian cysts controlled Menorrhagia controlled Menstrual cycle regularity improved Pelvic inflammatory disease incidence decreased Premenstrual syndrome reduced Protection against endometrial and ovarian cancer
Skin	Acne improved (with oestrogen-dominated pills)

Adverse effects

The adverse effects reported with combined oral contraceptive use are listed in Table 4.4. Some side-effects (e.g. amenorrhoea, spotting and break-through bleeding) may be reduced by changing to a preparation containing a different oestrogen/progestogen balance. Some side-effects may disappear with continued tablet taking. Any side-effect that persists should be investigated.

Combined oral contraceptives are associated with an increased risk of cardiovascular disease and associated mortality, including hypertension, venous thromboembolism (including deep-vein thrombosis and pulmonary embolism), myocardial infarction and stroke. This increased risk is due in part to the oestrogen content, and, therefore, the incidence of cardiovascular side-effects is probably lower with the newer low-dose oestrogen combined tablets. Nevertheless, the low-dose tablets cause an increase in blood pressure in many women, and also result in a small, but significant, increased risk of venous thromboembolism. Any increased risk of myocardial infarction and stroke is low in women aged under 35 years who do not smoke and who do not have pre-existing hypertension. The risk is highest in older women and those who smoke, although there is some evidence to suggest that older women who do not smoke may not have increased risk.

Other risk factors include a family history of arterial disease, diabetes mellitus, hypertension, obesity and migraine. Thrombosis may be more common when factor V Leiden is present, or in patients with blood groups A, B or AB. Specific

Table 4.4 Adverse effects reported with combined oral contraceptive use

System	Adverse effect
Cardiovascular system	Deep vein thrombosis Hypertension Myocardial infarction Oedema Pulmonary embolism Stroke
Central nervous system	Depression Headaches and migraine Increase or loss of libido
Endocrine system	Breast cancer Breast discomfort Stunted growth in prepubertal use Worsening of diabetes mellitus
Eyes	Corneal oedema Irritation from contact lenses Vision may deteriorate in myopic patients
Gastro-intestinal tract	Abdominal bloating Appetite increased Inflammatory bowel disease Nausea Vomiting (rarely)
Hepatic system	Changes to many liver enzymes Cholestatic jaundice Gall bladder disease Gallstones Hepatic adenomas
Skin	Acne Chloasma Photosensitivity Skin or hair changes
Urogenital system	Cervical cancer Menstrual irregularities (spotting, breakthrough bleeding, amenorrhoea)
Miscellaneous	Weight gain

risk factors for venous thromboembolism include a family history of venous thromboembolism, varicose veins and obesity. The risk of venous thrombosis varies according to the progestogen component of the combined tablet; a higher incidence has been associated with desogestrel and gestodene than with ethynodiol, levonorgestrel and norethisterone.

The effects of combined oral contraceptives on the incidence of malignant diseases are complex and contradictory. Overall, combined oral contraceptives are reported to slightly increase the risk of cervical cancer (although other factors may be involved) and breast cancer, but to protect against ovarian and endometrial cancer. In addition, there appears to be a negligible risk of liver cancer. The slight increase in risk of breast cancer that appears during use decreases after stopping, and is insignificant by ten years after discontinuation (Collaborative Group on Hormonal Factors in Breast Cancer, 1996a; Collaborative Group on Hormonal Factors in Breast Cancer, 1996b). The risk of cervical cancer increases with duration of use of combined oral contraceptives and high oestrogen dose.

Contra-indications

Contra-indications to the use of combined oral contraceptives are listed in Table 4.5.

Drug interactions

A number of potential and proven interactions between combined oral contraceptives and other drugs administered concurrently have been reported (*see* BNF, Appendix 1).

The most serious interactions occur with drugs that induce microsomal hepatic enzymes. Such drugs include anti-epileptics (e.g. carbamazepine, phenobarbitone, phenytoin, primidone and topiramate), the antifungal griseofulvin, antivirals (including nelfinavir, nevirapine and ritonavir) and the rifamycins, rifabutin and rifampicin. Both the oestrogen and progestogen components of combined oral contraceptives are metabolised by hepatic microsomal enzymes. Concomitant administration with an enzyme inducer will therefore reduce plasma concentrations of the oestrogen and progestogen and could lead to contraceptive failure. If the enzyme inducer (except a rifamycin, *see below*) is to be taken for only a short time, additional contraceptive precautions should be used while the woman is taking the course of enzyme inducer and for seven days afterwards (to allow recovery of

Table 4.5 Examples of absolute and relative contra-indications to the use of combined oral contraceptives

Absolute contra-indications[a]	Relative contra-indications[b]
Breast cancer	Age >35 years (avoid if >50 years)
Breast-feeding (until weaning or 6 months after birth)	Asthma
Cardiovascular disease (including previous or current thromboembolic disorders or high risk of them, and arterial disease or multiple risk factors for it)	Depressive disorders
Endometrial carcinoma	Diabetes mellitus
History of any serious condition affected by sex hormones (including haemolytic uraemic syndrome, chorea and otosclerosis)	Epilepsy
Lipid metabolism disorders	Family history of cardiovascular disease
Liver conditions (including cholestatic jaundice of pregnancy, acute infective hepatitis, porphyrias, liver adenoma, cirrhosis, chronic active hepatitis, disorders of hepatic excretion)	Gallbladder disease
Migraine (severe or focal or where there are other risk factors for cardiovascular disease)	Hyperprolactinaemia
Oestrogen-dependent tumours	Hypertension
Pemphigoid gestationis	Immobilisation
Pregnancy	Inflammatory bowel disease
Systemic lupus erythematosus	Major surgery
Thrombophlebitis	Migraine (see also absolute contra-indications)
Trophoblastic disease, recent (including hydatiform mole)	Obesity
Vaginal bleeding (undiagnosed)	Sickle-cell anaemia
	Smoking
	Varicose veins

[a] Conditions in which combined oral contraceptives should never be used

[b] Conditions in which combined oral contraceptives should not usually be taken or, if they are, careful monitoring is required

normal enzyme function). If these seven days run into pill-free (or inert-tablet) days, then the next pack should be started immediately. In women who are taking enzyme inducers (except the rifamycins) long term, it is recommended that either the woman should change to another method of contraception or preparations containing 50 µg of oestrogen should be used. It is recommended that these high-dose combined tablets should be taken continuously for three packs, followed by a pill-free interval of only four days. This method is referred to as 'tricycling'. Short courses of an enzyme inducer that produce more profound enzyme induction (e.g. rifabutin or rifampicin) require the continued use of additional precautions for four weeks after the course is finished. If rifabutin or rifampicin is to be taken long term, then an alternative form of contraception must be used.

Combined oral contraceptives themselves inhibit hepatic microsomal enzymes and may increase the effects of other drugs (e.g. alcohol, diazepam and prednisolone) taken concomitantly.

Some broad-spectrum antibacterials (e.g. ampicillin and tetracyclines) produce a disturbance of the gastro-intestinal flora on initiation of the treatment course. This reduces the enterohepatic recycling of the oestrogen component of combined oral contraceptives, thus reducing plasma-oestrogen concentrations; the progestogen component is unaffected. This effect is not thought to occur with narrow-spectrum antibacterials. The lower plasma concentrations of oestrogen lead to reduced contraceptive effectiveness. As the gastro-intestinal flora develop resistance to the antibacterial drug, the risk of reduced contraceptive effectiveness diminishes. The risk of contraceptive failure thus arises at the start of antibacterial treatment or upon changing long-term treatment. Additional contraceptive measures should be used for the duration of a short course of implicated antibacterials and for seven days afterwards. If these seven days run into pill-free/inert tablet days, then the next pack should be started immediately. If long-term antibacterials are started, additional contraceptive measures should be used for the first three weeks.

Other interactions can be predicted on the basis of the adverse effects of combined oral contraceptives (Table 4.4). Among the most important are: impaired glucose tolerance, which antagonises the action of antidiabetic drugs; depression, which may counteract the intended effects of antidepressant drugs; and raised blood pressure, which antagonises the effects of antihypertensive therapy. The effect of warfarin and other oral anticoagulants may be influenced by the concomitant use of combined oral contraceptives; the interaction is not predictable and both antagonism and enhancement of action have been reported.

The excretion of theophylline is impaired by combined oral contraceptives and may lead to toxic effects because of the narrow therapeutic range of the bronchodilator.

Progestogen-only oral contraceptives

Progestogen-only oral contraceptives are suitable for older women, for women over 35 years of age who smoke and for women of all ages in whom combined oral contraceptives are contra-indicated (Table 4.5). They are suitable for use by women who are breast-feeding. The failure rate with progestogen-only oral contraceptives in practice ranges between one and ten pregnancies per 100 woman years, which is higher than that for combined oral contraceptives. A complete list of the progestogen-only oral contraceptives available in the UK is given in BNF 7.3.2.

The choice of progestogen-only oral contraceptive for a first-time user is arbitrary; if the side-effects with one preparation are unacceptable to the patient, another preparation should be chosen until a suitable one is found.

Mode of action

The primary mode of action of progestogen-only oral contraceptives is to alter the ease with which sperm can penetrate cervical mucus. They also prevent proliferation of the endometrium so that it remains unfavourable for implantation of a fertilised ovum. Progestogen-only oral contraceptives prevent ovulation in only 15 to 40% of cycles, and the continued production of ova accounts for the decreased effectiveness of progestogen-only contraceptives compared with combined oral contraceptives.

Dosage and administration

Progestogen-only oral contraceptives are taken continuously (with no interval during menstrual bleeding) for as long as contraception is desired, starting the first course on the first day of a cycle. The daily occurrence of the cyclical changes in cervical mucus highlights the importance of regular dosage, which should be at the same time each day. If a dose is taken as little as three hours late, the contraceptive effect is not reliable. For the procedure for starting the first dose of the first course, and the action to be taken in the event of a missed dose, *see* Box 4.1b. Following childbirth, progestogen-only oral contraceptives may be started at anytime after three weeks postpartum. If they are started earlier, there is an increased risk of irregular bleeding. They have no effect on lactation. Progestogen-only oral contraceptives may be started immediately after a termination of pregnancy or miscarriage. Unlike combined oral contraceptives, progestogen-only contraceptives do not have to be stopped before major surgery.

Beneficial effects

Women taking progestogen-only oral contraceptives may experience improvement in the symptoms of premenstrual syndrome, dysmenorrhoea and breast tenderness.

Adverse effects

The range of side-effects from progestogen-only oral contraceptives is similar to that observed with combined oral contraceptives. However, unlike combined oral contraceptives, the available progestogen-only oral contraceptives carry less risk of thromboembolic and cardiovascular disease than combined oral contraceptives. As effects on carbohydrate metabolism are minimal, progestogen-only oral contraceptives may be used by insulin-dependent diabetics.

The most significant and common problem with progestogen-only oral contraceptives is a disturbance of normal menstruation patterns, which arises as a result of the effects of progestogen on ovarian function. Nevertheless, changes are not universal: some women may experience only minor deviations from their normal cyclical pattern; others exhibit spotting and breakthrough bleeding. Cycle irregularity tends to be worse during the early courses of progestogen-only contraceptives and gradually improves; it should not be taken as a sign of lack of contraceptive effectiveness. However, it may be sufficiently disruptive and persistent to lead women to seek other forms of contraception. Women can be reassured that previous patterns of menstrual regularity are normally resumed on stopping administration of progestogen-only contraceptives. Amenorrhoea may occur in some women and, once pregnancy has been excluded, is likely to indicate that ovulation has, in fact, been inhibited. Breast tenderness, headache and nausea may occur, although these symptoms generally abate during the first two or three months of administration.

Functional ovarian cysts can develop, producing significant pain and discomfort. Cysts tend to arise because of accumulation of fluid within follicles following abnormal ovulation. Pregnancies occurring in users of progestogen-only oral contraceptives are more likely to be ectopic than are pregnancies occurring in the general population.

Contra-indications

Some of the absolute and relative contra-indications to the administration of progestogen-only contraceptives are listed in Table 4.6.

Drug interactions

Progestogen-only contraceptives interact with enzyme-inducing drugs as described under Combined oral contraceptives, *above*. The effectiveness

Table 4.6 Examples of absolute and relative contra-indications to the use of progestogen-only contraceptives

Absolute contra-indications[a]	Relative contra-indications[b]
Arterial disease (severe)	Cardiovascular disorders
Breast cancer and other forms of sex hormone-dependent malignant diseases	Cholestatic jaundice (recurrent)
Hydatiform mole (recent)	Diabetes mellitus[c]
Liver adenoma	Functional ovarian cysts
Porphyria	History of ectopic pregnancy
Pregnancy	History of jaundice in pregnancy
Vaginal bleeding (undiagnosed)	Hypertension[c]
	Irregular menstrual bleeding at the menopause
	Liver disorders, active
	Malabsorption syndromes
	Migraine[c]
	Thromboembolic disorders[c]

[a] Conditions in which progestogen-only contraceptives should never be used

[b] Conditions in which progestogen-only contraceptives should not usually be used or, if they are, careful monitoring is required

[c] Suggested as relative contra-indications, although evidence of hazard is unsatisfactory

of progestogen-only contraceptives is not affected by broad-spectrum antibacterials.

Progestogen-only injectable contraceptives

Progestogens administered by intramuscular injection provide effective, convenient contraception that is easy to administer. They are as effective as the combined oral contraceptives, with the added advantage of having no 'user' failure. Two progestogens are available for injection: medroxyprogesterone acetate is for long-term use and can be considered as a first-choice contraceptive method; and norethisterone acetate, which is licensed for only two injections and is, therefore, only suitable as a long-term measure (e.g. while a couple are waiting for a vasectomy to become effective or after a woman has had a rubella vaccination).

Their mode of action is as for progestogen-only oral contraceptives, except that ovulation is always inhibited. Injectable progestogen-only contraceptives thus have the advantage that, unlike oral progestogen-only tablets, they also protect against ectopic pregnancy and functional ovarian cysts because they reliably inhibit ovulation. They provide effective contraception immediately if they are given during the first five days of a cycle. If an injection is given beyond this period, additional contraceptive measures must be used for seven days. Full counselling is essential to anyone wishing to receive an injectable contraceptive because the effects cannot be reversed for the duration of the activity of the drug.

Dosage and administration

Medroxyprogesterone acetate is given in a single dose of 150 mg during the first five days of the menstrual cycle and then repeated every 12 weeks. It may be administered following the birth of a baby, although heavy bleeding occurs in some women and it may be best to delay the first dose until five to six weeks postpartum. It is also recommended to delay the dose until six weeks postpartum if the woman is breast-feeding, to allow the infant's enzyme systems to develop fully; established lactation is not affected.

Norethisterone enanthate is given as a single dose of 200 mg during the first five days of the cycle or immediately after parturition, and may be repeated once eight weeks later. Norethisterone enanthate has not been reported to inhibit milk production. Traces of the hormone appear in the mother's milk, but are not considered to be harmful to the healthy neonate. However, neonates with severe or persistent jaundice should not be breast-fed.

Injectable progestogen contraceptives can be started immediately after a miscarriage or termination of pregnancy.

Adverse effects

The range of side-effects is as for progestogen-only oral contraceptives (*see above*). Menstrual irregularities are particularly common with injectable progestogen-only contraceptives and include:

- amenorrhoea in long-term use (more than one year)
- altered menstrual cycle (bleeding may be frequent, irregular or absent, and may persist for some time after discontinuation of the method)
- infertility following discontinuation of the method, which may last up to two years or more
- menorrhagia.

Contra-indications

As for Progestogen-only oral contraceptives, *see above*.

Drug interactions

Women who are taking enzyme-inducing drugs should have the frequency of injections increased from 12- to ten-weekly for medroxyprogesterone acetate and from eight- to six-weekly for norethisterone acetate. The effectiveness of injectable progestogen-only contraceptives is not affected by broad-spectrum antibacterials.

Research is ongoing into improving injectable methods of contraception; progestogen injections that are given monthly are available in some parts of the world.

Progestogen-only intra-uterine contraceptives

Progestogen-only intra-uterine contraceptives (sometimes referred to as intra-uterine systems (IUSs)) were developed as a result of attempts to improve the contraceptive effectiveness of intra-uterine devices (*see* Intra-uterine devices *below*).

The first of these (Progestasert®) incorporated progesterone into a T-shaped plastic frame from which the hormone was released through a permeable polymer membrane at the rate of 65 μg per day. However, a possible association with an increased incidence of ectopic pregnancies, and the inconvenience of having to replace the device annually, led to its withdrawal from the market in the UK (it is still available in some other countries). A second device (Mirena®) that has replaced Progestasert® in the UK is a similar T-shaped plastic device (impregnated with barium sulphate) that releases the progestogen (levonorgestrel) at a rate of 20 μg each day. The much lower concentration of released progestogen reduces the likelihood of the occurrence of systemic side-effects from the drug. Threads are attached to the base of the device that allow self-examination to confirm that the device is in place and allow its removal.

Progestogen-only IUSs have essentially the same mode of action as the progestogen-only oral contraceptives (*see above*), except that the progestogen is released locally; the physical presence of the system in the uterus may make a minor contribution to its contraceptive effect. Ovulation may be prevented completely or may continue normally. After one year, 85% of cycles are ovulatory. The failure rate is 0.2 to 0.5 pregnancies per 100 woman years.

Progestogen-only intra-uterine contraceptives provide contraception as soon as they are fitted and a rapid return to fertility after their removal. They reduce pelvic inflammatory disease (particularly in the youngest age groups, who are most at risk). After the initial few months, menstrual loss is reduced, as is dysmenorrhoea. However, IUSs provide no protection against sexually-transmitted diseases, including HIV.

Adverse effects

In the first three months, bleeding tends to be irregular and commonly results in semi-continuous spotting. This pattern generally improves and, in the long term, monthly blood loss is reduced. Hormonal side-effects during the initial period may include breast tenderness, headache and acne. However, progestogenic side-effects are less likely to be a problem compared with systemic progestogen-only contraceptives. Lower abdominal pain, back pain, vaginal discharge, depression and nausea have been noted in a small minority of women. Sometimes the IUS may be expelled or become displaced; rarely, perforation of the uterus or cervix may occur. Some women develop functional ovarian cysts, although these usually resolve spontaneously. There is a small risk of ectopic pregnancy in the event of failure of the IUS.

Contra-indications

Generally, as for standard IUDs and progestogen-only oral contraceptives.

Insertion

Pre-medication with oral analgesia, or local anaesthesia to the cervix, is required before fitting due to the width of the insertion tube. The IUS should be fitted ideally within the first seven days of a period. If fitted after this time, an additional contraceptive method should be used for the first seven days. To avoid expulsion of the device, it should not be inserted on the heaviest days of the period. Post-partum, an IUS may be fitted at about six weeks after vaginal delivery in women who are not breast-feeding and about eight weeks after a Caesarean delivery. It may be inserted immediately after a first-trimester miscarriage or termination. As with IUDs, the woman should check each month after the end of a period that the IUS threads come through the cervix. If the threads cannot be felt, the woman should be investigated immediately and another form of contraception must be used. The IUS may be left in place for five years. After insertion of the IUS, the woman should be seen after a few weeks, at six months, and then yearly. Removal of the IUS is usually performed during a period.

Interactions

Although enzyme-inducing drugs taken concomitantly will lower blood concentrations of progestogen, since the IUS action is primarily locally on the endometrium, the interactions are not considered to be clinically significant.

Other progestogen-only devices

Contraceptive implants provide long-acting, low-dose and reversible methods of contraception. A wide range of materials has been used. Levonorgestrel is the most widely used hormone to date, but newer progestogens may prove valuable in the future. Norplant® was the first implant to become available, launched in the UK in 1993. Although it remains in use in the rest of the world, it has been withdrawn in the UK. It consists of six thin flexible rods containing levonorgestrel, inserted subdermally in the upper arm under local anaesthesia. Specialised training is needed for the correct insertion of the implant and, if insertion is not performed correctly, removal may be complicated. The implant is effective for five years and can be removed at any time during this period. Fertility returns very quickly once the implant is removed. Adverse effects are as for other progestogen-only contraceptives (*see above*). Research is underway into another implant that consists of a single vinylacetate rod containing etonogestrel that is inserted subdermally.

Other implantable systems under investigation include injectable microspheres and microcapsules, and biodegradable implants.

Intra-uterine devices

The main impetus for the development of intra-uterine devices (IUDs) (Figure 4.2) was to provide women with a contraceptive method that had guaranteed effectiveness but demanded little or

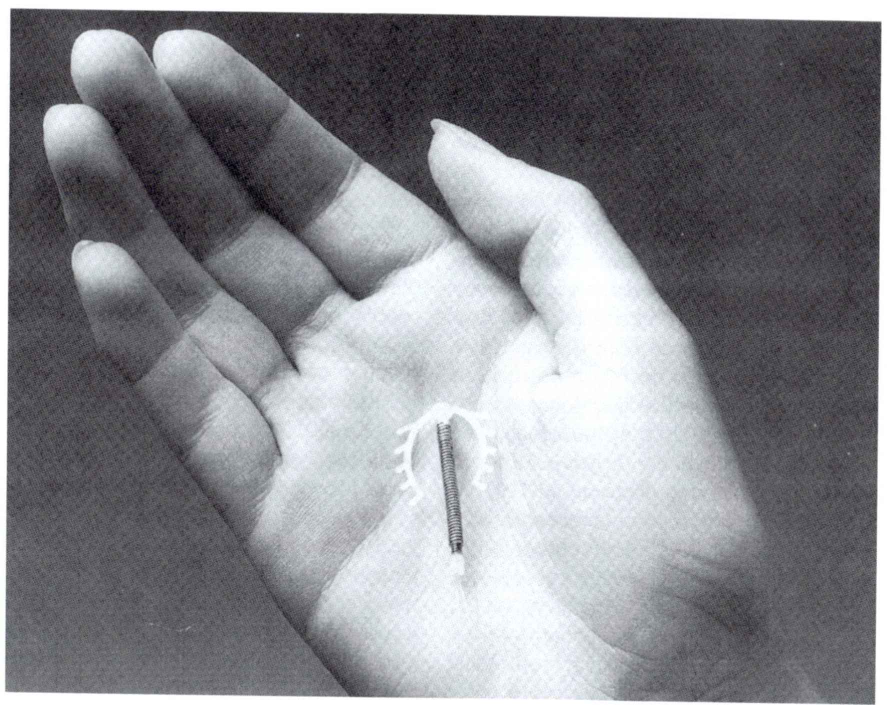

Figure 4.2 Intra-uterine device.

no attention after insertion. Other advantages to their use include: immediate effectiveness after fitting; non-interference with intercourse; and a high success rate in achieving reversibility of the contraceptive effect after removal. IUDs are especially useful for women who have had children but do not wish to use hormonal contraceptives, for those who find compliance with other contraceptive methods difficult and for older women who want an alternative to sterilisation. They are generally not suitable for nulliparous women, those at risk of sexually-transmitted diseases or those who suffer from heavy or painful periods.

The effectiveness of IUDs varies with the type of device. Modern IUDs have very low failure rates, ranging between less than one and three pregnancies per 100 woman years, with the lowest failure rates occurring in older women and after prolonged use.

For the use of IUDs in emergency contraception, *see* Emergency contraception *below*.

Mode of action

The contraceptive efficacy of IUDs is thought to involve an alteration in the uterine environment as a result of a pronounced foreign body reaction. The changes in uterine and tubal fluid that occur appear to impede the motility of sperm and transport of the ovum, and inhibit fertilisation. The release of copper ions from an IUD may potentiate these effects. IUDs may interfere with the implantation of a fertilised ovum, but this is no longer considered to be the prime mode of action.

Types of intra-uterine device

Inert devices

Advances in polymer science during the 1960s led to the manufacture of plastic (silastic) IUDs (the Lippes loop® and the Saf-T-Coil®). Inert devices are rendered visible on X-ray films by impregnating the plastic with barium sulphate. Although they are no longer available in the UK, the prolonged life of these inert devices makes it possible that some women may still be using them as a form of contraception, and may continue to do so until the menopause.

Bioactive devices

Bioactive devices were developed using the same basic structure as inert devices and are the most common form of IUD in use today. They were developed from the observation that adding copper to plastic IUDs significantly enhanced their contraceptive effect. Most of the currently used devices are shaped in the form of a letter 'T', and consist of a plastic carrier wound with copper wire or fitted with copper bands; some have a central core of silver to reduce the risk of copper fragmentation that can occur after prolonged use. As bioactive devices are more effective than inert devices, they can be made narrower, less cumbersome and less bulky. Consequently, the incidence of adverse effects caused by the physical presence of bioactive devices (*see below*) is less.

One or more nylon threads attached to the lower end of the plastic facilitate self-examination to confirm that the device is in place; they also permit its removal.

The total surface area (not the thickness) of the copper in proprietary devices is often indicated by the number incorporated in its name (e.g. there is 250 mm^2 copper in the Multiload® Cu250 device). Further modifications to bioactive devices have been tried in attempts to improve contraceptive effectiveness by using IUDs as delivery devices for progestogens (*see above* under Progestogen-only intra-uterine contraceptives).

Insertion and removal

Insertion

The timing of insertion and the technique of fitting an IUD are critical for its subsequent performance and need proper training. Although it is possible to insert devices at any time during the menstrual cycle, insertion up to day 9 appears to be part of the normal guidelines offered by some authorities. Most IUDs are inserted under aseptic conditions during the final days of menstruation or immediately after menstruation has terminated, since the cervical canal is slightly dilated at this time and the risk of insertion during an early, unconfirmed pregnancy is minimised. Fitting is generally avoided during the heaviest days of a woman's period. Following childbirth, an IUD may be inserted about six weeks after a vaginal delivery or eight weeks after a Caesarean delivery. Sometimes, an IUD may be fitted immediately after a vaginal delivery, provided that the woman is not breast-feeding; breast-feeding increases the risk of perforation. An IUD may be inserted immediately after a first trimester termination or miscarriage.

After insertion of copper-coated devices, menstrual irregularities, inter-menstrual bleeding and spotting, and dysmenorrhoea may occur. A watery, non-purulent vaginal discharge may be produced, but this is usually considered as normal. However, changes to the colour and consistency of the discharge require referral, commonly for antibacterial drug treatment. Some women may report abdominal pain and some bleeding immediately after insertion, and this can last for a few days. Pain may be controlled by simple analgesics. Prolonged abdominal discomfort may necessitate removal of the device. Women should be seen by the doctor six weeks and six months after insertion and then at yearly intervals.

Removal

The most common symptoms reported by women requesting removal of IUDs are pain and excessive bleeding (*see below*). These symptoms, which may occur together, are usually caused by incorrect positioning of the device or from the horizontal arms of the device becoming embedded in the walls of the uterus. Less frequently, pain and excessive bleeding may be caused by an infection.

Elective removal of an IUD may be carried out to permit attempts to become pregnant, at the menopause (normally 12 months after the last period) or when another method of contraception has been chosen. IUDs are usually removed during a period. If there is no desire to become pregnant, the device should not be removed in mid-cycle unless an additional contraceptive was used for the previous seven days, or if intercourse has not occurred during the preceding seven days. If the device has to be removed mid-cycle as an emergency (e.g. for severe pelvic inflammatory disease), consideration should be given to the use of post-coital contraception.

It is generally recommended that copper IUDs should be replaced every five years (although some manufacturers may recommend shorter time periods); some devices may be left in place for eight years. Any device inserted after 40 years of age may be left in place until the menopause. Ideally, an IUD should remain in place for as long as possible to reduce the risks of pelvic inflammatory disease and other complications that can occur after insertion. If an IUD fails and the woman is continuing with the pregnancy, then the device should be removed during the first trimester if possible.

Adverse effects

Pain and excessive bleeding

Lower abdominal pain may manifest as spasms and cramps, which can occur at any time during the menstrual cycle.

Increased blood loss may occur at menstruation, especially during the first couple of months. Menstrual blood losses of 70 to 80 mL are associated with inert devices and of 50 to 60 mL with copper devices. This compares with the average menstrual blood loss of 35 mL in women not fitted with an IUD. Bleeding and spotting may occur between each menses.

Ectopic pregnancy

There is a risk of ectopic pregnancy in the event of failure of the IUD. Most ectopic pregnancies occurring during IUD use occur in the Fallopian tubes, although they have been reported in other sites. The risk of ectopic pregnancy is increased in women with a history of pelvic inflammatory disease.

Pelvic inflammatory disease

There is an approximately four-fold increase in the risk of pelvic inflammatory disease in users of IUDs. The risk appears to be highest during the first three weeks after insertion. The increased incidence is thought to be a direct consequence of the presence of a foreign body in the uterine cavity, or may be associated with existing carriage of a sexually-transmitted disease. Ideally, pre-screening for sexually-transmitted diseases should be performed before fitting an IUD. Young nulliparous women appear to have a higher risk. Early detection of pelvic inflammatory disease is vital because, if untreated, it can cause infertility. Referral for treatment with broad-spectrum antibacterial drugs is essential; recurrent infection may necessitate removal of the IUD.

Perforation
There is an incidence of about one perforation of the uterine wall or cervix for every 1000 IUDs inserted; in extreme cases, the device may migrate over several weeks through the uterine wall and into the peritoneal cavity. Adhesions may develop with bioactive devices, or the IUD may perforate the wall of the bladder or gastrointestinal tract. In the event of perforation, the device must be promptly removed by surgery.

Lost threads and expulsion
The thread or threads attached to the base of an IUD hang down through the neck of the uterus into the vagina. Their presence acts as reassurance that the device is in place; they also provide a means of removal. Causes of the absence of detectable threads include: their upward disappearance beyond the external os into the uterus; penetration of the IUD through the uterine wall; shifting of the IUD out of position; or its expulsion. Missing threads may also indicate pregnancy. It is essential that women adopt alternative forms of contraception if the threads are no longer detectable because, even if devices have not been completely expelled, their contraceptive effectiveness is likely to have been reduced.

Total expulsion is uncommon, but the device may become sufficiently dislodged for the stem to protrude from the cervix. In such an event, the device should be removed by a doctor and, if desired, replaced by another IUD.

Expulsion of IUDs is most likely to occur at menstruation during the first three months of use, and may occur undetected. Expulsion is more common in nulliparous women, but the incidence decreases with age. Repeated expulsion is unlikely after insertion of a replacement device. Woman should be encouraged to check IUD threads regularly once a month after the end of a period.

Contra-indications

Some of the absolute and relative contra-indications to the use of IUDs are listed in Table 4.7.

Barrier methods and spermicides

Male condoms

Male condoms (sheaths, French letters or rubbers) are one of the oldest forms of contraception and are used all over the world. Condoms have the advantage of requiring no medical supervision. The condom is worn over the erect penis during coitus and acts as a contraceptive by collecting seminal fluid at its tip, thereby preventing the access of sperm to the female reproductive tract. Male condoms also inhibit the exchange of sexually-transmitted disease. Equally important, the use of condoms is one of the few methods of contraception in which the male partner can assume total responsibility. Condoms are commonly used as a sole form of contraception, although they may also be used as an additional measure, for example while a woman is learning to use a vaginal cap or diaphragm (*see below*) or during a course of a broad-spectrum antibacterial in women taking combined oral contraceptives (*see* Hormonal contraception *above*). Condoms are suitable for contraceptive use immediately after the birth of a baby.

The failure rate of condoms is about two to 15 pregnancies per 100 woman years, although their contraceptive effectiveness is better in older age groups. This increased effectiveness may be a result of reduced fertility and greater care in use.

Types of condom

The most commonly used male condom is made from natural latex rubber, hence its colloquial name. Male condoms made from latex that are manufactured to British Standards Institution (BSI) specification are tested as they come off the production line to ensure the absence of holes; samples are also tested for strength by inflation. Not all commercially available condoms are manufactured to these standards. Condoms made from latex rubber normally have a shelf-life of about five years when stored in a cool, dry place, although more rapid deterioration may occur in hot and humid climates.

Condoms may also be made from

Table 4.7 Examples of absolute and relative contra-indications to the use of intra-uterine devices

Absolute contra-indications[a]	Relative contra-indications[b]
Active pelvic inflammatory disease	Diabetes
Cervical abnormalities	Endometriosis
Confirmed or suspected pregnancy	Epilepsy
Distorted/small uterine cavity	Fibroids
History of bacterial endocarditis/severe infection	History of pelvic inflammatory disease
History of ectopic pregnancy or tubal surgery	Joint and other prostheses
Immunosuppressive therapy (established or marked immunosuppression)	Severe dysmenorrhoea
Malignancy of the genital tract	Women under 30 years of age, particularly if they have not had children
Prosthetic heart valve	Women of any age who have had a number of sexual partners and who may be at increased risk of sexually transmitted diseases
Severe anaemia	Women who are not in mutually faithful relationships
Sexually transmitted disease (untreated)	
Trophoblastic disease	
Undiagnosed abnormal vaginal bleeding	
With copper devices:	
Copper allergy	
Wilson's disease	
Medical diathermy	

[a] Conditions in which intra-uterine devices should never be used

[b] Conditions in which intra-uterine devices should not usually be used or, if they are, careful monitoring is required

polyurethane, a material that is double the strength of latex and, therefore, enables much thinner condoms to be made, which may have improved sensation during sexual intercourse. Polyurethane condoms have a longer shelf-life than latex condoms. There is currently no BSI standard for polyurethane male condoms. There are European standards for both latex and polyurethane condoms (represented by the CE Mark), although these do not represent such rigorous testing standards as the BSI standards.

Condoms can also be made from lamb intestines. However, such natural products conform less readily to the shape of the penis than synthetic products, and there is a greater tendency for them to slip off when the penis is retracted. Furthermore, the natural product is more expensive and it has not been conclusively demonstrated that it prevents the transmission of HIV infection.

Condoms are normally supplied in one size and are packaged flat by rolling onto the rim located at the open end. Variations of design and style, primarily to enhance the enjoyment of sexual intercourse, include the presence of ribbing and nodules over the surface; others may be coloured, perfumed or flavoured.

Some condoms incorporate a spermicide (*see below*), lubricant or both. The most commonly used spermicide is the nonionic surfactant, nonoxynol-9. The spermicide is coated over the inner and outer surfaces and is included as a precautionary measure against the accidental spillage of small amounts of seminal fluid. However, the concentration of spermicide used is not usually sufficient to be effective against the wholesale leakage of seminal fluid from a condom that has ruptured.

A lubricant (usually silicone-based) may be included to minimise friction between the penis and vagina on penetration, which may be a particular problem if vaginal secretions are minimal. A lubricant may also reduce the friction on the condom, thus lessening the chance of it slipping off. Any oil-based lubricants or vaginal or rectal preparations reduce the strength of condoms made from latex rubber and may render them less effective as a barrier method of contraception and as a protection from sexually-transmitted diseases, including HIV, and therefore must not be used. Polyurethane condoms are unaffected by oil-based preparations.

In the UK, the majority of condoms are bought from pharmacies, and it has been suggested that most are bought by women. Supermarkets and vending machines provide the other main purchasing outlets. Free supplies can be obtained from family planning clinics (*see* Contraceptive services *below*), but doctors cannot prescribe them at NHS expense on prescription forms, unlike most other forms of contraception.

Method of use

To maximise effectiveness, a condom should be fitted before there is any contact between the penis and vagina. The small amount of seminal fluid that may be discharged from the penis before ejaculation contains sufficient sperm to cause pregnancy (*see* Fertility and contraception *above*).

Great care should be taken in fitting and removal to prevent damage to the condom from sharp objects (e.g. fingernails or jewellery). The condom should be unrolled over the complete length of the erect penis, while keeping the closed end of the condom pinched between the forefinger and thumb; this allows an empty reservoir at the end of the condom to collect seminal fluid.

Ideally, the female partner should use a spermicide (*see below*), even if the condom has an integral coating of spermicide.

The condom should be held firmly by its rim at the base of the penis on withdrawal from the vagina, which should ideally take place as soon as possible after ejaculation. This helps to prevent the condom slipping off and reduces the risk of spillage of collected seminal fluid which may occur, particularly if the penis is withdrawn in a flaccid state. There should be no contact between the penis and vagina after removal of the condom following intercourse; if further intercourse is to take place, a fresh condom should be used. If the condom does rupture, emergency contraception (*see below*) should be arranged as soon as possible.

Beneficial effects

The most important advantage that the use of condoms confers is protection against sexually-transmitted diseases, including HIV. The possible association between sexually-transmitted diseases and genital cancer (e.g. cervical cancer) means that condoms may also reduce the risk of female malignancies. Male condoms may also protect the woman against pelvic inflammatory disease. Condoms can prolong the period of erection before ejaculation; the rim at the base of the condom may enhance the degree of erection by constricting the base of the penis.

Condoms may also be of benefit in instances where greater, not less, fertility is desired. It has been estimated that about one in five women may produce antibodies to sperm; the regular use of a condom over three to six months reduces the antigenic challenge of the sperm and decreases the concentration of circulating antibodies.

Disadvantages

Drawbacks with the use of male condoms include a perceived reduction in sensitivity in the sexual act. The method requires forward planning, it needs to be used carefully to be effective and it may interrupt intercourse. Allergy or sensitivity can occur to latex condoms and/or the spermicide.

Female condoms

The female condom is a lubricated, loose fitting polyurethane sheath that loosely lines the vagina and some of the vulva and acts as a barrier between sperm and egg, so preventing fertilisation. Its effectiveness rate is 85 to 95%. In the UK, the only female condom available is Femidom®. In addition to acting as a contraceptive, it also provides protection against sexually-transmitted diseases, including HIV, and may protect against cancer of the cervix and pelvic inflammatory disease. As with the male condom, the female condom has the advantage of not requiring any medical supervision.

Method of use

Female condoms are supplied in one size. They have two flexible rings: the inner ring acts as a guide during insertion and is pushed up behind the pubic bone; the outer ring lies flat against the body covering the vulva and helps prevent the condom being drawn down into the vagina during intercourse. It can be inserted at any time before intercourse and does not require additional spermicide. It can be used with oil-based products and, compared with male condoms, feels more normal for the partner.

Disadvantages

Careful insertion is required for it to be effective, and it can get pushed into the vagina during sex. Care must be taken that the penis is guided into the condom and not between the vagina and the condom. It should not be used by women with pre-existing vaginal or cervical infection.

Diaphragms

The diaphragm (vaginal cap or 'Dutch cap') is a thin, soft rubber dome that is inserted into the vagina and acts as a contraceptive by presenting a physical barrier to the passage of sperm by lying across the cervical opening. Sperm cannot gain access to the alkaline cervical mucus, but remain stranded and subsequently perish in the acidic environment of the vagina. Contraceptive action is improved by the concomitant use of a spermicide (*see below*) and diaphragms must always be used with a spermicide.

Average failure rates during the first year of use are about 2 to 15 pregnancies per 100 woman years. The failure rate is less in older women and in those experienced in use of this method.

Types of diaphragm

The diaphragm is a thin, soft rubber dome mounted on a metal rim; it is held in place in the vagina by the spring located in the rim. The metal rim of the diaphragm can be formed of a flat spring, a spirally shaped coil spring, or an arcing spring. The most commonly used version is the flat spring, which maintains a firmer shape than the coil spring and is relatively easy to manipulate when inserting. It comes in sizes 55 to 95 mm and is suitable for women with normal vaginas. The coil spring is more flexible (and consequently more difficult to control on insertion), but may be used in women with good vaginal muscle tone who find the flat spring diaphragm uncomfortable. It comes in sizes 55 to 100 mm. The arcing spring diaphragm combines the properties of both the flat spring and coil spring versions and squeezes into an arc for insertion. It comes in sizes 60 to 95 mm. It may be used in women experiencing difficulty in fitting either the flat or coil spring types or who have poor vaginal muscular support.

Method of use

There are considerable variations in anatomical dimensions between women and this requires that the correct size of diaphragm be selected by careful measurement. The largest size that is comfortable is selected, as the upper portion of the vagina enlarges during intercourse. Measurement requires an internal examination and is carried out by a doctor or family planning nurse. The diameter of diaphragms available in the UK ranges from 55 to 100 mm in steps of 5 mm; if the internal measurement lies half-way between available sizes of the flat spring diaphragm, the reduced tension within the coil spring model will usually provide a comfortable fit.

The diaphragm is fitted into the vagina between the posterior fornix and behind the pubic bone. It is held in place by the vaginal muscles, the tension of the ring and the pubic bone. If the diaphragm is inserted correctly, neither partner should be able to feel it. Women are usually issued with a temporary 'practice' diaphragm for several days to practise fitting and removal. Additional contraceptive cover during this period is essential. After the initial measurement and fitting, subsequent size checks are made at one week and three months; thereafter, re-measurement is necessary every 12 months (when the diaphragm should be replaced) and after a birth, miscarriage or termination of pregnancy, or changes in weight greater than 3 kg.

The diaphragm does not provide a total seal

around the neck of the cervix and it is therefore essential that two 5 cm strips of spermicide, in the form of a cream or gel, are coated onto both outer and inner surfaces immediately before insertion; spermicide may also be applied to the rim to facilitate insertion. Extra spermicide can also be used, and is essential if intercourse takes place more than three hours after insertion, or is repeated. Oil-based vaginal and rectal preparations will damage diaphragms made from latex rubber, and thus render them less effective as a barrier method of contraception.

The diaphragm is inserted into the vagina before intercourse and should remain in position for at least six hours after intercourse. The diaphragm should be removed within 30 hours of fitting (because of a small risk of toxic shock syndrome if left in place for longer), washed in warm water, dried and stored in a cool, dry place until next required. Before each use, the diaphragm should be checked for any holes or deterioration.

Beneficial effects

Using a diaphragm can protect against some vaginal infections (e.g. chlamydia and gonorrhoea), although less effective protection is afforded to others (e.g. herpes and syphilis). The presence of a physical barrier may also act to reduce the incidence of pelvic inflammatory disease and cervical cancer. It can be inserted at a convenient time before intercourse.

Disadvantages

The intimate examination needed for sizing and fitting may be unacceptable to some women. Additionally, the need for this to be carried out by trained personnel in a clinical environment may be a further demotivating factor in their use. The method requires careful use to be effective. Diaphragms provide no protection against some sexually-transmitted diseases, including HIV.

Urinary frequency and urgency, and urinary-tract infections, are more common in diaphragm users. These adverse effects occur primarily as a result of the upward pressure from the device on the urethra and the base of the bladder and are often due to poor initial fitting. Attention to cleanliness in their use is essential to prevent the introduction of *Escherichia coli* and other coliform bacteria from the perianal region. If recurrent urinary-tract infections occur, the size of diaphragm should be checked carefully and, if necessary, a smaller size or a cervical cap should be tried. Local soreness and ulceration may occur because of the pressure of the diaphragm within the vagina. In the event of vaginal soreness, women should be referred to the doctor or family planning clinic for reassessment and resizing. Allergy to the rubber or added spermicide can occasionally occur. A very few cases of toxic shock syndrome have occurred, mainly in women wearing the diaphragm for longer than 30 hours.

Contra-indications

Diaphragms are not suitable for use in women with very poor vaginal muscle tone or a shallow pubic ledge (a cap would be a suitable alternative). They also should not be used in women with vaginal abnormalities or who have had toxic shock syndrome. They should not be used if there is current vaginal, cervical or pelvic infection or recurrent urinary-tract infections.

Cervical caps

Cervical caps are smaller devices than diaphragms and come in different shapes and sizes. They fit directly over the cervix, thus preventing the passage of sperm into the cervical mucus. As with diaphragms, caps must be used with a spermicide. Caps are used as alternatives to diaphragms in women who have poor muscle tone and in some women with uterovaginal prolapse. Caps are unlikely to produce urinary symptoms and are unaffected by changes in body-weight. Compared with diaphragms, caps are less likely to reduce sensation in the vagina and may be more comfortable. However, because they are more difficult to fit than diaphragms, there is a greater tendency not to persist with the method. They appear to be used only rarely.

Types of cervical caps

Cervical caps are made from rubber. There are three types of cervical cap (Figure 4.3): the cavity rim cervical cap, the vault cap and the vimule cap. Each has a similar mode of action, but they differ slightly in shape. Cervical caps differ from diaphragms in that the rim is not reinforced by metal. Moreover, cervical caps are held in place mainly by suction, whereas diaphragms are retained by spring tension.

The cavity rim cervical cap (Preventif cervical rim) is a thimble-shaped device with a thickened rim and fits tightly over the cervix; this is facilitated by a groove on the rim. It is available in four sizes, with internal diameters of 22, 25, 28 and 31 mm.

The vault cap (Dumas cap) is a bowl-shaped, flat-domed cap similar in appearance to a diaphragm, although its rim does not have a metal spring. It is available in five sizes, ranging from 55 to 75 mm in 5 mm steps; in the UK, these five sizes are designated 1 to 5 and the numbering is moulded onto the rim.

The vimule cap has a bell-shaped dome and the open end is wider than its body. As a result, the cap covers the outer walls of the vagina as well as the cervix. It is made in three sizes: size 1 (small; 42 mm), size 2 (medium; 48 mm), and size 3 (large; 51 mm).

Method of use

Initial selection of cap size and type is made following careful internal examination, as for fitting of a diaphragm (*see above*). Caps should be replaced annually. Spermicide must be placed inside the dome before fitting. The timings for insertion, re-application of spermicide and cleaning are the same as for diaphragms. Spermicide must not be placed on the rim, as its presence may reduce suction. It is generally recommended that cervical caps should not be left in the vagina for longer than 30 hours. This timing allows for 24 hours of use, plus the six hours recommended before removal after last intercourse. If more than three hours elapse between insertion and sexual intercourse, further spermicide must be used. Caps should be checked for holes or deterioration before each use.

Newer types of cap are under investigation, with the aim of producing a cap that is easier to fit and that can be used without spermicides.

Spermicides

Spermicides should not be recommended as a sole method of contraception. They are primarily agents to be used with barrier forms of contraception (e.g. diaphragms, condoms); they may also be used with coitus interruptus. Their use may help to reduce the incidence of sexually-transmitted diseases, including HIV, and they may also increase lubrication in the genital tract.

Mode of action

Spermicides are surfactants that inhibit the uptake of oxygen by the sperm, reduce cell-wall surface tension and can alter the osmotic balance between sperm and their external environment. The viscosity of the inert basis may also prevent the progress of sperm. In addition, vaginal pH is altered, providing an inhospitable environment for sperm.

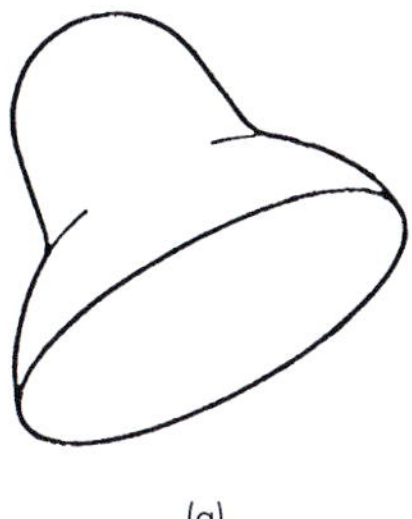

(a)

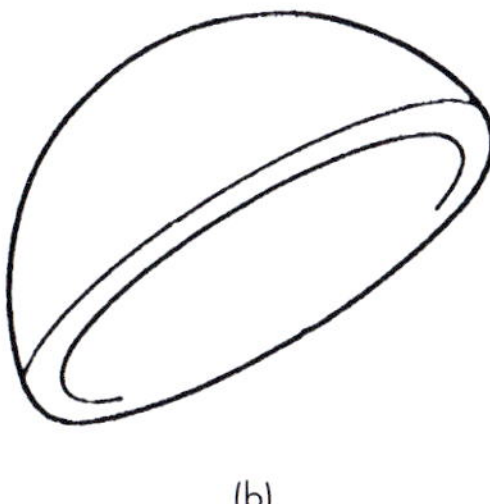

(b)

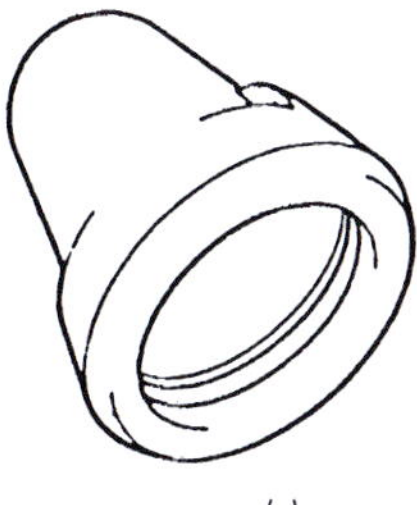

(c)

Figure 4.3 Cervical caps: (a) Vimule cap (b) Vault cap (c) Cavity rim cervical cap.

Types of spermicide

Spermicides are formulated as aerosol foams, creams, gels, pessaries and soluble films. A vaginal contraceptive sponge impregnated with nonoxynol-9 was formerly available. The creams and gels liquefy at body temperature and are rapidly distributed throughout the vagina. The foams are released from the pressurised container into an applicator that is inserted into the vagina. Pessaries and films take longer to disperse and are possibly less effective than creams, gels or aerosol foams. The most commonly used spermicide is nonoxynol-9 (used in varying concentrations); others include *p*-di-isobutylphenoxypolyethoxyethanol and octoxynol.

Method of use

Products are normally inserted as high as possible into the vagina just before intercourse, although pessaries and foaming tablets should be inserted at least ten minutes before.

Investigation is underway into the use of a new type of contraceptive sponge and into longer-acting spermicides.

Alternative methods of contraception

Coitus interruptus

Coitus interruptus (withdrawal method) is one of the oldest methods of contraception. It involves removing the penis from the vagina immediately before ejaculation. The method therefore requires considerable self-control and discipline at a time when sexual arousal is at its height. Despite considerable adverse criticism, particularly about the lack of 'completeness' of the sexual experience that coitus interruptus is said to produce, it can be effective and its use is clearly without harmful adverse effects. The failure rate of the method has been estimated as between 5 and 20 pregnancies per 100 woman years.

Failure of the method may be particularly high in inexperienced couples. One of the major problems is the lack of recognition that only small quantities of seminal fluid can contain sufficient sperm for conception to take place (*see* Fertility and contraception *above*), and that any delay in withdrawal of the penis may lead to the leakage of small amounts of seminal fluid immediately before the onset of ejaculation.

Greater confidence in the use of coitus interruptus may be possible if spermicides are also used. However, this may be unacceptable to people from certain ethnic and religious backgrounds.

Natural family planning

Natural family planning, or fertility awareness, is a method for achieving or avoiding pregnancy by observation of the natural signs and symptoms that occur during the course of the menstrual cycle which indicate the fertile and infertile phases.

Natural family planning may be regarded as the most acceptable form of contraception by couples who wish to feel in control of their own fertility. It may also be an advantageous method for those who are concerned about the use of appliances or drugs in controlling fertility, and for others who may not be allowed to use other forms of contraception for religious or ethical reasons. However, it must be clearly understood that a high degree of motivation and self-control is vital to ensure that intercourse is restricted to those times during each cycle when it is certain that there is no risk of conception. Women using this form of contraception must possess a reasonable understanding of the menstrual and ovarian cycles (*see* Fertility and contraception *above*) and require adequate teaching. There are a number of indicators that may be used to identify the fertile and infertile phases of the menstrual cycle. Combining more than one of the fertility indicators will provide more effective contraception. The indicators are described *below*.

Temperature

In this method, sometimes called the basal body temperature method, the body temperature is recorded throughout the menstrual cycle. Temperatures are measured with a fertility thermometer, which is calibrated between 35 and 39°C at 0.1°C intervals. Readings should be taken every day as soon as waking up, before getting out of bed and before drinking any hot fluids. Temperatures can be taken via the oral, rectal or vaginal routes, but whichever method is chosen, it should be used consistently and the thermometer should remain in position for three to five minutes. Temperatures are recorded on specially designed charts, and a clear increase in temperature of between 0.2 and 0.4°C can usually be seen about 12 to 16 days before the next period. This rise corresponds to the increased release of progesterone occurring after ovulation. Users of this method should clearly understand, however, that the infertile phase does not begin until three raised temperatures have been recorded above six previous lower recordings (excluding days 1 to 4), and is maintained until the onset of the next menses. Following this peak, unprotected intercourse can take place until the next menses.

The main difficulty in using this method arises because of natural fluctuations in body temperature. Increased temperatures can occur as a result of a mild infection (e.g. the common cold) or from drinking alcohol the previous night; reduced temperatures may follow administration of aspirin. One further difficulty is that there is no sustained temperature rise (i.e. indicating the end of the fertile phase) in an anovulatory cycle, which is paradoxically an infertile cycle throughout.

Cervical mucus

The cervical mucus method (Billings method or ovulation method) is based upon the physical changes that occur in the cervical mucus during the menstrual cycle. On its initial detection in the cycle, the mucus is thick, sticky and opaque and the opening of the vagina and vulva appear dry; further gradual changes occur in which the mucus becomes more copious, more slippery, less viscous and then almost clear immediately before ovulation, when the vulva is moist and wet. After the mid-cycle point, the mucus rapidly becomes cloudy again and then completely disappears or is virtually undetectable.

Mucus is observed on toilet paper at micturition or felt in the vagina. The time when the maximum amount of mucus is detected closely correlates with peak plasma-oestrogen concentration. At this stage, the mucus is often described as stretchy and slippery. To be an effective contraceptive method, intercourse should be avoided on the days between initial detection of mucus and four days after the peak mucus day is detected.

As in the case of the basal body temperature method, unrelated factors may modify the accuracy of the cervical mucus method. Vaginal candidiasis, and drugs used in its treatment, may reduce cervical secretions at the mid-cycle point, which may make accurate assessment of the occurrence of ovulation difficult.

Cycle length

Terms formerly used to describe this method include the 'rhythm' or 'safe period'. It is also called the calendar method. The length of the period between ovulation and the end of the menstrual cycle forms the basis of the calendar method. It requires a record of the length of menstrual cycles to be kept over at least a six-month period, and preferably over 12 months. Since this method makes no allowance for cycle irregularity, stress, illness or other factors, this method is no longer recommended as a reliable indicator of fertility.

Symptothermal indicators

This method (sometimes referred to as the multiple index method or double check method) uses a combination of basal body temperature monitoring and assessment of cervical mucus, plus several other indices which, with practice, women can use to detect ovulation. The most important of these additional indices is the determination of the position and firmness of the cervix, and the extent to which it is open. During the days immediately before ovulation, the cervix becomes softer to the touch and higher in position, and the cervical opening becomes wider. After ovulation, it descends, becomes firmer to the touch and the opening becomes smaller.

Other indices include mid-cycle ovulation pain, discharge or bleeding, breast sensitivity and mood changes.

Charts are available to record the combination of characteristics used in this method (Figure 4.4). Symptothermal methods must be taught by those who are experienced in their use, and interpretation of the indices must be carefully explained.

Fertility devices

Advances in technology and improved understanding of the reproductive processes have led to the introduction of a fertility device, Persona® (*see* Figure 4.5). This consists of a small, hand-held, computerised monitor and urine test sticks. The system detects hormonal changes related to fertility and defines the beginning and end of the fertile phase by measuring urine concentrations of oestrone glucuronide and LH. Urine is sampled using test sticks on designated days (indicated by a yellow light on the monitor) of the menstrual cycle (16 days in the first cycle, eight in subsequent cycles). After reading the test stick, the electronic monitor indicates fertile days by a red light and infertile days by a green light. This system has a failure rate of six pregnancies per 100 woman years. Persona® is not suitable for women whose menstrual cycle is shorter than 23 days or longer than 35 days, or for women who are breast-feeding. It should also not be used by women taking tetracycline or hormonal contraception, or by women with impaired liver function, kidney function or polycystic ovary syndrome. It is also not suitable for use by women who have experienced menopausal symptoms.

Sterilisation

Sterilisation is one of the most effective methods of contraception, and is usually irreversible. It is primarily selected by couples who have completed their family or, less commonly, for those

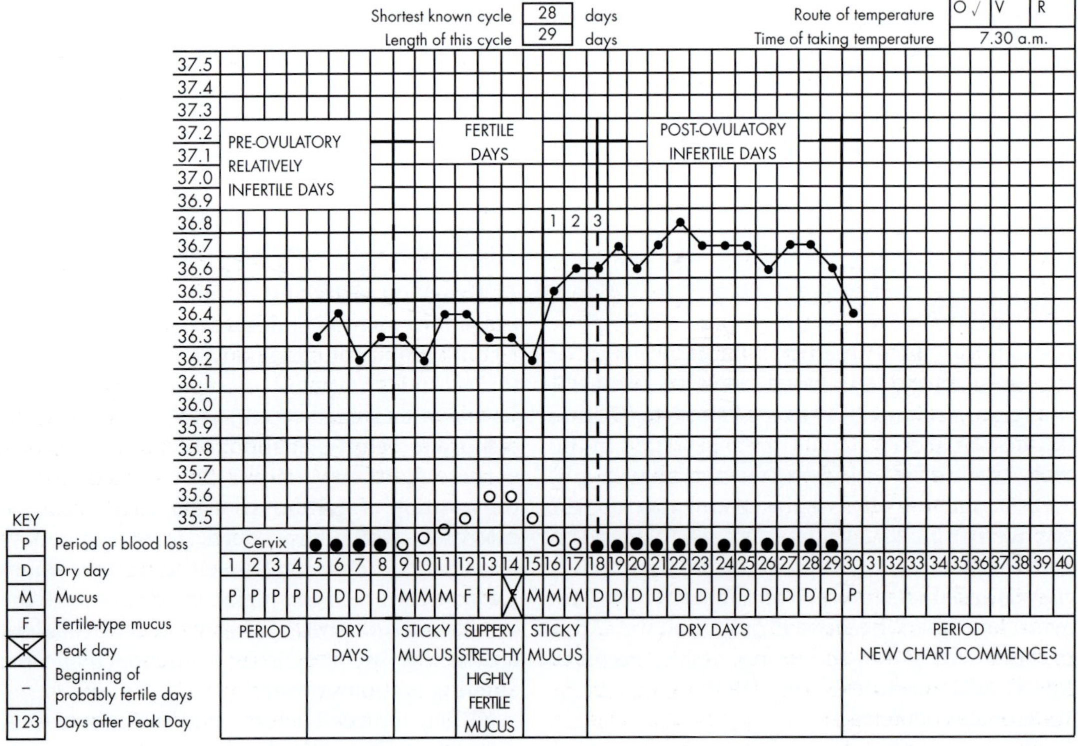

Figure 4.4 Example of a symptothermal chart.

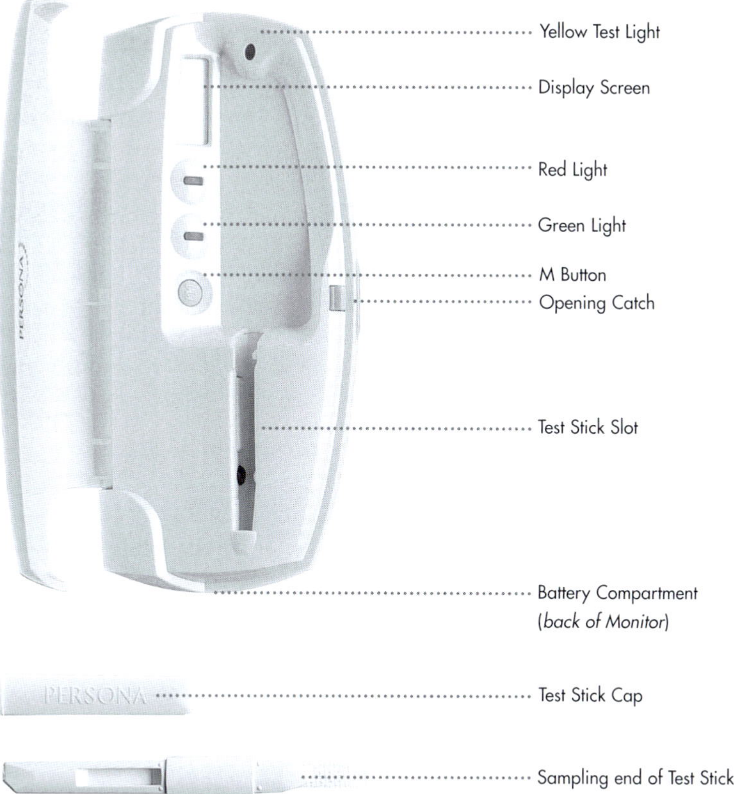

Figure 4.5 Persona fertility device (monitor and test stick). Reproduced with permission of Unipath.

who know that they will never want to have children. The average age at which sterilisation is selected as a means of contraception is falling. The number of vasectomy operations carried out has increased since they became available in the UK under the NHS in 1972. Surgical male sterilisation is carried out to stop the passage of the sperm along the vas deferens. Female sterilisation by surgical techniques is carried out to stop the passage of the ovum along the Fallopian tubes. Normally, neither procedure affects the production of male and female hormones responsible for secondary sexual characteristics. The failure rate of vasectomy has been reported to be extremely low (0.02 pregnancies per 100 woman years). Failure rates of between 0.1 and 3 pregnancies per 100 woman years have been reported for female sterilisation, although the true figure is likely to be nearer one pregnancy per 100 woman years. Some of the pregnancies that occur immediately after female sterilisation may be the result of a fertilised ovum present before the operation.

Male sterilisation is easy to carry out and involves minimal disruption to work or social activities. Female sterilisation takes longer to recover from, especially when carried out by laparotomy. However, female sterilisation is effective immediately, whereas it takes up to four months to confirm that male sterility has been achieved.

The importance to each partner of undergoing sterilisation must be discussed and stressed before surgery. Although the partner's consent is not required, it is clearly more desirable for both individuals to agree to the need for, and the objective of, sterilisation.

Male sterilisation

A vasectomy is usually carried out under local (occasionally general) anaesthetic. Surgery involves making a small incision in the upper portion of the scrotum and exposing the vas deferens, which carry sperm from the testes to the penis. Each vas deferens is cut and the cut ends ligated. Alternatively, a small portion of each tube may be removed and the cut ends replaced in different planes of the scrotal fascial tissue.

After surgery, scrotal swelling, bruising and discomfort will invariably occur and may last a couple of weeks. It is normally recommended that a scrotal support or tight-fitting underpants are worn during the day and at night for a week after surgery, and heavy manual work or vigorous sport should be avoided for at least a week. Scrotal haematoma with or without infection occurs in about 6% of men. It is easily treated with antibiotic therapy. Sperm granuloma, caused by leakage of sperm into the tissue between the cut ends of the vas deferens, and that produces a foreign body reaction can occur in about 30% of men. In some cases excision of the granuloma is required to relieve pain and inflammation, although other cases may be asymptomatic.

It is essential that men undergoing vasectomy are advised that the contraceptive effect does not develop immediately because of the presence of residual sperm in the distal portion of each vas deferens. Samples of seminal fluid are taken at least eight weeks after surgery, and vasectomy is considered effective when two consecutive negative semen samples are produced two to four weeks apart. Before confirmation of zero sperm counts, other forms of contraceptive cover must be maintained.

Various claims have been made for the reversibility of vasectomy. Although the surgical technique is relatively simple, fertility after vasectomy may be reduced in up to one-third of men because of the production of antibodies to sperm. Further reasons for lack of reversibility include: formation of scar tissue around the anastomosed vas deferens, which may act as a physical barrier to the passage of sperm; and immunological reactions developing at the site of accumulation of sperm, leading to their gradual destruction.

Female sterilisation

Blockage of the Fallopian tubes can be performed by laparotomy, mini-laparotomy or, more commonly, by the less invasive technique, laparoscopy.

Laparotomy is carried out under general anaesthetic and requires an incision of 5 to 8 cm in the abdominal wall. Mini-laparotomy involves a much smaller incision and permits a more rapid recovery, allowing patients to return home within one to two days. Laparoscopy is performed by inserting a fibre-optic tube, sometimes under local anaesthetic supplemented by analgesics, although general anaesthetic is more commonly used. The peritoneal cavity is inflated by gas and the tube is inserted through the abdominal wall to observe the Fallopian tubes. Recovery time is very short, with many women able to return home on the same day as surgery is carried out.

Once the Fallopian tubes have been reached, they may be blocked by excision and tubal ligation, by using clips or bands or they may be sealed by heat treatment (diathermy). Rest is recommended for the first days after surgery, with full activity resumed within one week for laparoscopy and within three weeks for mini-laparotomy. A longer period of rest is usually required after laparotomy. The only after-effect sometimes reported is the development of menorrhagia. Women should use contraception until their first period after sterilisation. If sterilisation does fail as a method of contraception, there is a higher risk that the pregnancy will be ectopic.

Emergency contraception

Most requests for emergency or post-coital contraception arise because intercourse has taken place without any form of contraceptive cover. This may include requests from women subjected to rape or from those undergoing treatment with potentially teratogenic agents (e.g. cytotoxic drugs and live vaccines) who have had unprotected intercourse. Other reasons for seeking emergency contraception include: loss of contraceptive cover caused by a damaged or displaced condom or diaphragm; failure of compliance with administration of oral contraceptives; or miscalculations in using natural family planning methods.

There are two methods of emergency contraception: the hormonal method (also known as the Yuzpe method) and insertion of an IUD.

Emergency contraception is intended to prevent implantation of a fertilised ovum in the uterus. Conception can occur if sexual intercourse takes place any time between days 9 and 17 of a 28-day cycle (*see* Fertility and contraception *above*). In theory, therefore, the use of emergency contraception should only be necessary for a limited timespan each month. In practice, however, the irregularity of many menstrual cycles makes it impossible to give definitive statements about when emergency contraception may be required. If there is any doubt about dates within the cycle, emergency contraception should be used.

Following treatment with an emergency contraceptive, women are requested to return to the doctor or family planning clinic after three weeks, or earlier in the event of any untoward symptoms. Follow-up permits the absence of pregnancy to be confirmed as well as contraceptive counselling.

It has been estimated that there is about a one in three chance of conception if intercourse takes place immediately before ovulation, but of those ova that become fertilised, at least one in three will fail to implant naturally. Implantation is a continuous process that is usually completed by seven to ten days. Any agent administered after implantation for the purposes of preventing pregnancy is termed a medical abortifacient, not a contraceptive.

Hormonal method

Although oestrogen-only and progestogen-only regimens have previously been used, combinations of the two agents are now recommended. Some progestogen-only regimens are still under investigation and have certain advantages (*see below*). The failure rate of hormonal emergency contraception is low, but it is less effective than insertion of an IUD.

Mode of action

The changes produced by the hormonal method depends upon the timing of administration during the menstrual cycle. If dosage is given sufficiently early in the cycle, ovulation may be prevented. Equally, however, ovulation may only be delayed and it is vital that a barrier contraceptive (*see* Barrier methods and spermicides *above*) is used during any future intercourse up to the time of the next menstrual period. Hormonal emergency contraception tends to cause an earlier than anticipated start to this subsequent menstruation; conversely, some women may have a later period than usual.

Administration at the time of, or immediately after, ovulation produces local tissue changes and disturbs the phased changes in the endometrium. This renders the local environment inhospitable to the ovum should it become fertilised and prevents implantation. Specific mechanisms of this effect are uncertain, but possible factors in preventing implantation include: blocking local oestrogen and progesterone receptors; disrupting the functions of the corpus luteum; interfering with the transportation of the ovum from the ovaries to the Fallopian tubes; and a direct action on the fertilised ovum. A few women have light bleeding shortly after taking hormonal postcoital contraception, but this should not be confused with a period. Alternative forms of contraception must be used until the next period.

Dosage and administration

Two tablets, each containing ethinyloestradiol 50 μg and levonorgestrel 250 μg, should be taken ideally as soon as possible after unprotected intercourse, but always within 72 hours of having intercourse, followed by a further two tablets 12 hours later (efficacy is improved the earlier treatment is started).

The high dose of oestrogen produces nausea in up to 50% of cases and vomiting in about 24%. If vomiting occurs within two to three hours of administration, the complete treatment regimen should be re-started, together with the addition of an anti-emetic or insertion of an IUD.

The most common reasons for failure of hormonal emergency contraception include:

delayed start to dosage; repetition of unprotected sexual intercourse; failure to complete the course as a result of poor compliance; or a sub-therapeutic plasma concentration of the hormones caused by vomiting. Increased dosages (three tablets per dose) are needed if the woman is taking enzyme-inducing drugs.

Adverse effects

In addition to nausea and vomiting, other adverse effects include headache, dizziness, breast discomfort and menstrual irregularities. However, the primary risk associated with hormonal emergency contraception is the potential for harmful effects on the fertilised ovum should contraception fail. There is a small, but statistically unproven, potential for high-dose oestrogens and progestogens to produce congenital malformations; ectopic pregnancy is also a possibility. However, such risks are normally thought to be outweighed considerably by the benefits of emergency contraception in preventing un-wanted pregnancies. This method is not appropriate as a regular form of contraception.

Contra-indications

Contra-indications to the use of hormonal emergency contraception include pregnancy, unprotected intercourse on several occasions during the same cycle and any condition for which oestrogen therapy is not recommended (e.g. history of thrombosis or focal migraine at time of presentation). There is no age limit for hormonal emergency contraception, even in smokers.

Progestogen-only methods

Several progestogen-only emergency contraception methods have also been used. Administration of two doses of levonorgestrel, each of 750 μg, given 12 hours apart and initiated within 48 hours of intercourse, has been shown to be as effective as the Yuzpe method. When the treatment is started within 72 hours of intercourse, this method is more effective than the Yuzpe method (Task Force on Postovulatory Methods of Fertility Regulation, 1998). This method has the advantage of much reduced nausea and vomiting. There are also few contra-indications to this method (only current or suspected pregnancy). Other progestogens are also under investigation. An anti-progestogen mifepristone is under investigation as a post-coital contraceptive; a single dose of mifepristone 600 mg is very effective and may have fewer adverse effects than the Yuzpe method.

Intra-uterine devices

The IUD method of emergency contraception should be used when: efficacy is a priority; there is an absolute contra-indication to the use of oestrogens; intercourse occurred within the previous five days; unprotected intercourse took place on several occasions during the same cycle; or tablets taken with the hormonal method have been vomited.

An IUD can be inserted to act as an emergency contraceptive up to five days after the expected date of ovulation (i.e. if intercourse occurs on day 8, an IUD may be inserted any time up to day 21 of a regular 28-day menstrual cycle). Copper IUDs are very effective and the failure rate has been shown to be very low. The progestogen-containing IUD is not effective as a post-coital contraceptive.

The mode of action and range of complications in the use of IUDs as emergency contraceptives are the same as in their more common use as regular contraceptives (*see* Intra-uterine devices *above*). The main advantage of their use over hormonal emergency contraception is that, when in position, IUDs provide continued contraceptive cover. If the device is not to be left in place it is removed towards the end of the next menstrual period.

Contra-indications to insertion of an IUD include: pregnancy; recent pelvic inflammatory disease; and a history of ectopic pregnancy. Special care is needed in cases of sexual assault or unsure histories of pelvic inflammatory disease or sexually-transmitted diseases. The woman should be screened for possible sexually-transmitted diseases and/or appropriate antibiotic cover given.

Contraceptive services

Pharmacists play an important part in providing contraceptive products and giving advice about contraception. However, this role must be considered within the context of the other family planning services. Widespread contraceptive services in the UK, even after the inception of the NHS in 1948, were primarily provided by voluntary organisations (e.g. the Family Planning Association). In the 1940s and 1950s, clinics run by voluntary organisations were predominantly used by married women. However, in the 1960s, changes in attitudes brought about by the development of hormonal contraception and the use of more effective IUDs led to increased demands for contraceptive services by both married and single women. Provision of free contraception for many women in the UK was first provided by the NHS (Family Planning) Act 1967. An expanded and completely free service was implemented following the NHS Reorganisation Act 1973. Since that time, free family planning has been available from hospitals, family planning clinics and general practitioners from 1975. Many genitourinary medicine clinics (also referred to as sexual health clinics or STD clinics) also provide contraceptive services, especially emergency contraception. Further family planning needs that cannot be satisfied from these services are met by voluntary organisations, which are partially funded by government grants.

Primary contraceptive services

General practitioner family planning services

General practitioner family planning services attract most of the women seeking contraceptive products, advice on contraception or both, and over 95% of doctors are registered to provide this service. However, not all general practitioners are trained to fit IUDs, diaphragms or caps. Contraceptives that can be prescribed in the UK are exempt from prescription charges. Male and female condoms are often not available from general practitioners.

Family planning clinics

Family planning clinics usually provide a more comprehensive service than that provided by general practitioners, and tend to offer more alternatives to the supply of oral contraceptives. In addition to providing the contraceptive products described in this chapter, other services available include well-woman clinics and screening procedures, and advice on sex and relationships, menstrual problems, infertility, and sterilisation. Many of the staff in family planning clinics are specifically trained for their advisory role. Moreover, all contraceptive devices, including condoms, are supplied free of charge.

Referrals are made from general practitioner services and family planning clinics to NHS hospitals for male and female sterilisation. However, many of these operations are now carried out by voluntary or private organisations because of long waiting lists, although patients usually have to pay for these services.

Family Planning Association

Information on contraceptive methods and services in the UK can be obtained from the Family Planning Association (FPA). Pharmacists can also approach the local health authority for information. The FPA produces literature, has an information and research centre, and operates a nationwide enquiry service for consumers and professionals.

The role of the pharmacist

For many years the medical profession disdained any association with contraception or contraceptive products, considering them to be a less than respectable form of medical treatment. The comprehensive involvement of the medical profession in contraception only resulted from the advent of prescription-only hormonal methods of contraception developed in the late 1950s and early 1960s (*see* Hormonal methods *above*).

In the late nineteenth century, condoms were obtained from pharmacies and surgical stores, and these outlets were particularly popular with members of the public who wanted easy access to effective birth control methods. This is still true today and pharmacists, with their associated professional image, are ideal suppliers of contraceptive products. The link between contraception and a respected profession helped to overcome many of the early objections to the use of contraceptives. Today, pharmacists provide a much needed complementary service for those who do not wish to use the comprehensive range of contraceptive services provided by the general practitioner family planning services and family planning clinics.

There are several reasons why those seeking contraceptive products or advice choose not to use the primary care services: some women may be reluctant to see a male doctor; clinics may not be used because women may lack awareness of their availability or location; there may be difficulties in transport to and from clinics; and frustration may occur at having to conform to an appointments system.

Advantages of pharmacists as suppliers of contraceptive products and a source of advice include: widespread locations, allowing ease of accessibility to the majority of the population; availability for up to seven days a week; anonymity of the pharmacist-client relationship; and no requirement for an appointment. Moreover, once contact has been established, pharmacists can act as a source of information about the availability of local family planning services.

The pharmacy may also be an ideal place for helping men develop awareness of their responsibilities in contraception. The current non-availability of condoms on prescription means that men will not usually seek advice from their doctors about contraceptive methods. The display of leaflets and products in the non-threatening environment of the pharmacy may encourage inexperienced or shy men and women to seek advice. A display of family planning leaflets can be ideally complemented by a clear statement that contraceptive advice can be obtained from the pharmacist, the individual's doctor or the local family planning clinic; the address of the local family planning clinic should also be displayed. There is a possibility that pharmacists may have a future role in providing emergency hormonal contraception.

References

Collaborative Group on Hormonal Factors in Breast Cancer (1996a). Breast cancer and hormonal contraceptives: collaborative reanalysis of individual data on 53 297 women with breast cancer and 100 239 women without breast cancer from 54 epidemiological studies. *Lancet* 347: 1713–1727.

Collaborative Group on Hormonal Factors in Breast Cancer (1996b). Breast cancer and hormonal contraceptives: further results. *Contraception* 54 (suppl): 1S–106S.

Committee on Safety of Medicines/Medicines Control Agency (1999). Combined oral contraceptives containing desogestrel or gestodene and the risk of venous thromboembolism. *Current Problems* 25: 12.

Drife J O (1983). What proportion of pregnancies are spontaneously aborted? *BMJ* 286: 294.

Task Force on Postovulatory Methods of Fertility Regulation (1998). Randomised controlled trial of levonorgestrel versus the Yuzpe regimen of combined oral contraceptives for emergency contraception. *Lancet* 352: 428–433.

World Health Organization (1997). WHO Scientific Group Meeting on Cardiovascular Disease and Steroid Hormone Contraceptives: summary of conclusions. *Wkly Epidem Rec* 72: 361–363.

World Health Organization Collaborative Study Group (1995). Venous thromboembolic disease and combined oral contraceptives: results of international multicentre case-control study. *Lancet* 346: 1575–1582.

Further reading

Belfield T (1999). *Contraceptive Handbook*, 3rd edn. London: Family Planning Association.

Clubb E, Knight J (1996). *Fertility – Fertility Awareness and Natural Family Planning*, 3rd edn. Newton Abbot: David & Charles.

Guillebaud J (1994). *Contraception: Your Questions*

Answered, 2nd edn. Edinburgh: Churchill Livingstone.

Guillebaud J (1997). *The Pill*, 5th edn. Oxford: Oxford University Press.

Loudon N, Glasier A, Gebbie A, eds (1995). *Handbook of Family Planning and Reproductive Health Care*, 3rd edn. Edinburgh: Churchill Livingstone.

Robertson W H (1990). *An Illustrated History of Contraception: A Concise Account of the Quest for Fertility Control*. Carnforth: The Parthenon Publishing Group.

World Health Organization (1987). Mechanism of action, safety and efficacy of intrauterine devices. *WHO Tech Rep Ser 753*.

World Health Organization (1988). *Barrier Contraceptives and Spermicides: Their Role in Family Planning Care*. Geneva: WHO.

World Health Organization (1990). *Injectable Contraceptives: Their Role in Family Planning Care*. Geneva: WHO.

World Health Organization (1994). *Contraceptive Method Mix: Guidelines for Policy and Service Delivery*. Geneva: WHO.

Useful addresses

Birth Control Trust
16 Mortimer Street
London W1N 7RJ
Tel: 020 7580 9360

British Pregnancy Advisory Service (BPAS)
Austy Manor
Wootton Wawen
Solihull
West Midlands B95 6BX
Tel: 01564 793225

Brook Advisory Centres
(Head Office)
165 Gray's Inn Road
London WC1X 8UD
Tel: 020 7833 8488

Family Planning Association (UK)
2–12 Pentonville Road
London N1 9FP
Tel: 020 7837 5432

International Planned Parenthood Federation (IPPF)
Regent's College
Inner Circle
Regent's Park
London NW1 4NS
Tel: 020 7486 0741

Margaret Pyke Centre
73 Charlotte Street
London W1P 1LB
Tel: 020 7436 8372

Marie Stopes International
153–157 Cleveland Street
London W1P 5PG
Tel: 020 7574 7400

Marriage Care
(previously Catholic Marriage Advisory Council)
Clitherow House
1 Blythe Mews
Blythe Road
London W14 0NW
Tel: 020 7371 1341

RCN Family Planning Forum
Royal College of Nursing
20 Cavendish Square
London WIM 0AB
Tel: 020 7409 3333

5

Smoking

Robin J Harman

In health promotion, possibly the greatest changes in attitudes since the publication of the first edition of the *Handbook of Pharmacy Health Education* (Martin, 1991) have been towards smoking. Tolerance to smoking in public places has declined significantly, with restaurants, public transport and shops all being examples of places where smoking is no longer usually considered acceptable. However, despite this, tobacco smoking remains the single greatest cause of preventable illness and premature death in the UK. More than 120 000 people a year die from smoking in the UK. In the European Union, the number of deaths from the use of tobacco is estimated to be in excess of 500 000 a year.

The UK government published its views on smoking, and the action it intends to take to reduce it, in a December 1998 White Paper entitled 'Smoking Kills' (DoH, 1998a). The title of the White Paper demonstrates the government's attitude to the issue. Much of the statistical data in this chapter derives from this White Paper and from Action on Smoking and Health (ASH), an organisation established in 1971 by the UK Royal College of Physicians.

Originally introduced into Europe in the fifteenth century from the New World, smoking was originally considered medicinally beneficial. However, only relatively small numbers of people took up the habit until the beginning of the twentieth century. It was only through the large increase in smokers during the first part of the 1900s that concerns about the health hazards associated with the habit developed from the 1950s onwards. This was largely due to epidemiological work, which demonstrated for the first time a link between the incidence of lung cancer and other respiratory diseases, and smoking of cigarettes.

The prevalence of smoking, trends and behaviour

Imagine the outcry should a jumbo jet aeroplane crash every day of the year, killing all 330 passengers and crew. Nevertheless, this is the toll of death in the UK from the use of tobacco: more than 120 000 people die each year in the UK due to its use, equivalent to about 13 people every hour of the day and night. This compares with the death of ten people in road traffic accidents each day of the year; the murder and manslaughter of on average about nine people each week; more than 11 people who commit suicide each day; and the death of three people each day from poisoning and overdosage.

In 1995, of a UK population of 58.6 million, nearly a quarter (12.1 million adults) were found to smoke cigarettes. There was an almost equal proportion of 30% of men and women in the population who were smokers. Although in 1972 the proportion of the population that smoked was 52% of men and 41% of women, the steady decline in numbers of smokers since that time may have stopped. The number of adult smokers rose in 1996 (the last year for which figures are available) (Office for National Statistics, 1997a) for the first time since 1972. This is possibly because the decline in smokers has been greatest in older age groups. The number of new young smokers is increasing, whilst longer-term smokers are being more successful in giving up the habit.

Other factors affect the prevalence and habits of adult smoking. It is almost four times more prevalent amongst male unskilled manual workers than among male professionals; the equivalent ratio in women is about three. Male smokers tend to smoke more high-tar cigarettes than women, and the proportion of high-tar smokers is higher in younger (16- to 19-year-old) than older smokers.

By comparison, in 1996, it was shown that 6% of men smoke cigars and 2% smoke pipes. This demonstrates a dramatic decrease in cigar smoking from the levels in 1974 when 34% of men smoked cigars and 12% of men smoked pipes. Less than 1% of women smoke cigars. (There are no figures for the number of women pipe smokers.)

One of the major concerns about the incidence of smoking is that nearly 25% of children aged 15 years are known to be regular smokers. This is all the more perplexing when it is illegal to sell cigarettes to children under 16 years of age (*see below*). Children are starting to smoke at an ever younger age: it was estimated in 1994 that more than one million cigarettes were smoked by children between 11 and 15 years of age (Office for National Statistics, 1997b).

The current legislation in the UK governing the sale of cigarettes to children under the age of 16 years is the Children and Young Persons (Protection from Tobacco) Act 1991. If the law is proven to have been broken, the person making the sale to the under-age child is liable to a fine of up to £2500. Retail outlets and cigarette vending machines must also be labelled to indicate it is illegal to sell cigarettes to children aged under 16 years.

There are also differences and changes in the ratio of male to female smokers with increasing age. Almost one-quarter of 14-year-old teenage girls smoke cigarettes, nearly twice the number of similarly aged teenage boys (13%). The numbers become slightly more equal in the 16- to 19-year-old group (32% females compared with 26% males). It is only in the 20- to 24-year-old group that the number of male smokers (43%) is greater than female smokers (36%).

Tobacco

The tobacco plants are *Nicotiana tabacum* and *N. rustica*. A specific grade and quality of tobacco is produced during the curing (drying) process by the different methods used. These include air-curing, flue-curing and sun-curing. In air-curing, tobacco leaves are dried by exposure only to air; hot air is applied in flue-curing. After drying, tobacco leaves are further conditioned, giving tobacco that generates smoke sufficiently mild to inhale. Each grade of tobacco has distinct properties. Different grades are selected for different tobacco products (e.g. pipe tobacco, cigars or cigarettes).

The primary objective from the use of all tobacco products is the absorption of nicotine. Acidic cigarette smoke contains nicotine in its ionised form, in which it is rapidly absorbed from the lungs. Little, if any, buccal absorption occurs on inhalation. By contrast, cigar and pipe smoke is alkaline. Nicotine exists in an unionised form, allowing high levels of buccal absorption in addition to rapid pulmonary absorption. An alkaline pH is created or exists in chewed tobacco, snuff and nicotine chewing gum to facilitate absorption of nicotine.

The sale of oral snuff in the UK is banned. Oral snuff comprised a small sachet held between the gum and cheek (snuff dipping). As a result of its mode of use, it was linked to oral and malignant disease, especially cancer of the mouth.

Cigarettes

The consistency of cigarette tobacco is achieved by blending different grades of tobacco. Cigarette characteristics (e.g. flavour, smell and burning profile) are modified by the use of a large number of additives which are selectively incorporated into the tobacco and the paper. Most commercially manufactured cigarettes also incorporate a filter. These were originally introduced to reduce tobacco wastage in the unsmoked portion. They were also considered to improve the cigarette's appeal to women by removing the development of soggy cigarette ends.

It has been by the use of filters, and their technology, that the largest impact has been made on lowering the amount of tar inhaled (*see below*). The tar content per cigarette, which is the quantity inhaled by the smoker, is graded and printed on the cigarette pack.

A low tar grading corresponds to 'safer' cigarettes. The amount of inhaled tobacco constituents, and especially tar, from cigarettes has steadily decreased over the years. This is despite no changes being made to the tobacco itself. Factors that have led to greater use of reduced tar products include:

- greater public awareness of the health risks of smoking (especially from higher tar cigarettes)
- improved manufacturing methods
- introduction of filters
- introduction of ventilation holes in filters (certain low tar brands)
- legislation requiring the labelling of tar content on cigarette packs, thereby providing manufacturers with an incentive to reduce tar content to appeal to smokers wishing to switch to low tar brands.

Low tar cigarettes pose a lower health risk than those classed as high tar. The use of low tar cigarettes may also help smokers to give up smoking entirely if they have previously switched from high to low tar brands. Although some smokers believe low tar cigarettes completely safe, they remain inherently unhealthy. A further problem with low tar cigarettes is that new smokers, and especially children, may find them less unpleasant if they are the first cigarettes smoked (*see above*) and reinforce the false belief that such cigarettes are relatively harmless.

Tobacco smoke

The two phases of tobacco smoke (gaseous and particulate) comprise more than 4000 compounds, of which the most important are carbon monoxide, nicotine and tar. The concentration of constituents inhaled by smokers from a cigarette depends on:

- brand of cigarette (e.g. low tar or high tar brand)
- physical characteristics (e.g. cigarette length; the type of filter, which affects the efficiency of tar removal; the porosity of the paper characteristics; and the packing density of tobacco)
- smoking behaviour
- temperature upon inhalation (the temperature is raised upon rapid, prolonged drawing on the cigarette).

Two types of smoke are generated during tobacco use:

- Mainstream smoke – smoke inhaled by the smoker. The lungs retain 85 to 99% of particulate matter and about 55% of carbon monoxide.
- Sidestream smoke (environmental tobacco smoke) – smoke emitted from the burning end of a cigarette. It is considerably diluted in the surrounding atmosphere, but is unfiltered and contains a much higher concentration of all tobacco constituents than mainstream smoke. The particulate phase, which contains tar and nicotine, ends up at the apex and in the central regions of the lungs.

It is likely, but unconfirmed, that variations exist to the pattern of pulmonary penetration of the two phases of tobacco. The gaseous phase, containing carbon monoxide, penetrates easily deep into the lungs, including the alveoli. This permits rapid absorption of constituents.

Carbon monoxide

The gaseous phase of tobacco smoke contains carbon monoxide, which is rapidly absorbed into the bloodstream. Its high affinity for haemoglobin creates carboxyhaemoglobin, which reduces the oxygen-carrying capacity of haemoglobin. The plasma carbon monoxide content increases through the day with each cigarette smoked. Depending upon the numbers smoked, saturation with carbon monoxide may be reached in the early evening; there is a gradual decline in levels during the night, but some may persist through to the following morning.

The precise consequences of inhaling carbon monoxide are not known. There are apparently no noticeable effects in healthy people, due to compensatory mechanisms to meet oxygen demands. However, in smokers with heart disease, these mechanisms may not prevent myocardial hypoxia.

Nicotine

Nicotine forms the major part of the particulate phase of tobacco smoke. It is rapidly absorbed following inhalation, from where it binds to acetylcholine receptors and passes the blood-brain barrier. It is initially rapidly distributed throughout the brain, but brain tissue levels fall quickly as the nicotine is circulated to other body tissues. Nicotine crosses the placenta and is found in amniotic fluid and the umbilical cord. Low levels are found in breast milk.

The effects of nicotine on body systems are mediated predominantly through the central and peripheral nervous systems. Dopamine release is stimulated in the brain. Other catecholamines, adrenaline and noradrenaline, are released from the adrenal medulla and from sympathetic nerves in blood vessels.

Nicotine is rapidly metabolised, mainly in the liver. Cotinine and nicotine-N-oxide are the primary metabolic products; both are inactive. Cotinine is used as a marker to determine nicotine intake and hence smoking behaviour. Due to its long half-life (ten to 20 hours), the metabolite can be detected and measured in blood plasma, saliva, urine and cervical mucus secretions. Some tobacco smoke constituents induce microsomal liver enzymes, increasing the breakdown of nicotine and its metabolites.

It is the plasma-nicotine concentrations which determine smoking behaviour, with cigarettes being smoked as necessary to produce the effects required by the smoker. If smoking is intermittent through the day, plasma-nicotine concentrations will vary significantly. Nicotine accumulates during the day and gradually declines at night. As with carbon monoxide levels, there may be a residual plasma concentration in the morning.

Tar

Tar droplets form almost all of the particulate phase of tobacco smoke. They consist of more than 1000 identified polycyclic hydrocarbons and a concentrated nicotine solution. Constituents of inhaled tar include:

- Acrolein
- Arsenic
- Benzene
- Benzo(α)pyrene
- Cyanide
- Formaldehyde
- Toluene.

The particle size of tar droplets (0.1–1.0 μm) allows their penetration to the alveoli, from where nicotine is rapidly absorbed. Almost all the particulate matter (85 to 99%) is retained in the lungs.

Smoking-related diseases

The effects of smoking on disease and mortality are well documented. By virtue of their market dominance, cigarettes and cigarette smoking are the greatest cause of smoking-related diseases. Whilst many people associate smoking only with lung cancer, there is an increasingly vast range and diversity of smoking-related diseases. More than 90% of lung cancer deaths can be attributed to smoking. The five-year survival rate from lung cancer for patients after diagnosis is less than 10%.

A summary of the potentially harmful effects of smoking is shown in Table 5.1. Mechanisms responsible for smoking-related diseases are difficult to determine, mainly due to the slow and long-term (over ten to 20 years) onset of the diseases.

It is a common belief that modern, low tar brands pose a reduced health risk compared with traditional high tar (plain and unfiltered) cigarettes. Although of a considerably higher incidence than in non-smokers, the risks of malignant disease (e.g. lung cancer, and cancer of the bladder, oesophagus or pharynx) are less than for smokers of high tar brands. The risk of respiratory system disorders may be marginally reduced, but risks of ischaemic heart disease and myocardial infarction remain the same in both groups.

Effects on the cardiovascular system

Smoking is linked to cardiovascular system disorders through the effects on haemostatic mechanisms. The agents having the most effect on the cardiovascular system are nicotine and carbon monoxide, which alter the following stages in haemostasis:

Table 5.1 A selection of the potentially harmful effects of smoking

Type of disease	Effects
Cardiovascular	Cigarette smoking doubles or trebles the risk of heart attack compared to non-smokers
	90% of all amputations of one or both limbs is due to peripheral vascular disease
Malignant	30% of all cancer deaths can be linked to smoking
	Other cancers linked to smoking: cancers of the mouth, lip and throat; of the pancreas and bladder; of the kidney and stomach; liver cancer; leukaemia
	Social class 5 males aged between 15 and 64 are three times as likely to die of lung cancer as men in social class 1
	Cervical cancer; social class 5 females are almost three times as likely to die of lung cancer as women in social class 1
	Smokers who use between 1 and 14 cigarettes daily have eight times the risk of dying of lung cancer compared with non-smokers
Musculoskeletal	Increased risk of development of osteoporosis
Reproductive	Smoking has been linked to increased sperm abnormalities and impotence
	Women who smoke and who take the contraceptive pill have ten times the risk of a heart attack, stroke or other cardiovascular disease compared with pill takers who are non-smokers
	Smoking leads to an earlier menopause (two to three years earlier)
	In pregnant women, smoking increases spontaneous abortion, haemorrhaging during pregnancy, premature birth; low birth-weight babies
Miscellaneous	An increased risk of sudden infant death syndrome (cot death) also occurs

- decreased prostacyclin concentration, which causes vasoconstriction and increased platelet aggregation
- increased carboxyhaemoglobin and fibrinogen concentrations
- increased concentration of free fatty acids
- increased plasma cell volume
- increased tendency towards platelet aggregation.

Nicotine may also directly damage blood-vessel endothelium linings.

Ischaemic heart disease

Ischaemic heart disease is the most important smoking-related disease. Other factors besides smoking (e.g. poor diet) need to be considered when assessing the overall risk of developing ischaemic heart disease. In pre-existing ischaemic heart disease, the role of smoking is shown more clearly. Smoking increases the demands of cardiac muscle for oxygen. However, this occurs in tandem with a reduced oxygen-carrying capacity of the blood, caused by the presence of carbon monoxide and the formation of carboxyhaemoglobin. The flow of blood to the coronary blood vessels increases to meet the extra demand. In healthy people, this compensatory mechanism is effective. However, if ischaemic heart disease exists, it is not possible to meet this demand. Ischaemia results, which leads to angina pectoris or myocardial infarction. Similarly, smokers have a reduced exercise tolerance in angina pectoris.

The number of deaths caused by smoking-related ischaemic heart disease is greater than for any other smoking-related disease, including lung cancer. The increased risk of developing ischaemic heart disease is reversed, becoming almost normal, within five years of giving up smoking. It has been estimated that mortality from myocardial infarction would be reduced by 25% if all smoking ceased. Giving up smoking is essential following myocardial infarction and reduces the risk of further infarction.

The risk of developing ischaemic heart disease and mortality rates from it increase with age.

Middle-aged smokers are at greatest risk. The difference in numbers of smokers between social and occupational groups also influences the risk of ischaemic heart disease within these groups. There is a much greater risk of ischaemic heart disease in manual workers compared with non-manual workers.

Hypertension

Although nicotine produces raised blood pressure after smoking a single cigarette or following administration of test doses of nicotine to healthy non-smokers, there is usually little difference in the blood pressure of smokers and non-smokers. Chronic smokers are usually lean, and the development of compensatory mechanisms stabilises expected pharmacological blood pressure increases. Smoking increases the risk of chronic hypertension progressing to malignant (accelerated) hypertension. It may also exacerbate diseases associated with hypertension (e.g. generating paroxysmal hypertensive attacks in phaeo-chromocytoma).

Atherosclerosis

As well as other factors (e.g. poor diet), atherosclerosis development can be related to smoking and, in particular, to the numbers of cigarettes smoked. As above, smoking probably affects haemostasis through nicotine-induced damage to blood-vessel endothelium.

Thrombosis

A further example of changes to haemostasis is seen in the increased ease by which blood coagulates in smokers. The risk of developing thrombosis is increased when combined with other risk factors (e.g. use of combined oral contraceptives). Thrombotic effects produced by smoking may also hamper the success of certain types of cardiovascular surgery and be responsible for the failure of arteriovenous shunts for haemodialysis.

Cerebrovascular disease

There is an increased likelihood of cerebral aneurysm, stroke and subarachnoid haemorrhage in smokers. In addition to the increased risk and development of atherosclerosis and thrombosis, and the effects of smoking on haemostasis, smoking reduces cerebral blood flow. Cessation of smoking gradually reduces the cerebrovascular risk.

Peripheral vascular disease

Smokers comprise at least 95% of patients presenting with peripheral vascular disease. Other conditions that also cause peripheral vascular disease (e.g. diabetes mellitus) increase the risk from smoking. The disease is probably mediated through haemostasis changes and peripheral vasoconstriction. The intermittent claudication which can accompany peripheral vascular disease may be caused by carbon monoxide producing carboxyhaemoglobin. Again, giving up smoking is the most effective treatment. Should surgical treatment be necessary for peripheral vascular disease, there is an increased failure of grafts in smokers.

Respiratory system disorders

Unsurprisingly, smoking is causally linked to many respiratory system disorders. Indeed, one of the earliest signs of smoking-related damage is decreased lung function, which is invariably followed by chronic cough ('smoker's cough').

The particulate phase of tobacco smoke produces most respiratory disorders, depositing irritants in the lungs, which narrow the bronchioles. Persistent smoking causes chronic obstruction of the airways and decreased lung function. Bronchial mucus secretion is increased in the presence of the irritants and the damage, causing the cilia lining the respiratory tree to cease to operate effectively to remove particulate matter. Pulmonary tissue inflammation also develops.

Chronic obstructive airways disease

Chronic obstructive airways disease (COAD) comprises the main group of respiratory system disorders caused by smoking. COAD is rarely seen in non-smokers. Chronic bronchitis is invariably caused by smoking through increased bronchial mucus secretion. (Care must be taken to eliminate possible causes other than smoking, including prolonged exposure to environmental pollutants.) Emphysema is caused by disruption of the pulmonary protease-antiprotease enzymes. Smoking increases the activity of the proteases indirectly by decreasing the actions of the antiprotease enzyme, alpha-1-antitrypsin.

Chronic bronchitis and emphysema are progressive diseases. However, if smoking is stopped before severe disability develops, lung function may improve. If smoking is stopped prior to the early development of COAD, there is a greater likelihood of lung function reverting to normal.

Respiratory-tract infections

Respiratory-tract infections (e.g. acute bronchitis) are more common in smokers than non-smokers, and many are recurrent. Infections probably occur as a result of the decreased ability of the lungs to remove foreign material, together with compromised lung function and capacity.

Malignant disease

Smoking has been shown to be the most important risk factor in the development of many malignant diseases, and the number of smoking-related malignant diseases is growing. Nicotine is not carcinogenic, but other carcinogens exist in tobacco smoke (e.g. nitrosated derivatives of nicotine formed during curing or during cigarette smoking).

Lung cancer

The incidence of lung cancer is highest amongst smokers, and the disease is causally related to smoking. Other factors (e.g. genetic predisposition) have been linked to the susceptibility to lung cancer, but smoking represents the largest risk factor. Although cigarettes are the most commonly used form of tobacco, lung cancer can occur with all forms of smoking. The types of lung cancer usually associated with smoking are epidermoid (squamous) cell and small (oat) cell carcinoma. The link between smoking and lung cancer is affected by:

- length of time that smoking has been practised and the age at which it was started
- depth of inhalation and the number of puffs taken with each cigarette
- number of cigarettes smoked daily.

Giving up smoking reduces the relative risk of developing lung cancer, although damage to lungs cannot be reversed.

Gastro-intestinal system disorders

Smoking is associated with the development of, and delayed healing in, peptic ulceration. After successful drug treatment of peptic ulceration, its recurrence is much more common in smokers. Although precise causative mechanisms are unknown, studies on the chronic effects of smoking on gastro-intestinal physiology show the following effects:

- increased gastric acid secretion
- increased reflux of bile into the stomach
- reduced synthesis and concentration of prostaglandin E_2 in the gastric mucosa.

Oral diseases

Blood-flow to the gums in smokers is reduced, and this may cause gingivitis and other oral inflammatory diseases (e.g. aphthous stomatitis and glossitis). Oral diseases are possibly caused by irritants in tobacco smoke and its high temperatures. Oral leucoplakia is also associated with smoking, and may lead to malignancy.

The effect of smoking on the appearance of teeth is dramatic. Teeth develop a yellow stain, which is extremely difficult to remove, and can be accompanied by characteristic breath odour. Dental caries has a higher incidence in smokers than non-smokers, although this may reflect smokers' reduced dental healthcare.

Obstetric disorders and effects on the foetus

Smoking reduces blood-flow to the mother's uterus. Nicotine and carbon monoxide freely cross the placenta, generating foetal hypoxia. Other effects on foetus physiology include:

- central nervous system dysfunction, produced by an increased foetal-lactate concentration
- increased heart rate, caused by release of catecholamines
- hypoxia, caused by the formation of carboxyhaemoglobin in the presence of carbon monoxide
- vasoconstriction, caused by nicotine and catecholamines.

Birth-weight and perinatal mortality

Mothers who smoke produce babies of a lower birth-weight than those born to non-smokers. The reduction in birth-weight may be due to the presence of hydrogen cyanide, which is converted to thiocyanate by vitamin B_{12}. Similarly, maternal thiocyanate concentrations increase and concentrations of vitamin B_{12} are reduced.

Perinatal mortality incidence is increased in smokers. More frequently occurring placental ageing and premature rupture of the membranes are thought to be causes.

Pre-term delivery

Babies of smoking mothers are commonly born one to three days earlier than those born to non-smokers. Foetal hypoxia and increased myometrial stimulation may be causes of pre-term delivery. Over-stimulation of foetal adrenal glands may also initiate earlier labour.

Spontaneous abortion

Spontaneous abortion is nearly twice as common in smokers than non-smokers. It usually occurs in late pregnancy, thereby precluding other causes (e.g. congenital abnormalities).

Placental malfunction

Pathological changes in the placenta occur from smoking and hypoxia. They may cause increased major antepartum haemorrhage, minor antepartum haemorrhage, and premature membrane rupture.

Pre-eclampsia and eclampsia

The incidence of pre-eclampsia and eclampsia is lower in smokers compared with non-smokers. This may be due to:

- capillary dilatation in muscles produced by nicotine
- tendency of smokers to be lean and less likely to gain weight during pregnancy
- increased levels of thiocyanate, which has antihypertensive properties.

When pre-eclampsia and eclampsia do occur in mothers who smoke, there is an increased risk of damage to the foetus.

Postnatal development

Smoking may slow the rate of intellectual development of the child until puberty. However, adult attainments appear unaffected. Smokers often discontinue breast-feeding due to insufficient milk. Infantile colic may be influenced by maternal smoking: its incidence is higher in breast-fed babies of mothers who smoke, whereas those babies of smokers who are bottle-fed appear to be unaffected.

Passive smoking

Passive smoking is commonly defined as the unwanted and involuntary exposure to, and inhalation of, tobacco smoke. It is also sometimes defined as exposure to environmental tobacco smoke, although this definition fails to describe unwanted and involuntary inhalation. Evidence has been increasing over the past two decades that passive smoking has harmful effects on health, although it is only recently that the extent and magnitude of increased risk has been partially quantified.

Based on a study in the USA (United States Environmental Protection Agency, 1992), it has been extrapolated that about 600 deaths from lung cancer and 12 000 cases of heart disease in the UK can be attributed to passive smoking by non-smokers. The greatest risks are for those continuously exposed to other people's smoke in the home or workplace. Again, as with attitudes to

smoking (*see above*), there has been a significant decrease in the tolerance by non-smokers towards the inhalation of smoke from cigarettes. This is underlined by the following:

- no-smoking policies at work and in public places
- increased public awareness of the health risks
- legislation prohibiting smoking in certain public places
- recognition by smokers of the risk of passive smoking
- social unacceptability.

Some non-smokers detest the smell of tobacco smoke and find even low atmospheric concentrations extremely irritating. The smell of ashtrays, in the absence of tobacco smoke, is also irritating to some non-smokers.

Exposure levels in passive smoking

The volume and concentration of sidestream smoke, which comes from the tip of a burning cigarette, determines exposure levels in passive smoking. (Sidestream smoke also affects smokers, who are therefore subject to a dual risk from smoking and passive smoking.) The extent of passive smoking in non-smokers can be assessed by measuring the plasma-carboxyhaemoglobin concentration; the carbon monoxide concentration in expired air; and cotinine concentrations in blood, saliva or urine.

Indoors, the extent of passive smoking is dependent upon the distance from smokers, the duration of exposure, the number of cigarettes smoked, size of the room and ventilation efficiency. It has been estimated that 85% of air in an enclosed room in which smoking takes place comes from sidestream smoke, which contains a higher number of possible harmful components than mainstream smoke. Passive smoking also occurs in open spaces, though obviously to a lesser degree.

The health risks of passive smoking are thought to be caused by constituents other than nicotine. The concentrations of nicotine found in non-smokers exposed to passive smoking is usually in the order of 1 to 5% of that in smokers. This concentration is accepted as being extremely small and insignificant in terms of the pharmacological effects of nicotine and relative health risk.

Effects of passive smoking on health

Children and adults may present to pharmacists with ailments, especially respiratory conditions, which could be related to the inhalation of tobacco smoke. Therefore, questioning about passive smoking, where applicable, should now form part of pharmacists' key questions.

Acute effects

Passive smoking produces dose-dependent acute effects in non-smokers. At low concentrations, non-smokers may experience irritation of the eyes and nose; at higher concentrations, effects include chest tightness, cough, headache, nausea and wheezing. However, some people are more susceptible to the acute effects of passive smoking than others.

In the presence of underlying disease in non-smokers, susceptibility to the acute effects of passive smoking is increased. Non-smokers with ischaemic heart disease may show a reduction in exercise tolerance. Asthmatic patients are generally sensitive to all the acute effects of passive smoking, and attacks may be precipitated. People who wear contact lenses are more susceptible to eye irritation and eye infection from passive smoking.

Chronic effects

The greatest concern with passive smoking is directed towards the chronic effects of passive smoking on the health of non-smokers, and especially children. It is likely that there is a dose-dependent relationship in the development of chronic effects.

An increased risk of heart disease in non-smokers can be linked to passive smoking, especially in women. Pulmonary illnesses that can arise include asthma, emphysema and respiratory-tract infections. Decreased lung function is indicated by a reduced forced expiratory volume in one second (FEV_1). The development of lung cancer is related to dose and length of exposure. The risk of developing other forms of malignant disease (e.g. breast and cervical cancer) may also be increased.

Passive smoking by children

It has been estimated that almost half of all children in the UK are exposed to tobacco smoke at home. Additionally, more than 17 000 children under five years of age are admitted to hospital in the UK each year because of the effects from tobacco smoke. This derives mainly from other members of the family (both close and extended) who smoke, as children cannot escape voluntarily from the smoky atmosphere.

The link between passive smoking and a wide range of childhood illnesses is now clearly established. The increased risk of acute and chronic respiratory-tract disorders in children exposed to passive smoking is reflected in such children having twice the chance of developing asthma. They also suffer more frequently from chronic cough and the occurrence of phlegm. Acute bronchitis and pneumonia is over one and a half times more common in a smoking environment in babies less than three years old. Parental smoking may cause up to 25% of cot deaths; it may also increase by up to 30% the risk of a child developing chronic middle ear effusion ('glue ear'), the commonest cause of deafness in children.

Prevention of smoking

The main objectives of any programme for the reduction of smoking in the population are to prevent smoking from being started and to assist smokers to stop smoking. Stopping individuals from starting to smoke is particularly important in teenagers (and increasingly younger children) who form one of the largest groups of new smokers each year (*see above*). Ensuring that they do not start smoking and become addicted to nicotine is likely to have the greatest effect on the incidence of smoking-related illnesses in both the short and long term.

One of the strongest disincentives to starting smoking is its increasing social unacceptability. As discussed above, smoking in public places, on public transport and in other communal areas (e.g. shopping centres and restaurants) makes it much more difficult for 'secretive' smoking or smoking by children away from parental supervision. Nevertheless, many people will be only too familiar with the sight of groups of children leaving school premises who carry out furtive (and sometimes less than furtive) lighting up of cigarettes. There is clearly a failure in the system which is intended to prevent youngsters even obtaining or possessing smoking materials.

Social unacceptability of smoking comes in other forms. Many people are becoming increasingly reluctant to accept the smell that permeates the atmosphere, clothing, breath and hair of smokers. Some non-smokers and former smokers are exquisitely sensitive and repulsed by the merest suggestion of the smell of tobacco. Personal relationships may also suffer, and indeed this facet of smoking has been frequently used in advertising campaigns to persuade people to give up or not to start smoking.

In the UK, the Health and Safety at Work Act 1974 specifies places where smoking is not permitted. Three examples are any areas in which food is prepared; garage forecourts, because of the risk from flammable materials; and by drivers of public service vehicles. From January 1996, EC legislation on health and safety required that where an organisation provides a rest area for its staff, a no-smoking area must always be provided.

Health warnings on cigarette packets are a legal requirement following the implementation of an EC Directive into UK legislation. The Tobacco Products Labelling (Safety) Regulations 1991 (part of the Consumer Safety Act 1987) specifies warnings which must appear on, and cover 6% of, the face of the packet; these are listed in Table 5.2. The tar and nicotine content of each cigarette must also be printed. Even smokeless tobacco products must be labelled with the statement 'Causes cancer'.

Tobacco companies, who, it is estimated, spend more than £100 million each year (1999 prices) on advertising, have argued that advertising does not act as an incentive for people to start smoking, but persuades current smokers to switch brands. (The £100 million does not

Table 5.2 Health warnings legally required on cigarette packets in the UK

Legal requirement	Warning
Always required on the front of the package	Tobacco seriously damages health
Warnings which must be printed on the back of the package, selected in strict rotation	Smoking kills Smoking causes cancer Smoking causes heart disease Smoking causes fatal diseases Smoking when pregnant harms your baby Protect children: don't make them breathe your smoke

include sponsorship, direct mailings or other forms of advertising.) The considerable sponsorship of many sporting events (e.g. Formula One motor racing and cricket tournaments) and non-sports events is similarly justified. However, an EC Tobacco Advertising Directive will ban all tobacco advertising by the year 2006.

Prior to this and the earlier Directive, which have to be implemented into national legislation, most advertising restrictions were covered by voluntary agreements between national governments and the tobacco companies. The most recent two UK voluntary agreements came into effect in 1995. One agreement covers sponsorship of sporting events; the other concerns the siting and content of advertisements. The most important measures are listed in Table 5.3; the timetable for the elimination of tobacco advertising in the EC is given in Table 5.4.

As described above, smoking involves both physiological and psychological dependence on nicotine. As in other forms of dependence, tolerance to the effects of nicotine also develops. Characteristic withdrawal symptoms arise, beginning within 24 hours and peaking after about seven days. Gradual relief from withdrawal symptoms can occur, although it may take a long period to do so.

Most smokers attribute their failure to stop smoking to the intense craving, which may persist for more than one year. It is usually intermittent and may be triggered by other people smoking, or at a time when a cigarette was previously smoked (e.g. after a meal). Nicotine replacement therapy (*see below*) will not completely eliminate craving, although other withdrawal symptoms are relieved. This implies that mechanisms other than nicotine addiction may influence the degree of craving.

Methods of giving up smoking

In common with all forms of drug addiction, smokers must pass through three stages to succeed in giving up: initial cessation, short-term maintenance and long-term maintenance. Nicotine withdrawal symptoms occur during initial

Table 5.3 Advertising measures covered by the two 1995 voluntary agreements in the UK between the government and the tobacco industry

- Removal of all permanent shopfront advertising by the end of 1996
- Reduced expenditure on billboard cigarette advertisements
- Elimination of all small poster advertising for cigarettes and hand-rolling tobacco, including those sited at bus-stops
- No poster advertising for any tobacco products within 200 m of school entrances
- 20% of each advertisement to be devoted to health warnings

Table 5.4 Timetable for elimination of tobacco advertising under the EC Tobacco Advertising Directive

Deadline	Advertising method
By 2001	Elimination of all advertising and promotion, except in the print media
By 2002	Elimination of all advertising and promotion in the print media
By 2003	Sponsorship of all events not organised globally to be stopped
By 2006	Sponsorship of all global events (individually agreed) to be stopped

cessation and short-term maintenance, and are the main reason for failure. In the long-term maintenance phase, nicotine withdrawal symptoms are absent, suggesting other less clear reasons for an individual's relapse to smoking.

Aversion and group therapy

Aversion therapy involves the development of a conditioned aversion to tobacco smoke and is available at smoking clinics. Therapy consists of smoking cigarettes in rapid succession (usually inhaling at six-second intervals), which results in the appearance of toxic effects of nicotine and irritant effects of tobacco smoke. These include burning mouth and throat, dizziness, nausea, numbness and tachycardia.

Good success rates are claimed for initial cessation and short-term maintenance. Long-term maintenance is influenced by a sense of achievement, overcoming craving and apparent health benefits (e.g. improved exercise tolerance and loss of smoker's cough).

Group therapy trains smokers to cope with nicotine withdrawal symptoms. Doing so in a group provides mutual support. Smokers are also made more aware of the harmful effects of smoking. Group therapy methods include relaxation techniques, stress management and activities to cope with craving (e.g. distraction). Good results are claimed for initial cessation and short-term maintenance, but not for long-term maintenance. One reason may be the tendency for smokers to forget or not practise the techniques after the course.

Nicotine replacement therapy

Nicotine replacement therapy (NRT) has become increasingly popular as an aid to stopping smoking. The first product widely used was nicotine chewing gum, but a range of products and formulations now exist. The choice of product depends upon the number of cigarettes smoked each day and the time at which the first cigarette of the day is smoked (*see* Table 5.5).

Nicotine chewing gum is available in strengths of 2 mg and 4 mg. Patient information leaflets with the product indicate a stepwise method of chewing the gum:

- chew slowly until the taste becomes strong
- rest the chewing gum between the cheek and the oral gum
- chew again when the taste has faded
- remove the gum after about 30 minutes chewing (once all the nicotine has been released).

Normally, about ten to 12 pieces of gum each day are used initially. (No more than 15 pieces per day should be used.) The same quantity of gum should be continued for about three months, after which the number of pieces

Table 5.5 Choosing the correct nicotine replacement therapy

Number of cigarettes smoked per day	Recommended product(s)
Less than 10	2 mg gum or inhalator
10 to 20	2 mg gum, 10 mg patch or inhalator
More than 20	4 mg gum and 16-hour patch
More than 20 and the first within 20 minutes of waking	4 mg gum and 24-hour patch

chewed each day should be gradually reduced to zero.

Chewing the gum too quickly will lead to quicker release of nicotine, producing increased salivation and some of the nicotine being swallowed, not absorbed. Minor side-effects have been reported, including a bitter taste (although flavoured chewing gums have been introduced), dizziness, headache, hiccups, indigestion, sickness and sore throat.

Nicotine patches are available in strengths of 5 mg, 10 mg and 15 mg. The patch is applied to a hairless area of the upper arm, chest, or thigh from which nicotine is absorbed subcutaneously. The 15 mg patch is applied for the first eight weeks of treatment, followed by two weeks of the 10 mg patch and then two weeks of the 5 mg patch. It is important to emphasise that smoking must be stopped completely when starting use of the patches. The patch should be applied on waking and left on for 16 hours. If nicotine addiction is particularly severe, requiring a cigarette within 20 minutes of waking, a 24-hour patch may be required.

A nicotine 'inhalator' comprises a cartridge that releases a vapour containing nicotine when inhaled through the mouth. The inhalator's use may be particularly beneficial for those smokers who feel the need to continue the hand-to-mouth movements associated with smoking. Each cartridge lasts about 20 minutes, compared with the five minutes that a cigarette usually lasts. Cessation of smoking is planned to take place over three months. Between six and 12 cartridges may be used initially and continued for eight weeks. In the following two weeks, the number of cartridges used should be halved, and then completely stopped by week 12.

Nicotine nasal spray is available only on prescription. It provides effects that are closest to the peaks and troughs of plasma nicotine that occur during smoking. However, its use may be terminated early because of coughing, nose and throat irritation, and watering of the eyes.

Non-nicotine medicine

Bupropion is a prescription-only medicine that was launched in June 2000. It acts by preventing the reuptake of dopamine and noradrenaline (norepinephrine) into central neurones, thereby reducing craving. It is intended to be used at a dose of 150 mg once daily for three days, then increased to 150 mg twice daily for two months. Smoking should be stopped during the second week of treatment.

The role of the pharmacist

Pharmacists are in an ideal position to counsel and assist in preventing smoking-related diseases. It has been suggested that a brief (less than five minute) and opportunistic discussion with a smoker who is thinking about giving up is often the most effective form of counselling. The discussion may prompt positive action either on the smoker's own initiative or with the assistance of NRT. The prominent display of health education leaflets and booklets in the pharmacy can also lead to such opportunities. Moreover, they can be taken away and read at leisure, reinforcing the pharmacist's professional advice.

All pharmacies should be no-smoking areas. As with all such policies, special facilities may be necessary for employees who are smokers. In 1987, the Pharmaceutical Society decided that pharmacies must not sell tobacco or tobacco products, including cigarettes containing tobacco. Pharmacists cannot sell non-smoked tobacco. To do so constitutes professional misconduct.

Pharmacists should also be alert to possible drug interactions with smoking. Pharmacodynamic and pharmacokinetic properties of drugs may be affected by, especially, nicotine. The polyaromatic hydrocarbons in cigarette smoke can induce microsomal liver enzymes, which may be important in smokers taking drugs with a narrow therapeutic index. Theophylline metabolism is enhanced in smokers, requiring an increased dose. Conversely, should smoking cease, a lowered dose may be needed to avoid toxicity. Other effects on drug action include:

- increased heparin metabolism
- increased clearance of warfarin, although prothrombin time appears unchanged
- reduced therapeutic effect of histamine H_2-receptor antagonists in gastric ulcer healing, and increased relapse rate.

Successfully stopping smoking

It is beneficial for smokers to have a structured programme for giving up. Practical steps can include the following:

- don't just cut down on the number of cigarettes smoked: stop completely
- choose a day to stop
- list the benefits of giving up smoking (e.g. health and financial; increased exercise capacity; improved taste of food; and reduced personal tobacco odour)
- motivate yourself
- avoid locations where smoking is likely (e.g. public houses)
- discard all smoking-related materials (e.g. cigarettes, lighters and ashtrays) on the day prior to stopping
- obtain the support of family and friends
- try and give up with a friend.

Self-motivation of smokers is vital in achieving success. One positive factor is that most smokers underestimate the cost of smoking and the financial benefits of giving up. Removal of the staining effect of tobacco smoke (e.g. on hands, clothes and virtually anything with which it comes into contact) may significantly enhance smoker self-motivation; the appearance of the mouth and teeth may also improve.

Weight gain is common on stopping smoking. Smokers, especially women, may be anxious about the extent. However, smokers are generally leaner than the general population. The benefits from giving up smoking overwhelmingly outweigh the risks associated with weight gain in smokers who give up. Any weight gain is usually not substantial and does not last; subsequently their weight will stabilise.

References

Department of Health (1998a). *Smoking Kills* (Cm 4177). London: HMSO.

Martin J, ed. (1991). *Handbook of Pharmacy Health Education*. London: Pharmaceutical Press.

Office for National Statistics (1997a). *Living in Britain: Results from the 1996 General Household Survey*. London: HMSO.

Office for National Statistics (1997b). *Smoking Among Secondary School Children in 1996*. London: HMSO.

United States Environmental Protection Agency (1992). *Respiratory Health Effects of Passive Smoking*. EPA/600/6–90/006F.

Further reading

Bower A, Eaton K (1999). Evaluation of the effectiveness of a community pharmacy based smoking cessation scheme. *Pharm J* 262: 514–515.

Department of Health (1998b). *Report of the Scientific Committee on Tobacco and Health*. London: HMSO.

Israel M (1999). Smoking cessation. *Pharm J* 262: 226–228.

Sinclair H (2000). Health promotion (I): smoking cessation. In: Bond C, ed. *Evidence-based Pharmacy*. London: Pharmaceutical Press.

Useful addresses

Action on Smoking and Health (ASH)
16 Fitzhardinge Street
London W1H 9PL
Tel: 020 7224 0743

Quitline
Victory House
170 Tottenham Court Road
London W1P 0HA
Tel: 0800 002200

6

Excessive alcohol consumption

Simon Wills

The use of alcohol is widely accepted in many different cultures, and is commonly a focus of social and business interactions. It is seen as relaxing and enjoyable, with the encouragement to drink recognised as being welcoming and friendly. Regular but low wine consumption has even been linked to a reduced risk of developing coronary heart disease when compared with the incidence in non-drinkers. However, when consumed to excess, alcohol is more likely to have harmful effects and lead to the development of health and social problems. The range of these problems is diverse and involves many social and medical factors. Alcohol is responsible for causing a wide range of diseases; social problems that may be attributed wholly or in part to alcohol consumption include road traffic accidents, violence, criminal offences, relationship problems and employment difficulties. In England and Wales, 33 000 premature deaths per year are associated with alcohol consumption.

However, total abstinence for the population is an impossible goal to attain, and the promotion of sensible drinking has been advocated as a more realistic target. Limits for safe alcohol consumption are difficult, if not impossible, to define accurately. Limits are therefore estimated (*see below*) and take into consideration the marked individual variation in the response to alcohol.

Excessive use

Excessive alcohol consumption on a regular basis can induce dependence (*see below*), and the term alcohol dependence syndrome has been put forward by the WHO to describe this state.

Awareness of the effects of excessive alcohol consumption is necessary to recognise and manage the health and social problems that may occur as a result, and to promote sensible drinking. However, there is widespread ignorance regarding the role of alcohol in health and social problems. Alcohol consumption is seldom viewed as harmful, except in alcohol dependence, and this perpetuates the popular belief that alcohol-related problems only occur in people who become dependent on alcohol. The influence of alcohol is governed by the amount and frequency of consumption, the rate of consumption, the drinker's state of mind, the environment, the reasons for consumption and whether other psychotropic substances have been ingested simultaneously. The precise levels responsible for causing specific problems are impossible to determine because of the marked individual variation in response to alcohol and a lack of data. Alcohol-related morbidity and mortality are frequently unrecognised and therefore not recorded. Alcohol consumption varies between men and women, and among different age groups. On average, men drink more alcohol on a regular basis than women, although in recent years, the gap has narrowed as consumption by women has increased. For both sexes, average per capita alcohol consumption is highest among those between 18 and 24 years of age, decreasing among the older age groups.

Causes of excessive alcohol consumption

The causes of excessive alcohol consumption are multifactorial, but closely integrated. The availability of alcohol is an important determinant of the per capita consumption of alcohol, which in turn influences the extent of alcohol-related health and social problems within a population. In some communities (e.g. orthodox Jews and Muslims), drinking alcohol is not socially or culturally acceptable, and this results in a lower incidence of excessive consumption.

It has been demonstrated that the tendency to excessive alcohol consumption, and in particular to becoming dependent, may be inherited, although the magnitude of a genetic contribution has not yet been determined. People with a family history of alcohol dependence are liable to develop the condition at an earlier age than those who do not have such a genetic disposition; it is also likely to be more severe and chronic. The data that support this finding are more conclusive in men than women. It is, however, possible that the children of parents who chronically abuse alcohol may be more likely to follow this example in later life simply as a result of learned behaviour. The effects of parental excessive alcohol consumption on their children are discussed *below*. Personality disorders may also lead to alcohol abuse, although they are not associated with all cases and cannot, therefore, be used as a reliable indicator.

Men are more likely to consume alcohol to excess than women, although the differences between the sexes is narrowing in this regard. Certain occupations tend to encourage excessive alcoholic intake either through increased availability (e.g. publicans) or is seen as the social norm (e.g. sailors).

Measurement of alcohol consumption

The term alcohol is used in this chapter to refer to the consumption of ethanol (ethyl alcohol), which is the major constituent alcohol of all alcoholic beverages. Methods available to quantify alcohol consumption include:

- conventional measures (e.g. pint of beer, bar measure of spirits or glass of wine)
- quantity of alcohol contained in beverages (in grams or percentage alcohol by volume)
- units of alcohol.

Conventional measures are frequently used to assess alcohol consumption. However, they do not provide a reliable indicator of the amount of alcohol consumed because of the wide variation in the alcohol content of different beverages. The quantity of alcohol expressed in grams or as the percentage alcohol by volume is the most accurate way of quantifying intake, but this can only be applied by those familiar with the use of these concepts: the general public find it cumbersome and difficult to use. For this reason, the unit system was developed. One unit is defined as 8 g or 10 mL of alcohol. It is the amount of alcohol contained in an average standard drink, and is equivalent to:

- half a pint of ordinary beer or lager
- one glass of wine
- one small glass of fortified wine (e.g. sherry or port)
- one single English bar measure of spirits.

The unit system for determining alcohol consumption is the simplest and most widely accepted method. It is easily related to conventional measures by the use of the defined standard drinks and enables quick and reliable estimation of alcohol consumption, especially when a number of different alcoholic drinks are consumed. Table 6.1 indicates the approximate alcohol content of different beverages, the corresponding value in units and their relationship to conventional measures. It should be emphasised, however, that the unit system only allows for estimated values of alcohol consumption. There is a wide variation in alcohol content between brands of the same type of beverage and considerable variation in the size of measures (e.g. wine glasses vary considerably in size); home measures are generally larger than those in licensed public places (e.g. measures of spirits at home may be the equivalent of three to four units of alcohol). The labelling of low-alcohol and alcohol-free drinks can create confusion, and it is more difficult to estimate the number of units consumed. This problem is discussed below. The easier unit system has led to a campaign to label all alcoholic drinks with the number of units.

Limits and habits of alcohol consumption

An estimate of weekly alcohol intake provides people who drink on a regular basis with a means

Table 6.1 Approximate alcohol content of various beverages[a]

Type of beverage	Measure	Alcohol content (%)	Alcohol content (grams)	Alcohol content (units)
Beer or lager				
Ordinary strength	pint	3	16	2
Export beer	pint	4	20	2.5
Strong beer or lager	pint	5.5	32	4
Extra strong beer or lager	pint	7	40	5
Cider				
Ordinary strength	pint	4	24	3
Strong cider	pint	6	32	4
Spirits	single English bar measure	32	8	1
Wine				
Table wine	glass	8 to 14	8	1
Fortified wine (e.g. port and sherry)	standard small measure	13 to 16	8	1
Vermouth	single bar measure	13 to 16	8	1
Liqueurs	standard small measure	15 to 30	8	1

[a] The average is quoted. Some beverages will have a higher alcohol content, and some a lower one.

of assessing their risk of developing alcohol-related health and social problems. Limits of alcohol consumption applicable to adult men and women are defined as:

- sensible limits
- potentially dangerous limits
- dangerous limits.

Sensible limits

Sensible limits of alcohol consumption are up to 21 units per week for men and up to 14 units per week for women. Consumption should be spaced out over the week rather than in one or two sessions of heavy drinking. There should also be occasional alcohol-free days. Within these sensible limits, the risk of developing alcohol-related health and social problems is low.

Potentially dangerous limits

Potentially dangerous limits of alcohol consumption are between 21 and 49 units per week for men and 14 and 34 units per week for women. The risk of alcohol-related problems increases as consumption rises. Drinking within these limits is associated with a moderate or intermediate risk of developing alcohol-related health and social problems.

Dangerous limits

Dangerous limits of alcohol consumption are above 49 units per week for men and above 34 units per week for women. These levels of alcohol consumption carry a high risk of alcohol-related health and social problems. It is rare for consumption to reach these levels without incurring alcohol-related health or social problems.

These limits of alcohol consumption represent a general guide for people to assess their level of intake. However, people generally have a range of drinking habits, and the response to alcohol is additionally governed by individual variation. Social drinking is within sensible limits: it is less than two to three units per day and does not cause intoxication. Heavy drinking falls within potentially dangerous limits and includes consumption of more than six units per day, but without immediate alcohol-related problems. Problem drinking describes alcohol consumption that has caused alcohol-related problems (e.g. drink-driving offences) and may occur at any level of alcohol consumption. There is considerable overlap between these categories, with people moving from one category to another (e.g. from social drinking to heavy drinking or problem drinking). Heavy drinkers or problem drinkers are not necessarily dependent on alcohol, but may progress to dependence.

Metabolism of alcohol

Alcohol is rapidly absorbed from the gastrointestinal tract, mainly from the stomach and small intestine. Alcohol is eliminated primarily by oxidation to acetaldehyde, catalysed by the enzyme alcohol dehydrogenase; a small proportion is metabolised to acetaldehyde by cytochrome P450 in the liver. The latter pathway is enhanced in heavy drinkers and is thought to account for the substantial tolerance (*see below*) that commonly develops. Acetaldehyde is further oxidised to acetate, which is a good source of energy for a number of tissues. However, metabolism of acetate utilises members of the vitamin B group, which may result in deficiency if there is inadequate dietary intake. Vitamin B deficiency, particularly thiamine deficiency, has been implicated in the aetiology of some alcohol-related diseases (*see below*).

Generally, for equivalent consumption of alcohol, women attain higher blood-alcohol concentrations than men, particularly at the time of ovulation or just before menstruation. The bioavailability differences of alcohol in women are thought to be caused by the higher proportion of fat in the bodies of women compared with men; there is therefore a lower water content in women compared with men. Alcohol is water-soluble and a lower water content therefore reduces the volume of distribution of alcohol, resulting in higher blood-alcohol concentrations. However, following intravenous administration of alcohol, blood-alcohol concentrations are similar in both men and women, indicating the possibility that other mechanisms may be responsible for, or contribute to, the higher blood-alcohol concentrations in women following oral intake.

In both men and women, alcohol is metabolised primarily in the liver. However, there is also some initial oxidation in the gastric mucosa, involving the enzyme gastric alcohol dehydrogenase, which may be responsible for reducing the amount of alcohol absorbed into the blood circulation. Differences in the degree of gastric metabolism of alcohol may account for, or contribute to, higher blood-alcohol concentrations in women. In men, there is greater gastric metabolism of alcohol, although it is reduced in alcohol dependence. In women, the gastric metabolism of alcohol is much lower and is almost negligible in alcohol dependence.

The maximum blood-alcohol concentration that may be attained is affected by the rate of absorption, which is in turn affected by several other factors. The rate of absorption of alcohol from the stomach is reduced by the presence of food, particularly fatty foods. Absorption rate increases as the concentration of alcohol in a drink increases, and the most rapid absorption occurs at about 20% alcohol by volume. However, when the concentration of alcohol exceeds 20%, the absorption rate starts to slow down again, and undiluted spirits are not absorbed as quickly as when diluted with water or mixer drinks. Carbonated drinks are absorbed more quickly than non-carbonated drinks. The faster a drink is consumed, the higher the blood-alcohol concentration achieved.

Small quantities of alcohol are excreted unchanged in the urine and from the lungs in expired air, and can also be detected in the saliva. There is a correlation between blood-alcohol concentrations and concentrations present in the saliva, urine and expired air. This fact is exploited in the estimation of blood-alcohol concentrations from small samples, particularly in suspected cases of drinking and driving.

At high blood-alcohol concentrations (above 100 mg/100 mL), the rate of elimination is constant and not dependent on the blood-alcohol concentration (zero-order kinetics). Blood-alcohol concentrations will, therefore, decline at a constant rate, which is usually in the region of 6 to 40 mg/100 mL per hour (the average is 15 mg/100 mL per hour). In relation to the number of units consumed, it can be crudely estimated that it will take about one hour for the body to remove one unit of alcohol. This can also be usefully translated into the time required for the body to eliminate a given quantity of alcohol (e.g. eight hours for eight units).

Acute effects of alcohol consumption

The acute effects of alcohol (acute intoxication) are caused by its depressant action on the central nervous system, although the precise mechanisms are complex. Alcohol seems to enhance the CNS actions of the inhibitory neurotransmitter GABA, and reduce the effects of excitatory neurotransmitters (e.g. glutamate). Alcohol-induced release of other neurotransmitters, such as dopamine, may be responsible for eliciting its pleasurable effects. The clinical features of acute alcohol intoxication (Table 6.2) are related to the blood-alcohol and brain-alcohol concentrations. The risk of accidental injury also increases with rising blood-alcohol concentrations.

It must be emphasised that there is a wide variation in the response to alcohol between individuals. Factors responsible for this variation include:

- tolerance to the effects of alcohol
- presence of food in the stomach
- blood-alcohol concentration
- gender
- medication.

Tolerance to the effects of alcohol

Tolerance develops with regular consumption. Heavy drinkers who have developed substantial tolerance may show little sign of intoxication at blood-alcohol concentrations that would cause severe intoxication in people who usually drink less (e.g. occasional drinkers).

Table 6.2 Acute effects of alcohol consumption in relation to the blood-alcohol concentration

Blood-alcohol concentration (mg/100 mL)	Acute effects
below 50	altered mood increased confidence relaxation sense of well being talkativeness
50 to 100 (inebriation)	impaired judgement inco-ordination loss of sensory perception loss of some social inhibitions slurred speech
100 to 300 (intoxication)	ataxia blurred vision loss of self-control slow reactions
300 to 500 (severe intoxication)	severe ataxia diplopia convulsions coma
above 500 (very severe intoxication)	loss of tendon reflexes hypothermia respiratory depression coma death

Presence of food in the stomach

The presence of food in the stomach reduces the rate of absorption of alcohol.

Blood-alcohol concentration

The effects of alcohol and the severity of intoxication are greatest when the blood-alcohol concentration is rising to its peak level compared with when it is falling. This may be caused by the development of tolerance within this short period of time. A rapid rise in blood-alcohol concentration will enhance the effects of alcohol to a greater extent than a slow rise.

Gender

The acute effects of equivalent alcohol intake are enhanced in women compared with men.

Medication

Other CNS depressants considerably enhance the effects of alcohol.

Alcohol-related problems

It is difficult to assess the amount of alcohol that may be responsible for producing specific health and social problems because many of these only occur after long-term abuse. Retrospective estimates of alcohol consumption are bound to be inaccurate, particularly as people who consume excessive amounts are often evasive about their intake.

Some people appear to be relatively unaffected by consumption of inordinate amounts of alcohol, whereas others readily develop problems. This suggests that there may be additional factors (e.g. nutritional deficiency, underlying disease or genetic susceptibility) that must also be considered.

Alcohol-related social problems

Social problems may arise as a result of alcohol abuse because it impairs judgement. Conversely, excessive alcohol consumption may be caused by social problems. It is likely, however, that alcohol is not solely responsible for the development of an individual's social problems, and other factors (e.g. personality disorders) may play an important role. Specific societal problems attributable to alcohol (e.g. violence between football fans, and drinking and driving) are increasingly recognised, although measures to reduce their incidence have had limited effect.

Family problems, particularly marital difficulties, are commonly encountered in association with unrestrained drinking; alcohol is a contributory factor to violence within the family. Children are likely to be severely affected by parental excessive alcohol consumption (*see below*), with neglect being the predominant feature. The expense of maintaining drinking habits contributes to poverty and debt, which may accentuate alcohol-related family problems.

Difficulties at work may arise as a result of drink problems and include absenteeism, accidents and inefficiency. Alcohol-related occupational problems can arise at any level, and managerial and leadership qualities may be diminished, resulting in poor overall performance of the company. Time spent away from work as a result of alcohol-related disorders contributes substantially to industrial costs.

Alcohol consumption and aggressive behaviour are often encountered together, although the association is complex and other factors may be involved. Perceived threat and provocation may contribute to aggression in a particular situation. Alcohol consumption may even cause a paranoid state (*see below*), which in some cases can be dangerous.

Drinking and driving increases the risk of accidents if the blood-alcohol concentration rises above 50 mg/100 mL; this threshold is lower for learners, inexperienced drivers and occasional drinkers. The blood-alcohol concentration above which it is illegal to drive is 80 mg/100 mL, although many believe that this limit should be lowered, perhaps to 50 mg/100 mL, or even less. However, evidence suggests that altering limits will not in itself affect the prevalence of drinking and driving. The increased likelihood of being caught and penalised has a more pronounced effect, and this might be achieved by random breath-testing of drivers, for example.

It has been estimated that drinking one unit of alcohol raises the blood-alcohol concentration by about 15 mg/100 mL in men and about 20 mg/100 mL in women. However, it is not possible to determine accurately the blood-alcohol concentration from the number of drinks a person has had, because the actual amount of alcohol absorbed and the rate of absorption are subject to wide individual variation. The only advice that can safely be given is not to drink at all before driving. It should also be pointed out that, on average, it takes one hour to eliminate one unit of alcohol from the body. Therefore, someone who has indulged in a heavy drinking session late into the night may still be over the legal limit for driving the following morning.

Intoxication with alcohol is also associated with an increased risk of: accidents and traumatic injury; crime; experimenting with street drugs; unwanted pregnancies; and acquisition of sexually-transmitted diseases. Most intentional overdoses with drugs are taken under the influence of alcohol.

Alcohol-related diseases

The relationship between alcohol consumption and development of disease has been largely derived from studies of alcohol-dependent people who regularly drink alcohol at a level above the sensible limits. Although the majority of serious alcohol-related diseases do occur in alcohol-dependent people, they are not exclusive to this group; some may arise in non-dependent heavy drinkers. Alcohol may not be the sole cause of a disease and other contributory factors (e.g. smoking or nutritional deficiencies) must be taken into consideration. There is a tendency for one major alcohol-related disease to dominate in the absence of any other sign of disease. Women are more vulnerable than men to the toxic effects of alcohol and are at greater risk of developing alcohol-related diseases.

Anaemias

Anaemias are common in long-term heavy drinkers, and result from the interaction of several factors, including poor diet, chronic blood loss, liver disease and a direct toxic effect of alcohol on bone marrow. Megaloblastic anaemia may arise, and is commonly seen in alcohol dependence associated with nutritional deficiency. It is caused by folate deficiency and a direct toxic effect of alcohol. Sideroblastic anaemia is associated with reduced serum-folate and erythrocyte-folate concentrations; a mixed macrocytic and microcytic anaemia, and liver disease may also be present. Iron-deficiency anaemia is frequently seen in alcohol-dependent patients, and haemorrhage (e.g. from oesophageal varices or gastritis) or poor diet may cause, or contribute to, this.

Cardiac disorders

A session of heavy ('binge') drinking may produce acute effects on the heart. These include ectopic beats, atrial fibrillation or ventricular tachycardia, and occur as a result of a direct toxic effect on cardiac tissue. In non-drinkers or occasional drinkers, acute effects usually occur at lower intakes than in people who have developed tolerance to alcohol as a result of regular drinking; susceptibility is also increased in the presence of established heart disease.

Alcohol-related cardiomyopathy (alcoholic heart muscle disease) occurs as a result of sustained heavy drinking. The mechanism is thought be a toxic effect on cardiac muscle due to defective cardiac protein synthesis or free radical damage. A dose-effect relationship between the amount of alcohol ingested and the development of dilated cardiomyopathy appears to exist, although the relationship is with the total lifetime alcohol consumption and not the present level.

Coagulation defects

Coagulation defects predispose the patient to life-threatening haemorrhage. Chronic alcohol abuse may impair platelet production, survival and function, producing thrombocytopenia. This resolves when alcohol is withdrawn although, initially, the platelet count may rise above the normal value.

Alcohol has no direct toxic effect on

coagulation factors. However, severe alcohol-related liver disease (e.g. cirrhosis of the liver or alcoholic hepatitis) suppresses the production of vitamin K-dependent coagulation factors, thus reducing the synthesis of prothrombin. Associated features include increased fibrinolysis and disseminated intravascular coagulation. This disturbance of haemostasis is not completely reversed by the administration of vitamin K.

Endocrine disorders

Hypoglycaemia may occur between six and 36 hours after binge drinking. The risk of developing alcohol-related hypoglycaemia is increased if alcohol is consumed on an empty stomach, following heavy exercise, or in the presence of nutritional deficiency and in diabetics on oral hypoglycaemics or insulin. In some cases, it may be severe and lead to hypoglycaemic coma. In patients with cirrhosis of the liver (*see below*), alcohol-related hypoglycaemia indicates a severe deterioration in liver function.

Excessive alcohol consumption is causally linked to the development of maturity onset diabetes mellitus (Type II or non-insulin dependent). Alcohol-related diabetes may be caused by chronic pancreatitis (*see below*) if extensive damage occurs. It may also arise as a result of cirrhosis of the liver.

Alcohol may cause a deterioration in sexual function, and these effects are thought to be mediated by impaired hypothalamic function, impaired metabolism of oestrogens by the liver or a direct toxic effect of alcohol on the testes or ovaries. There is a reduction in plasma-testosterone concentration in men and plasma-oestrogen concentration in women. Some disorders (e.g. temporary impotence or loss of libido) may be associated with a single session binge drinking; chronic alcohol abuse may produce permanent impairment. The disorders that may occur in men include gynaecomastia, impotence, loss of libido, loss of pubic hair, low sperm count, scrotal wrinkling and testicular atrophy. In women, alcohol-related sexual disorders include atrophy of the breasts and external genitalia, diminished flow of vaginal secretions, menstrual disorders and progressive masculinisation.

Alcohol causes an increase in the release of cortisol from the adrenal cortex. This is thought to be the mechanism responsible for causing pseudo-Cushing's syndrome in alcohol dependence. The clinical features resolve completely on abstinence.

A clinical syndrome resembling hyperthyroidism may arise in the presence of long-term alcohol abuse. The precise mechanism responsible is not known, although alcohol does not appear to have a direct effect on the thyroid gland. It is essential to distinguish this condition from true hyperthyroidism.

Gastro-intestinal disorders

Alcohol is a common cause of gastro-oesophageal reflux, which often leads to reflux oesophagitis; a characteristic symptom is heartburn. Alcohol also frequently causes acute gastritis, which may result in retching and vomiting, particularly in the morning after a night of heavy drinking; erosion of the gastric mucosa may produce mild haematemesis.

Oesophageal bleeding may occur as a result of reflux oesophagitis or ruptured varices; tearing of the oesophageal mucous membrane (Mallory-Weiss lesion) during retching and vomiting may also be a cause. Spontaneous rupture of the oesophagus (Boerhaave's syndrome) is an uncommon but life-threatening condition that may occur as a result of binge drinking.

Alcohol has been implicated as a cause of peptic ulceration, although there is little evidence to support this conclusion, or that moderate alcohol consumption may delay ulcer healing.

Excessive consumption of alcohol may cause diarrhoea as a result of increased intestinal motility and disturbed intestinal microflora.

A heavy drinking session may produce acute pancreatitis, and life-threatening complications include hypovolaemic shock, renal failure, liver failure and respiratory failure. Long-term abuse of alcohol is a major cause of chronic pancreatitis, and complications of extensive pancreatic damage include malabsorption and diabetes mellitus. It is thought that acute episodes of pancreatitis are usually superimposed on an underlying chronic condition.

Gout

Historically, alcohol consumption has been implicated in the development of gout and, while this still holds true today, the exact role of alcohol in the aetiology has not been determined. Gout is caused by hyperuricaemia, which may arise as a result of increased uric acid production or decreased uric acid excretion. Studies have shown that alcohol may play a part in both of these pathways.

Hypertension

Alcohol causes an immediate rise in blood pressure, and thus may exacerbate underlying hypertension or even be a primary cause; hypertension is commonly seen in heavy drinkers. The precise mechanism of alcohol-related hypertension is not known, although increases in plasma concentrations of cortisol, renin, aldosterone and vasopressin have been demonstrated following alcohol consumption; the increased sympathetic activity produced by alcohol may also contribute. However, these pressor effects are seen after the increase in blood pressure has occurred and, therefore, do not account for the immediate rise.

Blood pressure returns to normal when alcohol consumption ceases, although it may not be necessary to stop drinking completely in all cases; reduction to sensible limits may be all that is required.

Liver disease

Varying types of liver disease are commonly associated with excessive alcohol consumption, although the precise aetiological mechanisms are unknown. Alcohol-related liver disease in women tends to occur following a shorter period of alcohol abuse compared with men, even when lower quantities of alcohol are consumed, and is often more severe with a poor prognosis.

Fatty degeneration is characterised by the presence of large fat droplets within liver cells, producing an enlarged liver. It is common in heavy drinkers and is probably dose-related. It is not necessarily harmful, and is usually reversed if alcohol consumption is stopped or reduced to sensible limits.

Acute alcoholic hepatitis is associated with sustained excessive consumption and is more serious than fatty degeneration, although it does not develop in all heavy drinkers. Features include hepatomegaly with necrosis and fibrosis of varying degrees. This condition may be a precursor to cirrhosis of the liver. It can remain unchanged for years or, in some cases, recovery may occur despite continued drinking. However, medical advice should always be to stop drinking immediately, in which case the disease is usually reversible. Chronic active hepatitis may also occur as a result of chronic alcohol consumption.

Cirrhosis of the liver is a serious disorder caused by chronic excessive alcohol consumption, although it occurs in only 10 to 30% of heavy drinkers. The first clinical signs usually present between 50 and 70 years of age. It is characterised by the destruction of parenchymal cells, loss of their normal lobular structure with widespread fibrosis and regeneration of the remaining cells to form nodules. Complications may arise as a result of portal hypertension and include ascites, jaundice, oesophageal varices, renal failure and hepatic encephalopathy. About 15 to 30% of these patients develop hepatocellular carcinoma, which has a poor prognosis. Alcohol-related cirrhosis of the liver may be accompanied by varying degrees of fatty degeneration or acute alcoholic hepatitis, or both, in patients who continue drinking.

Cirrhosis of the liver is a progressive disorder, although it can be arrested if alcohol consumption is stopped, and the liver may then be able to compensate for some of its lost functions.

Malignant disease

Alcohol consumption and development of malignant disease have been tentatively linked but, as data are limited, the precise role of alcohol has not yet been identified. Alcohol itself is probably not carcinogenic, but may act by accelerating the development of malignancy. However, some alcoholic drinks do contain carcinogens (e.g. nitrosamines and polycyclic hydrocarbons); acetaldehyde, a metabolite of alcohol, is carcinogenic. The risk of developing alcohol-related cancer appears to be dose-related. It is probably also related to the type of alcoholic drink consumed, since some studies show that whilst chronic ingestion of one type of drink predisposes to a cancer, others do not.

Malignant diseases that may be associated with excessive alcohol consumption include breast cancer, oropharyngeal cancer, laryngeal cancer and malignancies of the gastro-intestinal system, particularly oesophageal cancer. Hepatocellular carcinoma (primary liver cell cancer) is linked to alcohol consumption because about 80% of cases develop in the presence of cirrhosis of the liver (*see above*). It has a higher incidence in men than women and a poor prognosis.

Nervous system disorders

Long-term consumption of alcohol above sensible limits is associated with a wide range of nervous system disorders, which are thought to be mediated by nutritional deficiency or a direct toxic effect of alcohol on nervous system tissue, or both.

Memory loss is characterised by the loss of short-term memory ('blackouts') and is commonly seen following binge drinking. Memory of the events that occurred during the binge is usually diminished or absent, despite full consciousness and awareness being maintained at the time.

Chronic alcohol abuse is associated with regular episodes of memory loss, which may last several hours or even days. Awareness, consciousness and relatively normal behaviour may be maintained during this time. In some cases, patients travel long distances, but are unable to recall the experience.

Wernicke's encephalopathy is caused principally by alcohol-related thiamine deficiency. The predominant symptoms are ataxia, confusion and paralysis of the eye muscles; peripheral neuropathy (*see below*) may also be present and there is often some degree of memory impairment. Stupor and coma may occur in the late stages before death. In many cases, symptoms are non-specific and the condition is not diagnosed until post-mortem. Parenteral administration of thiamine elicits a rapid response and arrests progression of the disease, although some abnormalities may persist.

Korsakoff's psychosis is caused mainly by alcohol-related thiamine deficiency, and is thought to be the chronic form of Wernicke's encephalopathy. The two are sometimes referred to as Wernicke–Korsakoff's syndrome as a result of this association. Wernicke's encephalopathy may be the acute phase and Korsakoff's syndrome the chronic phase of the same illness.

Short-term memory is grossly impaired and patients are unable to recall events for longer than a few seconds or minutes after they have occurred. General intellectual ability remains relatively unaffected although there is a disordered sense of time and place. Patients remain alert and often fabricate very plausible, but inaccurate, details of incidents to fill in the memory gaps (confabulation); they believe their accounts to be true. Memory of past events usually remains intact. The condition may improve a little if sobriety is maintained over a period of years.

Cerebellar degeneration may occur after prolonged alcohol abuse, and is characterised by progressive ataxia. The main manifestation is an unsteady gait with little or no effect on the arms. The cause is not known, although nutritional deficiency, especially of thiamine, has been suggested. Wernicke's encephalopathy with peripheral neuropathy is also commonly present. There is some improvement with abstinence and administration of thiamine.

Peripheral neuropathy is commonly encountered with chronic abuse of alcohol, and is most likely to be caused by deficiency of members of the vitamin B group, especially thiamine; there may be a direct toxic effect of alcohol. It is characterised by distal axonal degeneration, producing paraesthesia and pain in the feet; subsequently, the hands may also become affected. Muscle weakness and wasting may eventually develop distally in the arms and legs, and tendon reflexes are lost.

Cerebrovascular disorders may be caused by alcohol abuse. Strokes or subarachnoid haemorrhage in young men may follow alcoholic binges. The mechanism may be either the hypertensive effects of alcohol or disturbed haemostasis.

Seizures may occur due to alcohol withdrawal, after a stroke or be due to a head injury sustained whilst intoxicated.

Nutritional deficiency

Nutritional deficiency and chronic excessive alcohol consumption are inextricably linked (especially in alcohol dependence), and factors that may be responsible include:

- utilisation of alcohol as an energy source
- dietary neglect, often associated with financial constraints
- impaired storage, utilisation or excretion of nutrients
- malabsorption.

Alcohol is a source of energy, but alcoholic drinks do not contain appreciable quantities of other nutrients. One gram of alcohol yields 0.029 MJ (7.0 kCal) of energy; therefore one unit provides 0.232 MJ (56.0 kCal) of energy. This extra source of energy with a normal diet will contribute to the development of obesity. If dietary sources of energy are gradually replaced by alcohol, bodyweight remains static as long as the total energy requirements are being met. If the diet is further reduced, the total intake of energy may be insufficient, leading to weight loss and more severe nutritional deficiency.

Chronic excessive alcohol consumption is commonly associated with an inadequate and irregular intake of food and an unbalanced diet; people who live alone are at increased risk. Heavy drinking also results in loss of appetite, because the immediate energy demands are being met by alcohol and because the various gastro-intestinal side-effects of alcohol tend to dissuade patients from eating. The stomach also feels bloated following beer drinking. Drinking alcohol on a regular basis is an expensive habit to maintain, and financial constraints may mean that priority is given to alcohol over food. Alcohol may also cause malabsorption, and nutrients affected include folic acid, pyridoxine, thiamine and vitamin B_{12}. Members of the vitamin B group are used as coenzymes in the metabolism of alcohol and, in the presence of an inadequate intake, there may be insufficient amounts to meet normal metabolic requirements.

Psychiatric disorders

Alcohol abuse is associated with psychiatric disorders or emotional disturbances, although it may be difficult to determine cause and effect. In either case, it is vital to refrain from further alcohol consumption. Behavioural disorders commonly arise as a result of problem drinking, with irresponsible and unreliable behaviour particularly evident. Alcohol withdrawal (*see below*) and thiamine deficiency (*see above*) can produce a range of strange behaviour and psychiatric problems. Anxiety, insomnia and phobias are also common in problem drinkers.

Sustained drinking may induce depression, although it is not known what role alcohol plays in the aetiology. Alternatively, people may start drinking because of low self-esteem, lack of confidence or feelings of guilt or worthlessness, which are all symptoms of depression. Alcohol-related depressive disorders represent a high risk of suicide. There is an association between manic-depressive illness and alcohol consumption, although the relationship is unclear and complex. The manic phase may contribute to excessive drinking as a result of elation and hyperactivity; conversely, alcohol may be used during the depressive phase to help improve mood. Excessive consumption is, therefore, frequent and regular and may lead to alcohol dependence.

Paranoid states, especially pathological jealousy, are commonly associated with alcohol abuse. Sexual jealousy and an unfounded belief in a partner's infidelity may arise. A common state of paranoia, which often occurs following a session of heavy drinking, is the belief that other people (usually passers-by) are making derogatory and insulting remarks.

Skeletal myopathy

Acute alcoholic myopathy may arise after a session of heavy drinking, particularly in alcohol-dependent patients. It is probably caused by hypokalaemia (and perhaps hypomagnesaemia) following vomiting, diarrhoea and aldosteronism. The muscles of the thigh and the upper arm are most usually affected, and symptoms include pain, swelling and weakness. In severe cases, there may be extensive destruction of muscle fibre, which may lead to renal failure. Chronic skeletal myopathy is associated with long-term alcohol consumption, although the relationship is with the total lifetime alcohol consumption rather than the current level. Atrophy of proximal muscles produces weakness and flaccidity; other symptoms may include low back pain and leg cramps.

Alcohol and specific groups

The effects of alcohol vary considerably with age and sex, and influence the development of alcohol-related health and social problems. Groups that require special consideration are children, the elderly and pregnant or breast-feeding women.

Children

Alcohol consumption by children

The effects of alcohol on children arise from their own alcohol consumption and that of their parents/carers. At this age, the dangers of alcohol consumption by children arise from acute intoxication and its sequelae rather than alcohol dependence.

Children under five years of age possess very little alcohol dehydrogenase and so, compared with adults, the capacity for alcohol metabolism is relatively limited. The symptoms of acute intoxication are more severe as a result, and because children have not learned how to deal with the effects of intoxication. Hypothermia may be encountered and is thought to arise as a result of impairment of temperature regulation systems. Respiratory depression may also occur in severe intoxication and requires close supervision and, in some cases, respiratory support. Hypoglycaemia is a serious effect of acute alcohol intoxication in children and is most likely to occur when alcohol is consumed in the morning before eating.

Infants and young children are particularly at risk of accidental poisoning as a result of their inquisitive natures. In the home, alcohol is generally considered to be relatively harmless and, unlike other potentially dangerous substances, bottles of alcoholic drinks are often kept within sight and easy reach. Young children are also keen copiers and are likely to drink what they have seen their elders drinking. Accidental poisoning may occur when they consume alcohol in the morning following a social event held in the home by their parents the night before. There may be remnants of alcoholic beverages in glasses or bottles left within reach. Older children, especially those approaching their teenage years, are usually familiar with alcohol, its effects and use in social situations. However, they may misjudge the potency of alcohol.

Adolescents are invariably aware of alcohol. Experimentation is the most important cause of severe acute intoxication in young teenagers. Equally, alcohol forms an important part of being sociable for many older adolescents. Regular alcohol consumption may start at a young age and, although long-term alcohol-related diseases may not be a problem, social and psychological effects may become apparent. Violence, crime and other behavioural problems are commonly caused by alcohol. There has been much concern that some alcoholic drinks are being marketed with young, under-age adolescents in mind. These drinks are often very sweet, attractively packaged and fruit-flavoured.

Excessive alcohol consumption by adults

Regular excessive alcohol consumption by parents has serious implications for the emotional or psychological development of children. The home environment is frequently tense and children develop feelings of uncertainty, neglect, rejection and isolation, as a result of which they may become socially and emotionally labile. Drunken parents may also physically abuse their children.

Children may be blamed by their parents as the cause of their drink problem. Children are likely to believe this to be true because of their lack of knowledge and understanding. It should be emphasised, however, that children respond to parental excessive alcohol consumption in a variety of ways: whereas some children develop social and psychological problems, others remain unaffected.

Children may find it difficult to cope with parental alcohol-related health and social problems, and are often put under enormous pressure. In some cases, older children may have to take responsibility for younger siblings. Children often hide their own emotional and psychological problems, and those of their parents, from outsiders and pretend that home life is normal. They may have learning difficulties at school, and their childhood days are generally less happy. Parental alcohol abuse may lead to delinquency in their children; these children are also liable to consume alcohol regularly, and drug misuse may be an additional feature.

The elderly

Elderly people are more vulnerable to the toxic effects of alcohol than younger people, which may be because the elderly attain higher blood-alcohol concentrations for an equivalent consumption of alcohol. This effect can be attributed to the ageing process, which results in a reduction of lean body mass, lower water content and increased proportion of fat compared with younger people. Delirium tremens is associated with a higher mortality in the elderly; alcohol is also commonly involved in suicide attempts. Causes of excessive alcohol consumption in the elderly are numerous and include bereavement, boredom, loneliness, social isolation and illness.

The elderly have a greater tendency to hide drink problems than younger people, and are more likely to consume alcohol throughout the day rather than indulge in sessions of heavy drinking. Non-specific alcohol-related disorders are commonly caused, or exacerbated, by excessive alcohol consumption in the elderly and include hypothermia and poor hygiene.

The effects of drug interactions involving alcohol are more important in the elderly as a result of the frequent use of one or more medicines. The choice of medication should be carefully assessed if excessive alcohol consumption is a problem.

Pregnant and breast-feeding women

Foetal alcohol syndrome

Alcohol freely crosses the placenta and similar blood-alcohol concentrations are seen in the foetus as in the mother. There is evidence that alcohol consumption during early pregnancy adversely affects foetal development. The condition is referred to as the foetal alcohol syndrome (FAS) and varies in severity, depending on the level of alcohol consumption. Heavy drinking during pregnancy (e.g. more than four to five units per day) increases the risk of development of the complete FAS. This syndrome is characterised by developmental defects producing facial abnormalities, mental retardation and central nervous system disorders (e.g. epilepsy, spasticity and lack of co-ordination). There is also growth deficiency both *in utero* and following birth. Other disorders that may arise include cardiac disorders, urogenital disorders, musculoskeletal defects and haemangiomas. Not all symptoms are apparent at birth, and the extent and severity of FAS may not be realised for some years. Although the physical manifestations of the FAS typically abate with age, late manifestations can include behavioural disorders and intellectual defects.

The likelihood of developing FAS cannot be predicted from alcohol consumption alone, because not all women who drink heavily during pregnancy give birth to infants exhibiting signs of developmental abnormalities. The detailed role of alcohol in the aetiology of FAS is unknown and women at highest risk cannot yet be identified. Similarly, a safe level of alcohol consumption during pregnancy has not been established, so it would seem wise for all women planning to become pregnant to avoid alcohol completely. Complete abstinence until delivery would be the ideal, but it is considered by some authorities that such restrictive advice may be too severe to be heeded.

Regular heavy drinking in late pregnancy can occasionally cause withdrawal reactions in the neonate.

Alcohol in breast milk

The consumption of alcohol before breast-feeding may result in adverse effects in the infant, although these are extremely rare and only likely to occur at high maternal blood-alcohol concentrations. Alcohol in breast milk has been found to cause a slight decrease in psychomotor development of breast-fed infants, although this appears to be clinically insignificant. The concentration of alcohol in breast milk closely parallels maternal blood-alcohol concentration, but the resultant blood-alcohol concentration in the infant is usually low. Maternal blood-alcohol concentrations would have to be very high indeed to result in sedation in the infant. Despite this, babies have a minimal capacity to clear alcohol from their bodies so it would seem wise to be cautious. In addition, consumption of moderate to high amounts of alcohol seem to impair milk ejection from the breast, so regular consumption of these quantities may prevent breast feeding. Even small amounts seem to reduce the quantity of milk taken by the infant.

An occasional drink during breast-feeding is not thought to be of any clinical significance to the baby, but pharmacists should advise breast-feeding women that they should restrict their intake of alcohol. If consumed, it should be shortly after breast feeding, and then further feeding avoided for two hours after each unit of alcohol if effects upon the infant are to be minimised.

Alcohol-dependence syndrome

Continued excessive alcohol consumption may eventually result in the alcohol-dependence syndrome, which is most often seen in men in their mid-forties, although it can occur earlier. In women, alcohol dependence is associated with the early onset of nervous system disorders, which tend to occur following a shorter period of dependence and at lower levels of consumption than in men, and with an increased risk of death. There is also a greater tendency for permanent nervous system abnormalities in women following successful treatment of dependence and abstention from further alcohol consumption.

Alcohol-dependence syndrome is characterised by the manifestation of withdrawal symptoms when the blood-alcohol concentration falls. Other features include:

- consumption of alcohol to relieve alcohol withdrawal symptoms (relief drinking)
- consumption of alcohol on a daily basis
- development of substantial tolerance to the effects of alcohol
- inability to stop consumption
- priority given to alcohol consumption above all else (e.g. social interaction, work and health).

Tolerance to the acute effects of alcohol is substantial in alcohol dependence, and can occur up to a point where the dependent person may be able to tolerate blood-alcohol concentrations that would be associated with severe intoxication in the average person. A common misconception held by alcohol-dependent people is that since the amount of alcohol consumed does not result in acute intoxication, it is not having a detrimental effect. In the late stages of dependence, tolerance may be reduced to the point where the acute effects of alcohol consumption return to those seen in the average person.

Alcohol withdrawal symptoms

Alcohol withdrawal symptoms characteristically appear on waking and are relieved by drinking. Their severity and intensity are highly variable.

Initial acute withdrawal reactions start within a few hours of the blood-alcohol concentration reaching zero and peak between 24 and 36 hours later. Symptoms may also appear as the blood-alcohol concentration falls, especially if the decline is rapid. The characteristic symptoms are apprehension, raised blood pressure, insomnia, irritability, nausea and retching, sweating, tremor and weakness. Additionally, hallucinations may occur, usually within 48 hours of stopping alcohol intake; they are generally visual in nature, although auditory hallucinations may also be experienced. Convulsions may occur in a small proportion of patients after seven to 48 hours of stopping alcohol, and are usually generalised tonic-clonic (grand mal) convulsions. In rare cases, status epilepticus may occur, although other causes (e.g. hypoglycaemia, subdural haemorrhage or CNS infection) must be considered. Arrhythmias may occasionally be associated with alcohol withdrawal, although these may be caused by other alcohol-related disorders (e.g. hypokalaemia and electrolyte imbalance). Heart failure may be precipitated, particularly if alcohol-related cardiomyopathy is present.

Delirium tremens is a serious and life-threatening manifestation of alcohol withdrawal, and begins within four days of stopping or reducing alcohol consumption; it may last for three to seven days. It is not common, occurring in only about 5% of patients. It is characterised by severe agitation and irritability, confusion, disorientation, impaired perception, insomnia and nightmares, delusions, nausea and vomiting, fever, profuse sweating, dehydration, electrolyte imbalance, gross tremor, hypertension and arrhythmias. As in acute withdrawal reactions, hallucinations in delirium tremens are commonly visual in nature, although auditory hallucinations may also occur. Feelings of extreme fear and apprehension arising from the hallucinations may lead to aggressive or suicidal behaviour. Most deaths are caused by fever, arrhythmias or co-existing illness (e.g. infection); the elderly are at increased risk of fatal delirium tremens.

Management of the alcohol-dependence syndrome

Recognising alcohol dependence early can lead to successful treatment before any alcohol-related diseases develop. However, alcohol dependence is not always easy to detect. Persuading patients that they may be dependent on alcohol and require treatment may be even more difficult.

Alcohol-dependent patients are usually secretive about their drinking behaviour, even when they know they are dependent. They may deny being dependent and may even believe that they can stop whenever they want to. Patients may want to stop drinking alcohol but are unable to, and asking for help is often a difficult first step for them. This may arise as a result of the social stigma associated with alcohol dependence.

Clinically, alcohol dependence can be identified in two ways. Firstly, patients may present with alcohol withdrawal symptoms. Secondly, patients may present with signs and symptoms of alcohol-related health and social problems. However, other clues to the presence of alcohol dependence include:

- emotional and psychiatric disturbances (e.g. anxiety, aggression, depressive disorders or insomnia)
- facial appearance (e.g. bloated face, facial flushing and bloodshot eyes)
- family history of excessive alcohol consumption
- frequent requests for medical assistance (e.g. for gastro-intestinal disorders)
- gynaecomastia
- hand tremor and red palms
- social problems (e.g. marital problems and work problems, especially inefficiency and Monday morning absences)
- tachycardia
- trouble with the police (e.g. drinking and driving, assault and drunkenness)
- untidy appearance and smelling of alcohol.

Alcohol-dependent patients are commonly affected by anger, frustration, guilt and isolation. Anger is often directed towards members of the family, and patients frequently blame close relatives for the alcohol dependence. Family members often try not to antagonise the patient and, in some cases, may believe that the problem is not serious. These and other social, emotional and psychological problems that may contribute to excessive alcohol consumption must be identified and addressed in association with the management of alcohol dependence. Examples of these problems include financial difficulties, bereavement, marital problems and social isolation.

The management of alcohol dependence involves a short-term phase, during which alcohol consumption must be stopped, and the more difficult long-term modification of drinking behaviour.

The short-term phase produces alcohol withdrawal and requires control of the resultant symptoms. The management of withdrawal (sometimes referred to as detoxification) is based on the extent and severity of the withdrawal symptoms. Communication with patients who are intoxicated or experiencing severe symptoms may be difficult. The drinking habits of the patient are first identified where possible, although details about alcohol consumption are often more reliably obtained from relatives or friends. The extent and severity of previous episodes of alcohol withdrawal (when known) are a reliable guide to predict the outcome on the present occasion, although successive episodes of withdrawal may increase in severity. Care should be taken to determine an accurate account of any medication or non-prescribed drugs of abuse that are taken. Opioid or benzodiazepine withdrawal as well as alcohol withdrawal can be difficult to manage. Regular medication should not be discontinued during detoxification, to prevent deterioration of underlying medical conditions (alcohol-related or otherwise).

Alcohol withdrawal, in all its forms, is associated with considerable psychological distress for the patient, and management should be directed towards optimising comfort and safety. The environment should be supportive, calm and non-threatening. Patients may also require assistance with walking, personal hygiene, changing their clothing and adjusting their bedclothes. Disorientation is a common feature of alcohol withdrawal and support is necessary to overcome it.

Alcohol detoxification is always managed in a hospital or specialist detoxification unit. This ensures that the patient can be cared for, and that medication is taken. Patients presenting with symptoms of delirium tremens should preferably be managed by specialists. In most cases, drug treatment for about one week is necessary to control the symptoms. Recovery can occur safely in the absence of drug therapy, but this is rarely advised because the severity of withdrawal is usually not predictable.

Benzodiazepines (e.g. chlordiazepoxide and diazepam) or chlormethiazole are commonly used in the management of alcohol withdrawal; the most widely used are benzodiazepines. All these drugs have sedative properties, which is their primary advantage. They do not cure excessive alcohol consumption, neither do they prevent withdrawal; they simply suppress many of the symptoms and so make withdrawal more bearable. Large doses are used on the first day (e.g. 60 to 100 mg of chlordiazepoxide, or 9 to 12 chlormethiazole capsules), in four or more divided doses. (Smaller doses are used in the elderly.) These large doses are gradually reduced on subsequent days until the drug is stopped after seven to ten days. It is important that alcoholics are not sent home on 'maintenance' doses of these drugs, as this serves no purpose and may be dangerous if consumed with alcohol. It also predisposes to later benzodiazepine dependence.

Clonidine or sodium valproate have also been used with some success, instead of benzodiazepines, for detoxification, but they are not widely used in the UK.

All patients must be given thiamine during the withdrawal period, to treat deficiency. If symptoms of Wernicke's encephalopathy are present, large doses of intravenous thiamine are needed. Dehydration caused by sweating, fever or increased muscular activity must also be corrected. Electrolyte imbalance (e.g. of potassium, magnesium and phosphate) and co-existing infection also require treatment. When patients are discharged, they can be given multivitamin preparations or thiamine to take at home.

The longer-term phase of alcohol withdrawal involves helping the patient to establish modified drinking behaviour, or abstinence, and concentrates on rehabilitation with appropriate management of any contributory factors (e.g. anxiety). Coping with everyday problems without alcohol plays an important part in the rehabilitation process.

Drugs may also be used in some cases to help patients abstain from alcohol, but should be accompanied by counselling and general supportive measures. Acamprosate is indicated to maintain abstinence in alcohol dependent patients by reducing the craving for alcohol (Anonymous, 1997a). It seems to affect the balance of neurotransmitter actions in the human brain in a similar way to alcohol itself, facilitating the actions of GABA and inhibiting the actions of some excitatory amino acid neurotransmitters. Acamprosate should be started as soon as the acute phase of withdrawal/detoxification has been completed. The drug does not interact with alcohol, so treatment should be maintained even if the patient does experience a minor relapse. Treatment is usually continued for one year.

Naltrexone is a long-acting opioid antagonist that, like acamprosate, seems to reduce craving for alcohol (Anonymous, 1997b). It appears to block the pleasurable effects of drinking, and can be given after detoxification to prevent a resumption of excessive alcohol intake.

Disulfiram is occasionally used to discourage alcohol consumption by producing an unpleasant reaction (e.g. facial flushing, tachycardia, and nausea and vomiting) if alcohol is consumed concomitantly. However, its use is gradually being abandoned.

The aim of the long-term phase is to help patients achieve lifestyle modifications that will allow them to cope with, or eliminate, the pressures responsible for their former drinking problem. Recreational activities, particularly those not related to alcohol consumption, are useful to establish modified drinking behaviour. It should be emphasised to patients and their families that relapses and setbacks, although sometimes frequent, do not imply an incurable state. Encouragement is essential for patients to have another attempt at stopping or reducing alcohol consumption. In some cases, specialist care may be necessary following several failed attempts, or if the risk of alcohol-related disease is increasing or social problems become more evident. Self-help groups and organisations (*see below*) concerned with the problems of excessive alcohol consumption are of value in helping patients modify their drinking behaviour. Such groups are staffed by people with extensive knowledge of the problems associated with excessive alcohol consumption, and who may formerly have had drinking problems themselves. Self-help groups should be recommended at an early stage to all people with suspected or identified alcohol dependence.

Promotion of sensible alcohol consumption

The prevention and control of excessive alcohol consumption by advocating total abstinence would not be acceptable to the majority of people and, in most cases, is not necessary. Promotion of sensible alcohol consumption is a more realistic goal. Health education should aim to make clear the relationship between alcohol consumption and the development of health and social problems, although it is recognised that, as this may not be sufficient in itself to reduce levels of consumption, additional methods may be necessary.

As illustrated above, factors influencing alcohol consumption and, more importantly, excessive alcohol consumption are wide-ranging and diverse. The WHO has identified the following areas that could be targeted to promote sensible alcohol consumption:

- increased availability of low-alcohol and alcohol-free drinks
- modifications in lifestyle
- health education (of both the public and the professions)
- pricing policies to increase the 'real' price (i.e. the price in relation to disposable income) of alcoholic drinks
- regulation of production
- reducing the availability (e.g. restrictive licensing laws)
- restrictions on advertising
- treatment and counselling.

Campaigns should be co-ordinated between all relevant agencies (e.g. government departments, the medical, nursing and pharmaceutical professions, voluntary organisations and health education authorities). There is wide regional variation in the services available: some authorities do not have a policy on alcohol consumption, and the burden is allowed to fall entirely on voluntary organisations. In the UK, government involvement in the promotion of sensible alcohol consumption is directed by the Ministerial Group on Alcohol Misuse, which recommends policy measures. Initiatives recommended by this Group include:

- alcohol education to form part of the national school curriculum
- the appointment of regional alcohol co-ordinators
- the exclusion of anyone who looks under 25 years of age from alcohol advertisements

- funding Alcohol Concern to aid local organisations dealing with excessive alcohol consumption
- reducing the ease with which convicted drink-drive offenders may regain their driving licences
- making the sale of alcohol to under-age children illegal, even if done unwittingly, combined with increased fines
- national 'Drinkwise' days to promote sensible drinking
- enquiries about alcohol consumption to form part of the general lifestyle enquiries made by health-care personnel.

Low-alcohol and alcohol-free drinks

The image of non-drinkers as being 'antisocial' is one of the main reasons for regular alcohol consumption (especially in young people). However, this stigma is gradually disappearing with the development and marketing of low-alcohol and alcohol-free drinks, and the increasing social acceptance of not drinking alcohol. Perversely, however, alcohol-free drinks are not necessarily any cheaper than alcoholic drinks and are not always widely available or encouraged. It is important that the current position is reversed, especially with respect to the young, who are particularly vulnerable to social pressures.

Adolescents, especially those at school, may not go out specifically to drink, but rather to meet friends. If alcohol is available in these situations, it is likely to be consumed. A change in social environment may have a greater influence on the drinking habits of young people than campaigns warning of health risks. Similarly, widespread promotion of low-alcohol and alcohol-free drinks to drivers could have a significant impact in reducing the number of alcohol-related road-traffic offences and accidents. Selecting appropriate drinks to avoid consuming excessive amounts of alcohol can be difficult because the labelling of low-alcohol and alcohol-free drinks can be confusing, and sometimes inaccurate. It is important to emphasise, therefore, that the label on all such products should be studied carefully to determine the alcohol content, which is usually stated as percentage alcohol by volume. However, in certain situations (e.g. in licensed premises or at parties), this may be difficult.

Drinks labelled as alcohol-free would be expected to have no alcohol in them. However, they may contain a small quantity of alcohol (less than 0.05% by volume) and would therefore not be suitable for people who avoid alcohol on religious or cultural grounds. De-alcoholised beverages would also be expected to contain no alcohol. However, not all the alcohol may be removed, and up to 0.5% alcohol by volume may be found.

Drinks labelled as low-alcohol represent the most confusing area. The term 'low' is taken to mean that the alcohol content is lower than in regular beverages. Generally, low-alcohol beers and lagers have an alcohol content of less than one-fifth of the regular beers or lagers (i.e. an alcohol content below 1% by volume). Wines of normal strength contain up to 14% alcohol by volume; low-alcohol wines may contain up to 5% alcohol by volume. This concentration of alcohol is higher than many regular beers and lagers, and if several glasses are consumed, may increase blood-alcohol concentrations above the legal limit for driving.

The terms 'reduced alcohol' and 'greatly reduced alcohol' have no specific relationship to the content of alcohol in the drink, and such beverages may contain substantial quantities of alcohol. The terms light or 'lite' commonly mean the same as low-alcohol. However, these terms are also used to mean a low calorie drink, which may have the same alcohol content as a regular alcoholic beverage.

The role of the pharmacist

Pharmacists have an important part to play in developing and enforcing local guidelines for treating alcohol withdrawal. Pharmacists can recommend that GPs consider prescribing thiamine and/or vitamin supplements to those with known alcohol dependency where compliance is likely. Pharmacists should discourage GPs from prescribing 'maintenance' doses of benzodiazepines or chlormethiazole following completion of an alcohol detoxification programme.

Pharmacists are experts on drug interactions and, therefore, familiar with the interactions between medicines and alcohol. This topic should be included in counselling on the appropriate use of medicines and when checking prescriptions for known alcoholics. A summary of potential drug-alcohol interactions is included in the BNF (Appendix 1). Further details on the importance or management of individual interactions can be obtained from a local Medicines Information Centre. In addition to alcohol, the pharmacist should also be alert to the fact that some people who consume excessive amounts of alcohol may also be drug abusers. The presence of alcohol-related disease (e.g. liver disease) should be borne in mind when considering drug contraindications.

Pharmacists can make an impact on reducing excessive alcohol consumption by becoming actively involved in national and local campaigns promoting sensible drinking. Individual pharmacists can have an even greater impact by giving advice, where appropriate, about sensible alcohol consumption. Use of available health education material is essential to complement the professional advice, and the pharmacist should also be aware of the self-help groups, support organisations and detoxification facilities available locally.

Talking to a patient or customer about their level of alcohol consumption may initially be difficult. It should be regarded in the same light as any other enquiries about lifestyle (e.g. smoking) and will soon become an established routine. To assess the individual risk attached to alcohol consumption, it is important to estimate a person's average weekly consumption. However, alcohol consumption is frequently underestimated, particularly by those who consume excessive amounts. It may be helpful to suggest that the patient keeps an 'alcohol diary' to record each alcoholic drink, noting the amount, time, place and situation (e.g. business, social or alone). There is little to be achieved from talking to people who are drunk, and it may be necessary to wait until a more appropriate time when the person is responsive.

Pharmacists should be alert to the possibility of specific symptoms being possible signs of alcohol-related disease or alcohol withdrawal (*see above*). Drinking and driving is a particularly serious social consequence of alcohol consumption. It should be emphasised that driving ability is significantly impaired by lower blood-alcohol concentrations than those set as the legal limit for driving. It is better to stress that alcohol should not be consumed at all if driving. It is also important to mention that some low-alcohol drinks contain a substantial amount of alcohol, and may in themselves cause an impairment of driving ability; some may even increase the blood-alcohol concentration above the legal limit for driving.

References

Anonymous (1997a). Acamprosate for alcohol dependence. *Drug Ther Bull* 35: 70–72.

Anonymous (1997b). Naltrexone: an option for alcohol-dependent patients? *Drugs Ther Perspect* 10: 5–8.

Further reading

See also the Further reading section of Chapter 7.

Anonymous (1998). How important are drug-alcohol interactions? *Drugs Ther Perspect* 11: 13–16.

Ashworth M, Gerada C (1997). Addiction and dependence II: Alcohol. *BMJ* 315: 358–360.

Cook C H C, Hallwood P M, Thomson A D (1998). B vitamin deficiency and neuropsychiatric syndromes in alcohol misuse. *Alcohol Alcohol* 33: 317–336.

Ferner R E (1998). Interactions between alcohol and drugs. *Adverse Drug React Bull* No. 189: 719–722.

Hall W, Zador D (1997). The alcohol withdrawal syndrome. *Lancet* 349: 1897–1900.

Hart C L, Smith G D, Hole D J, *et al.* (1999). Alcohol consumption and mortality from all causes, coronary heart disease, and stroke: results from a prospective cohort study of Scottish men with 21 years of follow up. *BMJ* 318: 1725–1729.

Harvey J (1995). Detecting the problem drinker. *Medicine* 47–50.

Hughes K, MacKintosh A M, Hastings G, *et al.* (1997).

Young people, alcohol, and designer drinks: quantitative and qualitative study. *BMJ* 314: 414–418.

Mayo-Smith M F (1997). Pharmacological management of alcohol withdrawal: a meta-analysis and evidence-based practice guideline. *JAMA* 278: 144–151.

Rimm E B, Klatsky A, Grobbee D, *et al.* (1996). Review of moderate alcohol consumption and reduced risk of coronary heart disease: is the effect due to beer, wine or spirits? *BMJ* 312: 731–736.

Sabroe S (1998). Alcohol and cancer. *BMJ* 317: 827.

Saitz R, Mayo-Smith M F, Roberts M S (1994). Individualized treatment for alcohol withdrawal: a randomized double-blind controlled trial. *JAMA* 272: 519–523.

Williams D, McBride A J (1998). The drug treatment of alcohol withdrawal symptoms: a systematic review. *Alcohol Alcohol* 33: 103–115.

Useful addresses

See also the Useful addresses section of Chapter 7.

Accept Services UK
724 Fulham Road
London SW6 5SE
Tel: 020 7371 7477

Al-Anon Family Groups including Alateen
61 Great Dover Street
London SE1 4YF
Tel: 020 7403 0888

Alcohol Concern
Waterbridge House
32–36 Loman Street
London SE1 0EE
Tel: 020 7928 7377

Alcoholics Anonymous (AA)
PO Box 1
Stonebow House
Stonebow
York YO1 7NJ
Tel: 01904 644026

7

Drug abuse

Simon Wills

The abuse of illicit, prescribed and over-the-counter (OTC) drugs has been a recurring problem throughout the twentieth century, and seems set to continue. The cost of drug abuse to society is difficult to determine because of the paucity of adequate data, but there can be little doubt that, in terms of serious health and social problems, the costs are substantial. The need to prevent, control and treat drug abuse and dependence has been given additional impetus by the spread of diseases, such as AIDS and hepatitis B and C, through the sharing of injection equipment by users of intravenous drugs. Attempts to eradicate drug abuse over the past century have not met with success, and many agencies now concentrate on counselling and education of users, or potential users, and harm minimisation, whilst offering a range of detoxification, substitution and support services, where appropriate.

The problems associated with the use of the social drugs tobacco and alcohol are covered in Chapters 5 and 6 respectively. The illicit use of ergogenic drugs by athletes is discussed in Chapter 8, Sport and Exercise.

There have been many attempts to define drug misuse or abuse. The terms 'misuse' and 'abuse' are often used interchangeably; the former is preferred in some quarters since it appears to be less judgemental. However, 'abuse' is still probably more widely used. It is difficult to provide a wholly accurate definition of drug abuse that covers all of the issues and criteria associated with it; but it is important to distinguish between abuse and dependence, which are quite separate issues. Abuse occurs before dependence is possible. Abuse has the following characteristics:

- the drug is taken for a non-medical purpose
- the desired effect is a psychoactive effect, altered body image or intoxication
- the drug may be taken once, occasionally or more often
- administration is often initiated or continued despite knowledge of potential or actual adverse effects.

In the UK, a 'problem drug user' has been succinctly defined by the Advisory Council on the Misuse of Drugs as 'a person who has physical, psychological, social or legal problems associated with drug abuse'. Problem drug use encompasses all levels and stages of drug abuse, and not only that which has resulted in drug dependence; it covers experimental use through to uncontrolled regular use. However, the definition of a 'problem' is subjective, and what constitutes a 'problem' to one person may well be 'no problem' to another.

Factors contributing to the commencement of drug abuse are wide-ranging, and no single cause can be identified as the most important. Drug abuse can be linked to the relief of unpleasant feelings and experiences, which may include anxiety, depression, lack of self-identity, frustration, diminished self-esteem and boredom; drugs may be used in these instances to provide pleasure, happiness or a means of escape. Peer pressure, curiosity, personality traits and social deprivation can be contributing factors, and increased availability is also associated with increased utilisation. An unstable family life, or problems with relationships, may be associated with abuse. Drug abusers are often stigmatised, which may perpetuate relationship problems as individuals often try to conceal their habits from family and friends because of social unacceptability. Disclosure of drug-related problems can lead to alienation.

Drug abuse is generally considered to be associated with younger people. Although experimentation does more commonly occur at a young age, and certain drugs are particularly abused by young people (e.g. volatile substances and 'Ecstasy'), drug abuse can occur at any age. Abuse is also more frequent in men than women, although the number of women using drugs is increasing.

The many potential adverse consequences of drug abuse include accidents, absenteeism, impoverishment, crime, acute or chronic side-effects, delinquency, marital problems, suicide, unemployment, homelessness and infection.

The Misuse of Drugs Act was passed in 1971 to provide control over illicit drug abuse. The Misuse of Drugs Regulations 1985 were also introduced under the Act. The legislation is detailed in *Medicines, Ethics, and Practice: a Guide for Pharmacists*, issued by the Royal Pharmaceutical Society of Great Britain regularly to all UK pharmacists (RSPGB, 2000). The Advisory Council on the Misuse of Drugs was set up under the Act, and its function is to advise the government on measures to prevent and deal with problems arising from the abuse of drugs.

Drug dependence

The World Health Organization (WHO) recommended use of the term 'drug dependence' in preference to the more pejorative 'addiction', and offered the following definition:

> a state, psychic and sometimes also physical, resulting from the interaction between a living organism and a drug, characterised by behavioural and other responses that always include the compulsion to take the drug on a continuous or periodic basis in order to experience its psychic effects, and sometimes to avoid the discomfort of its absence. Tolerance may or may not be present. A person may be dependent on more than one drug.

Physical dependence

Drug abuse can lead to a state of physical dependence, which is typically characterised by the development of neuroadaptation and tolerance, as well as withdrawal symptoms on stopping use. Neuroadaptation is the ability of nerves to adapt at a cellular level to the presence of a drug; it is thought to be at least partly responsible for the development of tolerance and the characteristic withdrawal symptoms on stopping drug use.

Drug tolerance may be defined as a state of decreased responsiveness to the pharmacological actions of a drug as a result of previous use of that drug, or a related drug. The central nervous system responds to a progressively smaller extent when the drug is given repeatedly; higher doses are then required to produce the same effect. Tolerance can range from a small reduction in subjective effects to complete absence of the pharmacological action of a drug. It can develop slowly or rapidly; rapid development of tolerance is sometimes called acute tolerance or tachyphylaxis. The use of a drug that produces physical dependence often confers cross-tolerance to pharmacologically-related drugs. It is important to realise that, just because tolerance has developed, it does not mean that the dose will necessarily be increased. Long-term users of caffeinated drinks or prescribed benzodiazepines, for example, do not in most cases continue to escalate their intake, despite tolerance to the agent's effects. At street level, tolerance may prompt the desire to take bigger doses, but intake is often limited by the individual's ability to pay or otherwise obtain supplies.

Withdrawal symptoms, or abstinence syndromes, typically occur when drug use is stopped in an individual who has developed physical dependence. However, these reactions can also occur if the dose is suddenly decreased to a significant extent, or if an antagonist is given. Withdrawal symptoms are characteristic for different groups of chemically-related drugs; they also tend to be opposite to the normal effects that the drug produces in the user. For example, a stimulant drug such as amphetamine tends to produce depressant withdrawal symptoms (e.g. lethargy and depression); a CNS depressant (e.g. temazepam) produces excitatory withdrawal symptoms (e.g. anxiety and sleeplessness). Withdrawal symptoms can be terminated by re-administration of the drug (or a chemically-related one). In some cases, withdrawal can be ameliorated by administering drugs that provide a certain amount of symptomatic relief, allowing the individual to cope more easily.

The relationship between tolerance, neuroadaptation and withdrawal symptoms is complex and not fully understood. Withdrawal symptoms can occur in the presence of little, if any, apparent tolerance, particularly in the early stages of dependence. Conversely, profound tolerance can occur in the absence of withdrawal symptoms: there is always a proportion of chronic users of any dependence-producing drug who do not experience withdrawal reactions.

Psychological dependence

This can be associated with almost all drugs of abuse. It is a feeling that the drug is necessary to enable the normal functioning of an individual, or is essential to enable the individual to reach a certain higher level of functioning that is desirable. Learned behaviour and personality characteristics are two of a wide range of psychological factors that contribute to the development and maintenance of drug dependence. Learned behaviour influences the further use of a drug for its desirable effects following initial use; this process is termed positive reinforcement, where the pleasant effects increase the likelihood of further use of the drug. At the same time, the development of withdrawal symptoms acts as negative reinforcement, being the unpleasant reaction which happens if the drug is not taken. Learned behaviour can also be related to the environment. Triggers which initiate craving (e.g. the sight of injecting equipment or friends who use drugs) act as environmental reminders of drug use, and thus as reinforcers. Personality characteristics are involved in the development and maintenance of drug dependence, although there is not an identifiable 'dependence personality'. After an initial exposure, some individuals may feel a need to use drugs as a response to adverse circumstances.

Social factors

The sense of identity associated with being an 'addict' or 'junkie' may contribute to personal acceptance and identification as part of the 'drug scene'. In this environment, drug dependence may be reinforced as a result of common experiences and a shared way of living. The daily acquisition and administration of drugs becomes a part of everyday life. The self-image of users is also important: a person who views their own drug use as a life-long, intractable dependence is more likely to maintain the habit.

Management of drug dependence

There are two basic pharmacological options in managing drug dependence acutely: substitution therapy, with a prescribed alternative to a street drug (e.g. methadone for heroin users); or medicated drug withdrawal (detoxification). In addition, a variety of drugs may be needed to treat or prevent withdrawal symptoms. The pharmacological options for management of drug dependence are described, as appropriate, under each drug or group of drugs below (*see* Drugs of abuse *below*).

Supportive therapy and counselling are essential at all stages when treating drug dependence, and should be introduced as early as possible. Self-help and community groups may provide useful assistance and advice in the management of drug dependence; some of these are listed below (*see* Useful addresses *below*).

Routes of administration and associated adverse effects

Drugs are abused by three main methods: inhalation, injection and oral ingestion. The route of administration can determine the type and severity of medical complications associated with drug abuse, which can also be related to the presence of adulterants. Additionally, the route of administration may influence the risk of dependence.

Inhalation

Inhalation of a drug enables absorption from the respiratory tract, and this can be almost as rapid as from intravenous injection. Inhalation takes place in one of three ways: by smoking, vaporisation or nasal inhalation of powder. Smoking requires combustion of the drug or a carrier substance (often tobacco), and can cause inflammation of the lung tissue and reduced lung function. Forced inhalation of drugs is associated with the development of pneumothorax, pneumomediastinum and pneumopericardium. Drugs that are commonly smoked include cannabis and heroin.

Vaporisation requires a source of heat to turn the drug into a vapour which can be inhaled: crack cocaine and heroin are abused in this way. Some drugs are so volatile that vaporisation occurs at room temperature (e.g. alkyl nitrites and many solvents).

Intranasal inhalation of a dry powder ('snorting') may cause irritation of the highly vascular nasal mucosa. Hyperaemia, rhinorrhoea and sinusitis may result. Prolonged intranasal administration of cocaine may cause necrosis and perforation of the nasal septum. Amphetamine powder can also be inhaled nasally in this manner.

Injection

Parenteral administration of a drug may be by the intravenous route ('mainlining', 'shooting up'), subcutaneous injection ('skin popping') or intramuscular injection. Intravenous injection enables rapid plasma-drug concentrations to be achieved, often resulting in a sudden feeling of intense euphoria, known variously as a 'rush', 'buzz', 'high' or 'flash'. This method of administration is associated with the widest range of adverse effects. Injection requires that the various powders, tablets or capsules supplied be converted into a solution and then filtered to remove insoluble particles.

Infected (hot) abscesses occur following injection because sterile methods of administration are not possible: even when clean needles and syringes are used, the street drug itself is not sterile. In addition, the injector is likely to use tap-water and a homemade filter, neither of which is sterile. In the case of heroin injection, an acidic environment is often created within the drug suspension to aid dissolution; this is provided by adding non-sterile acids (e.g. citric acid powder). Furthermore, most injectors do not sterilise the surface of the skin prior to injecting through it. A range of other infections can occur as a result of injecting street drugs. These may result directly from the injection, or they may develop later from an infected abscess. Potential infections include skin infections, endocarditis, septicaemia and joint or bone infections. Bacteria or fungi may be responsible, and often the causative organisms are atypical, thus alerting the clinician to the possibility of drug abuse. Finally, micro-organisms may be introduced into the body as a result of using shared needles and syringes which have become contaminated with the blood of infected users. Hepatitis B or C and human immunodeficiency virus (HIV) infection are the most serious infections which can be spread in this way.

Tissue reactions may result from the irritant properties of some drugs, to adulterants in illicit substances, or excipients in tablets and capsules that have been prepared for injection. Local irritation and trauma on intravenous injection can lead to thrombophlebitis; if a vein is missed on injection, sterile abscesses may form. Inadvertent injection into an artery can cause vasospasm and lead to gangrene of the tissues supplied by the artery (e.g. the fingers or leg). Unintentional injection into nerves can cause paraesthesia or hyperaesthesia; paralysis may also occur.

Subcutaneous administration may cause chronic suppurating skin infections at the injection sites, which can lead to amyloidosis and nephropathy. Only anabolic steroids are given by the intra-muscular route because they are mostly formulated in oil.

Injection of poorly soluble adulterants or excipients may cause adverse reactions, especially granulomatous lesions in organs such as the lungs and kidneys. A wide range of pharmacologically active adulterants are used, including quinine, strychnine, local anaesthetics, ketamine and other street drugs. These all have their own potential to cause adverse effects.

Oral ingestion

Oral administration is a potential option for most street drugs. It is convenient, discrete and requires no special equipment. Despite this, it is not very popular because the desired effects develop much more slowly than when given by other routes, and peak concentrations also are lower. This gives a 'blunted' effect compared with injection or inhalation. The only street drugs usually given by the oral route are LSD and 'Ecstasy'. However, many prescription and OTC drugs which are abused are taken orally.

Drugs of abuse

The range of drugs that have abuse potential is extensive. It is impossible to discuss all of them in detail, and only those commonly encountered or those causing the most public concern are discussed below. Information on the potential adverse effects of the various drugs upon human pregnancy are summarised in Table 7.1, but the reader should refer to more detailed sources for information on this subject.

Alkyl nitrites

Alkyl nitrites are not used therapeutically, although amyl nitrite was formerly used as a vasodilator in angina pectoris and in the emergency treatment of cyanide poisoning. In 1996, the Royal Pharmaceutical Society of Great Britain successfully prosecuted a supplier of alkyl nitrites for breaching the Medicines Act 1968, as alkyl

Table 7.1 'Street' drugs in pregnancy

Drug	Effects on foetus	Neonatal withdrawal reactions reported
Amphetamines and 'Ecstasy'	Ecstasy is neurotoxic in adults and may be in babies too, but this has not been studied. Some evidence for an increase in foetal heart disease, but little data. Microcephaly, prematurity and intra-uterine growth retardation.[a]	Possible
Cannabis	Probably does not cause malformations. Weak link to childhood cancer and to delayed maturation of CNS, but not proven.	No
Cocaine	Vascular brain damage to the foetus is rare, lack of data to support a link with other malformations. May cause spontaneous abortion, prematurity and intra-uterine growth retardation.[a]	No
LSD	Generally assumed not to be teratogenic, but has been inadequately studied to justify this optimism.	No
Opioids (heroin and methadone)	Probably do not cause malformations. Intra-uterine growth retardation and prematurity.[a]	Yes – common
VSA	Possible links to facial deformities, spontaneous abortion, low birth weight and prematurity needing further study.[a]	Possible

[a] Links between most street drugs and prematurity or intra-uterine growth retardation may simply reflect the impact of the mother's lifestyle upon pregnancy. Several studies, involving pregnant cocaine-using women particularly, have shown that if adequate antenatal care is given to users, their babies are indistinguishable from controls in terms of size.

nitrites are classed as medicinal products and should not be freely on sale to the public. This test case does not seem to have made much difference to the wide availability of these substances in pubs and clubs. Abuse, possession or supply of alkyl nitrites does not contravene the UK Misuse of Drugs Act.

Identification and street names

Amyl nitrite and butyl nitrite are usually referred to at street level as 'poppers'. They are marketed in small glass bottles under a variety of brand names such as 'Rush', 'Rave' and 'Ram'. The alkyl nitrites are colourless or clear yellow, volatile liquids with a characteristic smell of 'old socks'.

Method of administration

The liquid vapour is inhaled rapidly through the nose, usually directly from the bottle.

Actions

Nitrite inhalants are rapidly absorbed following inhalation to produce a sudden, but short-lived euphoria known as a 'rush'. Other effects include smooth-muscle relaxation and vasodilatation. The nitrite inhalants are used to produce altered consciousness and for their stimulant action. However, their use as a 'sex aid' is predominant, especially by male homosexuals. Purportedly, nitrites improve sexual performance and enjoyment by heightening libido, prolonging erection, relaxing rectal smooth muscle and dilating the anal sphincter.

Side-effects

Common, acute side-effects include headaches, flushing, dizziness, hypotension and reflex tachycardia. Nitrite inhalants have also been reported to cause syncope, acute psychosis, raised intraocular pressure, transient hemiparesis, methaemoglobinaemia and coma. Nitrites seem to have adverse effects upon the mammalian immune response, and it has been suggested that the use of them could facilitate the development of opportunistic infections and Kaposi's sarcoma in homosexual men with HIV infection. However, evidence to support this is inconclusive.

It is particularly important that patients taking sildenafil (Viagra®) do not use alkyl nitrites. Severe life-threatening hypotension could occur if the two drugs are taken concomitantly.

Dependence and management

Dependence has not been described, probably on account of the irregular pattern of use by most adherents, and the very short duration of action.

Amphetamines, 'Ecstasy' and related stimulants

Amphetamine, a synthetic compound, was first available for medicinal use in the 1930s as a nasal vasoconstrictor. Its stimulant and appetite suppressant properties were realised, and amphetamine was used for a range of disorders (e.g. depression, obesity, impotence and migraine). During the 1960s, use of amphetamines became restricted to obesity and depressive disorders. Medicinal use is now largely restricted to narcolepsy and hyperactivity in children, under specialist care only.

As a result of the extensive availability of amphetamines, abuse was inevitable and became widespread. Amphetamines were used to enhance energy, concentration, and mental and physical performance. Sportsmen and sportswomen began to use amphetamines to improve athletic performance, although this is now prohibited (*see* Chapter 8, Participation in sports and exercise).

In the late 1960s, there was widespread abuse of intravenous methamphetamine. Voluntary restrictions were imposed by prescribers, and supplies of methamphetamine were withdrawn by manufacturers, but abuse then switched predominantly to amphetamine sulphate. The Pharmaceutical Society of Great Britain advised pharmacists not to supply amphetamine sulphate as some doctors, wittingly or otherwise, were still writing prescriptions. This action was widely approved and helped stem abuse of amphetamine sulphate. As the awareness of the abuse of amphetamines grew, voluntary restrictions were placed on prescribing and the availability of amphetamines was drastically reduced.

Identification and street names

These drugs include:

- amphetamine ('whizz', 'speed', 'uppers')
- methamphetamine ('meth', 'crank', 'crystal', 'ice')
- 3,4-methylenedioxymethamphetamine ('Ecstasy', 'E', 'XTC', 'MDMA', 'Adam') and related drugs ('eve', 'MDA', 'DOM')
- prescription amphetamines (e.g. dexamphetamine, methylphenidate)
- OTC sympathomimetics (*see* OTC medicines *below*).

Methods of administration

- amphetamine is usually inhaled nasally or injected; it is occasionally smoked
- methamphetamine is usually vaporised and then inhaled
- Ecstasy is taken orally
- methylphenidate tablets are usually crushed and injected when abused
- OTC sympathomimetics are usually taken orally, but some forms can be injected.

Actions

Amphetamines and related stimulants are sympathomimetics and have similar effects: they stimulate the central and peripheral nervous systems. Amphetamines produce CNS stimulation by promoting the release of the neurotransmitters dopamine, noradrenaline and serotonin (5-HT). In addition, amphetamines inhibit neuronal re-uptake of these neurotransmitters and some may act as direct agonists on catecholamine receptors. As a group, they differ mainly in their potency, although some preferentially affect certain neurotransmitters (e.g. Ecstasy seems to exert a wider range of serotonergic actions in the CNS). The text which follows concentrates mainly on amphetamine, but the effects of related stimulants can be taken to be largely the same, although they may be less intense. Any significant differences between the various derivatives are discussed.

At low doses, amphetamines cause increased alertness, prevention of fatigue, mood elevation (including increased self-confidence and concentration), elation and euphoria; there is also increased activity and talkativeness. The need for food and sleep is postponed until use is discontinued. Physical performance is improved as a result of decreased fatigue. Amphetamines may be taken to reduce fatigue and improve social performance. High doses may make the user feel that they have infinite power.

Cravings for the intravenous amphetamine 'rush' may lead to repeated administration to sustain the effects; this is commonly referred to as a 'speed run'. Intravenous administration may continue for up to a week, until supplies are exhausted or adverse effects of amphetamines develop (e.g. excessive fatigue and paranoia). Intravenous amphetamines may be used in combination with other drugs. Ecstasy, for example, is commonly taken with LSD, alkyl nitrites or amphetamine. Nasal inhalation induces a similar amphetamine 'rush' to intravenous administration, but is less intense.

Ecstasy is nearly always taken orally, and in intermittent fashion. It is intimately associated with various popular youth music and dance cultures, and is typically taken over the weekend at large private parties and in night clubs. Ecstasy provides stamina, which facilitates continuous dancing for long periods. It may also enhance the appreciation of music, but it is mainly taken for its emotional and 'spiritual' effects. The drug seems to promote emotional closeness, personal insight and feelings of tranquility.

Side-effects

Amphetamines can produce a range of side-effects. The onset of drug action is often heralded by a series of characteristic 'fight or flight' effects, typical of sympathomimetics. These include tachycardia, sweating and headache. Other acute symptoms include restlessness, dizziness, tremor, irritability, insomnia, fever, confusion, panic attacks and anxiety. An amphetamine psychosis has been described, which may be difficult to distinguish from acute paranoid schizophrenia.

Auditory and visual hallucinations may occur, and feelings of persecution may be present. Recovery is usually attained within a few days, although occasionally a chronic condition develops. There is also a risk of violent behaviour. The doses that induce particular side-effects are not predictable. Toxic effects on the cardiovascular system include palpitations, cardiac arrhythmias, anginal pain, hypotension or hypertension, and circulatory collapse. Effects on the gastro-intestinal system include dry mouth, anorexia, nausea and vomiting, diarrhoea and abdominal cramps. Excessive doses can produce convulsions, coma or death.

Following a 'speed run', users may sleep for 24 to 48 hours and, on waking, extreme hunger is experienced. This may be followed by severe depression and fatigue (the 'crash' or 'coming down'), leading to further amphetamine use.

Ecstasy has been particularly associated with a range of side-effects related to body temperature and fluid balance. In the hot environment of a party or night club, prolonged dancing causes thirst and profuse sweating with concomitant loss of electrolytes. If the lost fluid is replaced by water or other low-electrolyte drinks, this can result in hyponatraemia. Ecstasy can also stimulate thirst and promote fluid retention in the kidney. In extreme cases, hyponatraemia may result in irreversible brain damage and coma, and deaths attributed to this have been reported in the media and medical literature. Ecstasy may also cause death or serious harm by another mechanism: intensive exercise in the presence of Ecstasy may sometimes trigger hyperpyrexia, a condition where the body temperature rises uncontrollably to a dangerously high level. This may cause convulsions, or be associated with rhabdomyolysis, in which skeletal muscle breaks down into its constituent proteins. Hyperpyrexia and rhabdomyolysis can combine to cause disseminated intravascular coagulation, kidney failure and acidosis.

Perhaps the most serious potential side-effect of Ecstasy is, as yet, incompletely understood. Animal studies have demonstrated that the drug destroys serotonin-containing neurones in the CNS. This occurs in primates as well as other mammals, and although the nerves do grow back, the growth is incomplete and neural connections are broken. Human studies have demonstrated that the turnover of serotonin metabolites in the cerebrospinal fluid of Ecstasy users is much higher than normal, and that the density of serotonin binding-sites in the brain is much reduced. This suggests that the changes observed in animals may also occur in humans. The consequences of this are unknown, but it has been postulated that the damage may ultimately lead to memory impairment, anxiety, depression or other emotional disorders.

Dependence and management

Prolonged use of amphetamines may cause psychological dependence, characterised by the compulsion to seek further supplies of the drug. However, amphetamine use can be occasional and may not always lead to dependence. Ecstasy is an example of an illicit amphetamine derivative that is nearly always taken episodically, so that dependence and withdrawal are unlikely to develop.

Tolerance to the euphoric and anorexic effects of amphetamines can occur; cross-tolerance between amphetamines and related stimulants, including cocaine, is also exhibited. However, tolerance does not develop to the psychotic adverse effects of amphetamines, and a toxic psychosis may occur after weeks or months of continued use. This usually requires inpatient treatment under the care of a psychiatrist.

Withdrawal symptoms following amphetamine use include apathy, depression, craving and anxiety. Withdrawal, which may continue for some weeks, may be severe in the early stages. Other symptoms include excessive hunger and eating, suicidal thoughts secondary to depression and prolonged sleep.

In some areas of the UK, dexamphetamine has been prescribed as a substitution therapy, to reduce withdrawal symptoms and craving and to aid amphetamine users to discontinue the drug. It is not envisaged that dexamphetamine should be prescribed as a form of long-term maintenance therapy. The published data available on this practice are very limited, and the UK Department of Health currently recommends that only experienced specialists should prescribe dexamphetamine. Most chronic amphetamine users are not prescribed dexamphetamine, but may need to be prescribed antidepressants.

Antimuscarinic drugs

Antimuscarinic drugs are not generally available at street level, but can be abused by patients who have been prescribed them for a legitimate medical indication. They are widely used in the treatment of parkinsonism and to reduce the extrapyramidal side-effects of antipsychotic drugs.

Identification

All drugs with antimuscarinic actions are potentially abusable. These drugs include:

- procyclidine, orphenadrine, benzhexol, benztropine
- hyoscine, atropine and plants containing them (e.g. *Datura stramonium*)
- drugs with antimuscarinic side-effects (e.g. amitriptyline, some antihistamines).

Method of administration

Almost always oral, although injection of some individual drugs with antimuscarinic properties may be locally prevalent (e.g. cyclizine).

Actions

Antimuscarinic drugs commonly produce euphoria and, in some instances, hallucinations and disorientation. Other effects described by users include relaxation, a sense of well-being and increased sociability. The stimulant properties of antimuscarinic drugs may result in individuals feeling more energetic. It is known that some illicit drugs (e.g. cannabis and opioids) act in part by decreasing cholinergic activity.

The extent of antimuscarinic drug abuse is not known, although it appears to be most common in patients being treated with antipsychotic drugs, who may go to great lengths to secure additional supplies of medication. Patients on antipsychotic therapy may fake extrapyramidal symptoms, or their intensity, in order to obtain antimuscarinic drugs. Requests for prescriptions or supplies to replace 'lost drugs' or drug supplies running out more quickly than expected may also be an indication of abuse. Patients may also be reluctant to stop antimuscarinic drug treatment or have the dose reduced. In some cases, patients may stop taking their antipsychotic medication and increase the dose of antimuscarinic drug, in order to achieve a feeling of euphoria and well-being.

Side-effects

Blurred vision, flushing, tachycardia and memory impairment (especially affecting recent memory) may occur following antimuscarinic drug abuse. The use of high doses of antimuscarinic drugs may result in the development of a toxic psychosis. It is characterised by profound visual hallucinations, illusions, distortion of the sense of time, dehydration, excessive thirst and feelings of persecution.

Dependence and management

Physical and psychological dependence can occur with antimuscarinic drugs. Tolerance develops, with the need to increase doses to achieve a similar degree of mood elevation. Withdrawal symptoms have been described occasionally and include myalgia, profuse sweating, gastro-intestinal disturbances, anxiety and sleep disturbance; rebound extrapyramidal effects may occur in patients receiving antipsychotic drugs, or motor function deterioration in patients with parkinsonism.

If termination of their prescribing is deemed necessary, withdrawal in patients who are abusing antimuscarinic drugs should ideally be gradual, although the rate of withdrawal is dependent on individual circumstances. Supportive therapy may be beneficial.

Barbiturates

Barbiturates were widely prescribed until the 1960s, when their dependence potential and the often fatal consequences of overdosage were fully realised. Barbiturates have a narrow therapeutic margin, beyond which life-threatening toxicity may occur. They have been involved in many overdose fatalities. However, the introduction of benzodiazepines in the early 1960s provided a safer alternative and the prescribing and abuse of barbiturates has declined dramatically.

Identification and street names

These drugs include: phenobarbitone, amylobarbitone (Amytal®), quinalbarbitone (Seconal®), butobarbitone (Soneryl®), amylobarbitone with quinalbarbitone (Tuinal®). When they were used more widely at street level, a variety of slang names were popular, including 'barbs', 'downers' and 'sleepers'.

Methods of administration

Barbiturates are usually taken orally, especially by those dependent on them as a result of prescription. However, use by injection is also encountered, especially in those who inject other drugs. Injection of barbiturate solutions poses particular problems as a result of their alkalinity, which renders them highly irritant to tissues.

Actions

Barbiturates augment the action of the inhibitory CNS neurotransmitter gamma-aminobutyric acid (GABA), and are thus general CNS depressants. They have anxiolytic and sedative properties; memory and thought impairment may also occur.

Side-effects

At higher doses, intoxication produces slurred speech, unsteady gait and progressive lack of muscle co-ordination. Other possible effects include dizziness, ataxia, nystagmus and headache; paradoxically, excitement and confusion may also arise. Toxic doses result in CNS and respiratory depression. Hypothermia may occur, with fever on recovery. Cardiorespiratory collapse is the commonest cause of death following overdose. A hangover effect can occur with long-acting barbiturates, and is similar to that following alcohol use.

Dependence and management

Barbiturates can induce both physical and psychological dependence. Tolerance develops rapidly because of the induction of liver microsomal enzymes, which increases the rate of barbiturate metabolism. However, tolerance to the sedative effects tends to develop more rapidly compared with depressant actions on vital centres, and this increases the possibility of serious toxicity as doses are increased. Cross-tolerance between the barbiturates, benzodiazepines and alcohol may be exhibited.

Withdrawal symptoms associated with abrupt cessation of barbiturate use are similar to those experienced with benzodiazepine use (*see below*), although the symptoms and course of events may be more severe and intense.

Ideally, withdrawal from barbiturates should be managed under medical supervision, although this may not always be possible. A long-acting barbiturate, usually phenobarbitone, is substituted for the abused drug and a reducing regimen instigated.

Benzodiazepines

Benzodiazepines were developed in the early 1960s as a safer alternative to barbiturates, and were initially claimed to have little or no abuse or dependence potential. However, within a decade it was realised that indiscriminate prescribing had created very large numbers of dependent patients. The UK Committee on Safety of Medicines (CSM) issued the following advice on the prescribing of benzodiazepines:

- benzodiazepines are indicated for the short-term relief (two to four weeks only) of anxiety that is severe, disabling, or subjecting the individual to unacceptable distress, occurring alone or in association with insomnia or short-term psychosomatic, organic or psychotic illness
- the use of benzodiazepines to treat short-term 'mild' anxiety is inappropriate and unsuitable
- benzodiazepines should be used to treat insomnia only when it is severe, disabling, or subjecting the individual to extreme distress.

Additional advice to augment the CSM advice includes:

- non-drug alternatives should be tried first
- all new patients should be warned of the potential for dependence
- for anxiety or insomnia, most patients should be encouraged to take benzodiazepines 'when required', and not feel that these drugs must be taken every day
- prescriptions should be reviewed regularly and discontinued as soon as possible.

The Council of the RPSGB recommends that pharmacists should take every opportunity to discuss any problems they encounter in the use of benzodiazepines with the medical practitioner concerned. Taking into account the CSM guidelines, pharmacists are advised to counsel patients who are receiving prescriptions for benzodiazepines where, on the evidence available, it is considered appropriate to do so.

More recently, as the number of patients dependent on prescribed benzodiazepines has fallen, the number of individuals abusing them at street level has increased markedly. Abuse at street level is thought to be created almost entirely via diversion of legitimate medical supplies of benzodiazepines. The amounts reaching the street might be reduced by doctors' practices adopting policies which include:

- avoiding prescription for those with a history of drug abuse
- not prescribing benzodiazepines to temporary residents and being careful about prescribing to patients that are new to a practice
- documenting evidence of benzodiazepine abuse so that other prescribers will be aware of the problem
- prescribing non-benzodiazepine alternatives where abuse is suspected
- non-abusers may sell their medication on the street, so all prescriptions must be regularly reviewed.

Abuse of temazepam caused such concern in the UK that liquid and gel-filled capsules were withdrawn from the market, and temazepam itself was re-scheduled from Schedule 4 to Schedule 3 under the Misuse of Drugs Regulations in 1996.

Identification

All benzodiazepines are potentially abusable, including: temazepam, diazepam (Valium®), lorazepam (Ativan®), chlordiazepoxide (Librium®), nitrazepam (Mogadon®), flunitrazepam (Rohypnol®).

Methods of administration

Benzodiazepine dependents take these drugs orally. Those who abuse them at street level often inject ground-up tablets or capsule contents in water. Some abusers take benzodiazepines orally.

Actions

The benzodiazepines are used therapeutically for their anxiolytic, hypnotic, anticonvulsant and muscle relaxant properties. Like barbiturates, they work by augmenting the action of the neurotransmitter GABA.

Benzodiazepine abuse may be associated with concurrent use of other drugs, especially opioids. Benzodiazepines are sometimes used at street level to reduce the effects of opioid withdrawal and, in some cases, to relieve stress and emotional disturbances. The effects of intravenous benzodiazepines are described by drug users as exhilarating, and include excitement and talkativeness; aggression, hostility and anti-social behaviour may also occur.

Mention should be made of the use of flunitrazepam for so-called 'date rape'. This drug has reportedly been used to spike women's drinks by men, mainly in the USA. The sedation caused, coupled with benzodiazepines' amnesic effects, enabled perpetrators to have sexual intercourse with affected women against their will. In theory, given the right circumstances, any one of the benzodiazepines might be put to a similar use. The Rohypnol® brand of flunitrazepam has now been reformulated so that a blue dye is released when attempts are made to dissolve the tablet in a drink.

Side-effects

Side-effects of benzodiazepines include sedation, amnesia, drowsiness, lightheadedness, confusion and ataxia. Other reported side-effects include headache, vertigo, hypotension and gastro-intestinal disturbances. Benzodiazepines may also cause paradoxical effects, including increased anxiety and perceptual disorders. Long-term benzodiazepine administration may impair psychomotor function and cognition. Ataxia and confusion, especially in the elderly, may result in falls and accidents.

Of the benzodiazepines, temazepam is most likely to be injected by abusers, but all commonly used benzodiazepines can be and are injected. Temazepam can be irritant on injection, and, apart from the general problems associated with injecting an oral preparation (*see* Routes of administration and associated adverse effects *above*), injection can also be associated with blackouts.

Dependence and management

Benzodiazepine dependence commonly occurs as a result of inappropriate prescribing. All health authorities, NHS Trusts and Primary Care Groups should work to an agreed set of prescribing guidelines for benzodiazepines. Long-term use of benzodiazepines is associated with dependence, and withdrawal symptoms develop in about one-third of prescribed users. Long-term users are predominantly women, and there may be associated physical illness, depression or history of other psychoactive drug use. The elderly are also more susceptible to the side-effects and long-term consequences of benzodiazepine use.

Withdrawal symptoms associated with discontinuation of benzodiazepine use may occur following as little as four to six weeks' treatment. Therefore, monthly repeat prescriptions are usually inappropriate and put patients at risk of developing dependence. Dependence on benzodiazepines commonly consists of both psychological and physical dependence. It is also believed that benzodiazepines are no longer effective for the treatment of anxiety or insomnia after only a few weeks continued use: intermittent short courses are preferred.

Withdrawal symptoms associated with abrupt discontinuation of benzodiazepines include insomnia, anxiety, confusion, tremor, convulsions and delirium. Other symptoms include muscle spasm, psychosis and gastro-intestinal upset. The symptoms are of varying intensity, but are generally more severe and begin more quickly with short-acting benzodiazepines (e.g. lorazepam) than long-acting benzodiazepines.

Substitution with diazepam is the usual first step in the management of benzodiazepine withdrawal. Diazepam is chosen because its very long half-life tends to make withdrawal less intense and more tolerable. A reducing regimen is then agreed with the user. Sometimes, a fixed dosage reduction at agreed intervals is used (e.g. dose reduction by one-eighth every two weeks). Alternatively, patients can negotiate size and frequency of dosage reductions with the prescriber, or be given control over their own detoxification, if sufficiently motivated. In these situations, patients allow themselves to become 'comfortable' at a reduced dose before initiating a further reduction. The precise schedule will depend upon individual circumstances. The time required for withdrawal can vary from a few weeks to several months, depending on the dose, the duration of benzodiazepine use and the patient's desire to stop. Some withdrawal symptoms may persist for months. Supportive therapy and counselling are helpful; the willingness of the patient to discontinue benzodiazepine use is essential.

Cannabis

Cannabis (Indian hemp) is derived from the shrub, *Cannabis sativa*. The plant grows in hot, dry conditions; suitable climates exist mainly outside Europe, and major supplies originate from the West Indies, India, Pakistan, Afghanistan, the Middle East, the Far East, Africa and parts of North and South America. Cannabis consists of male and female plants, both of which contain a group of compounds known as cannabinoids. A series of cannabinoids (over 60) have been isolated from the plant. The one responsible for most of the psychoactive effects is delta-9-tetrahydrocannabinol (THC), which is found in all parts of the plant except the seeds; the highest concentration of THC is found in the flowering shoots of the female plant. The THC content is variable and depends on the conditions and place of growth, and storage; cannabis plants grown in natural sunlight in the UK have a low THC content as a result of an unfavourable climate. However, indoors, growers may go to great lengths to provide a suitable climate artificially.

The large-scale use of cannabis has, for many years, fuelled a campaign to legalise its use in the UK, on which the debate is continuing. Some of the arguments for legalisation of cannabis use are:

- moderate use is not harmful
- far more dangerous substances (e.g. alcohol and tobacco) are legal
- costs of not legalising cannabis use (e.g. police and court time) exceed those of legalising use
- current laws are openly flouted
- an individual should have the freedom to use cannabis if he or she wishes
- legalising its use will not cause an increase in the number of users.

Some of the arguments against legalisation of cannabis use are:

- legalisation of cannabis will convey a negative message with respect to drug abuse generally
- cannabis use may proceed to abuse of other drugs
- social and health problems associated with cannabis use (e.g. crime, promiscuity, effects on driving and psychosis) preclude legalisation
- cannabis use is associated with anti-establishment and anti-society culture
- the effects of more widespread use of cannabis are unknown
- legalisation runs counter to society's traditional protective role.

It would appear that only a minority of cannabis users go on to use other drugs, and the presence of particular personality traits is more likely to predispose users to sequential drug use.

Identification and street names

A wide variety of names are used on the street. Some of the most popular names for the herb include 'grass', 'dope', 'weed', 'blow', 'bhang', 'pot', 'ganja', 'puff', 'soap', 'bud' and 'kif'. The resin is usually known as 'hash', but is also known by most if not all of the names that are applied to the herb. Cigarettes containing cannabis are usually known as 'joints', 'reefers' or 'spliffs'.

Although a range of cannabis preparations exist, there are three main forms of cannabis:

- herbal cannabis (marijuana), which consists of the dried leaves and flowering tops of cannabis plants. The concentration of THC, the principal psychoactive ingredient, is typically 0.5–2.5%
- cannabis resin (hashish): the resin extracted from the flowering tops and leaves; the concentration of THC may be up to 10%
- cannabis oil (hash oil): a liquid extract of cannabis resin having a high THC content (up to 60%).

Cannabis herb is usually obtained as the dried plant, or it may be compressed into blocks. Compressed herb commonly includes the whole plant; female plants represent the better quality product. Cannabis resin varies in its appearance, depending on the country of origin. The resin is commonly formed into blocks, sticks or cakes, which may be soft and pliable or hard and dry, crumbling into a powder. It is typically brown in colour, with a fudge or toffee-like texture.

Methods of administration

Cannabis is nearly always either smoked or vaporised. The dried herb can be smoked alone, but it is usually mixed with tobacco. Cannabis resin or oil is also smoked with tobacco. Pipes in all shapes and sizes are also used to smoke cannabis. They often have a long stem, through which smoke is inhaled, to reduce the burning effect of the hot smoke by allowing it to cool. Pipes may be designed to allow the smoke to pass through water and cool before inhalation ('hubble-bubble' pipes). The resin can be vaporised by a technique known as 'hot knifing': a heated knife is passed into a block of resin and held up so that the vaporised material can be inhaled.

The technique employed in inhaling cannabis preparations is designed to ensure maximal absorption. The smoke or vapour is inhaled deeply and the breath held (usually for 20 to 30 seconds), which facilitates absorption of the highly fat-soluble cannabinoids. The effects are rapid following inhalation, appearing within minutes.

Cannabis is never injected, but is occasionally taken orally, usually in the form of sweets or cakes to disguise the unpleasant taste. The onset of action is much slower (between 30 and 120 minutes), but the duration of action is more prolonged.

Actions

The effects of cannabis are dependent on the dose, route of administration, personality, expectations, previous experience and the environment in which it is taken. Cannabis may cause euphoria, relaxation, disinhibition, increased social interaction and laughter. Sensory perception tends to become enhanced (e.g. leading to an increased appreciation of music or art). The perception of time is altered, causing it to appear to pass more slowly. Increased appetite is common.

Side-effects

The initial effects of cannabis may be heralded by dizziness, nausea, facial flushing, dry mouth and tremor. Tachycardia and reddening of the eyes are common during intoxication, and are probably due to vasodilatation; vasodilatation may also produce orthostatic hypotension. Emotional lability, dysphoria, paranoia, anxiety and panic attacks can occur, and are probably more likely in naïve users. Short-term memory loss is common; some users become drowsy. Vigilance, co-ordination, judgement and reaction times are diminished, all of which could impair task performance (e.g. driving). Ataxia can occur.

High levels of use may cause an acute psychosis, which is characterised by confusion, delusions, hallucinations and emotional disturbances; it may occur with small doses in susceptible individuals. Cannabis psychosis commonly lasts from a few hours to days, and almost invariably resolves within a week of stopping cannabis use. In the presence of regular, heavy cannabis use, cannabis psychosis may occur repeatedly. In some cases, psychosis may continue for prolonged periods. However, it has not been established whether cannabis use can lead to the development of a chronic and persistent psychosis.

Chronic cannabis use may lead to impaired lung function, chest infections, wheeziness, a persistent cough and lung cancer. Cannabis contains a higher concentration of polyaromatic hydrocarbons than tobacco, which are thought to be responsible for carcinogenicity.

The effects of cannabis on male or female sexual function are controversial and unclear. A reduction in the number and motility of spermatozoa has been reported, but this has not been definitely linked to male infertility.

Cannabinoids are fat-soluble and therefore rapidly distributed to adipose tissue. They are released slowly into the bloodstream, and metabolites can be detected in the urine for several days after only a single use of cannabis.

Dependence and management

Dependence is not generally considered to be a major feature of cannabis use. Tolerance to the initial psychological effects and tachycardia may occur, especially with chronic use. Most individuals who use cannabis tend to do so periodically, and so cannabis use can usually be stopped without any untoward effects. Psychological dependence may occur, but there is increasing recognition that some regular heavy users of cannabis may develop a withdrawal syndrome upon discontinuation. Symptoms include anxiety, restlessness, insomnia and depression; physical signs may also occur (e.g. tremors and weight loss). Drug treatment for some of these symptoms may be appropriate, but supportive therapy and/or counselling are at least as important.

Cocaine

Cocaine is an alkaloid obtained from the leaves of the coca plant *Erythroxylum coca* and other *Erythroxylum* spp. The coca plant is indigenous to Bolivia and Peru, although it is cultivated in other countries as a result of the rapid expansion in the illegal world trade of cocaine during the 1970s. South American Indians chew coca leaves for the relief of fatigue and hunger, and as part of religious ceremonies. It is intended, primarily, to improve work performance and induce a feeling of well-being in an environment which may be harsh. The leaves usually contain less than 2% cocaine, which results in low plasma-cocaine concentrations. This form of use releases cocaine slowly and avoids rapid increases in plasma-cocaine concentrations. Consequently, the problems associated with cocaine abuse are not often seen in the native populations of South America.

Cocaine has been used as a local anaesthetic since the 1860s, and was marketed in various forms for both medicinal and non-medicinal purposes during the latter part of the nineteenth century. Coca-Cola, for example, contained cocaine until the coca component was removed in 1903.

As a drug of abuse, cocaine was formerly linked to high-income groups and 'elite society', because of its expense. It was portrayed as a 'rich man's drug' and its use was seen as glamorous. However, cocaine use has now spread to other sections of society.

Identification and street names

Cocaine is available in two forms. Cocaine hydrochloride is a white or off-white powder, known variously on the street as 'coke', 'Charlie', 'snow' or 'C'. However, cocaine as the free base is also available and this is the form referred to as 'crack'. Crack cocaine is supplied as small white or off-white lumps known as 'rocks', 'bits' or 'nuggets'.

Methods of administration

Cocaine hydrochloride is predominantly administered by the intranasal route. This usually involves placing a quantity of cocaine hydrochloride powder on a small mirror or other hard smooth surface. The powder is then formed into a thin line known as a 'snort' or 'hit' with a razor blade, and inhaled into a nostril through a thin tube, straw or rolled-up paper. Intravenous injection of cocaine hydrochloride is less common. The production of cocaine base from the hydrochloride salt can be accomplished relatively easily by individual users at street level, and is called freebasing.

Crack cocaine is nearly always heated and inhaled; it can be mixed with cigarette tobacco and then smoked, or heated in a water pipe or on a piece of aluminium foil and the vapour inhaled. The vascular network of the lungs allows rapid absorption.

Users may indulge in binges ('runs'), in which repeated doses are taken in quick succession for prolonged periods until either the supply of cocaine or the money to buy it is exhausted. Cocaine hydrochloride is sometimes injected in combination with heroin (a 'speedball').

Actions

Cocaine blocks neuronal re-uptake of dopamine and noradrenaline in both the central and peripheral nervous systems. Increased availability of these neurotransmitters is thought to account for the euphoria, which is commonly described as the 'cocaine high'. Depletion of neurotransmitters, and consequently reduced availability, is thought to be responsible for the subsequent dysphoria, which is referred to at street level as a 'crash'. The euphoric effects of cocaine base are more intense than those from cocaine hydrochloride, but the dysphoria is more intense too.

The euphoria is characterised by CNS stimulation, which gives rise to intense pleasure and a sense of well-being, accompanied by increased physical and mental capacity. Other effects include appetite suppression, tremor, tachycardia, insomnia, hyperactivity, mydriasis and, perhaps, increased interest in sex. After taking cocaine, there is usually some dysphoria, characterised by depression and anxiety, and this can impel further use of cocaine.

The onset and duration of effect depends largely on the route of administration. Smoking cocaine base or the intravenous injection of cocaine hydrochloride results in a rapid onset of action, typically within 15 to 60 seconds, and lasts about 20 minutes. In contrast, intranasal administration is associated with a much slower onset of action, and an effect which lasts up to 1.5 hours.

Side-effects

High doses may cause hallucinations, anxiety, panic attacks, restlessness, profound insomnia, agitation, convulsions and gastro-intestinal disturbances. Prolonged insomnia may lead to confusion and exhaustion. Severe depression may occur following the use of cocaine, especially the base. When large doses have been used, or after a period of prolonged and continued use, dysphoria may develop into cocaine psychosis as a result of high plasma-cocaine concentrations. It may be characterised by the presence of hallucinations (auditory, olfactory, tactile or visual), delusions and paranoia. Formication (feelings of insects crawling on the skin) may also occur, and is sometimes called 'cocaine bugs'. Fever may occur as a result of the disturbance of temperature regulating systems and increased muscle activity. Nausea and vomiting can occasionally develop.

The repeated use of cocaine hydrochloride by inhalation into the nose may cause ulceration and perforation of the nasal septum as a result of vasoconstriction. Smoking cocaine can exacerbate respiratory illness, and commonly causes non-cardiac chest pain of unknown aetiology.

Cocaine can cause hypertension and tachycardia; these are thought to be contributory factors in the development of cocaine-induced myocardial infarction or ischaemia. However, cocaine may also precipitate cardiac arrhythmias and coronary artery vasospasm. Arrhythmias related to cocaine use include sinus tachycardia, ventricular tachycardia, ventricular fibrillation and ventricular asystole; they may be life-threatening.

Death as a result of respiratory failure may occur in rare cases if vital medullary centres become depressed in the dysphoric phase. Death may also be caused by cerebral haemorrhage or convulsions.

Dependence and management

Psychological dependence has long been associated with cocaine use, and appears to be more intense and common in heavy users. The risks of developing psychological dependence to cocaine appear to be higher following intravenous use and smoking compared with intranasal use. In contrast, the chewing of coca leaves by the native population of South American countries does not appear to induce psychological dependence, and these people have little difficulty in discontinuing use. The evidence to support the development of physical dependence is less definite. Cocaine does elicit tolerance to its euphoric effects, and withdrawal reactions do seem to occur, but their recognition has been hampered by the fact that symptoms are rarely physical.

Tolerance to the euphoric effects of cocaine base is characterised by an inability of abusers to derive pleasure and enjoyment from use of the drug. This can develop quite quickly (over a matter of hours) during a 'cocaine run' or when cocaine use becomes a daily habit. Cross-tolerance occurs between cocaine and amphetamines.

Withdrawal symptoms associated with cocaine use may develop insidiously or suddenly. The effect is referred to as a 'crash' when it occurs acutely. Initially, the individual may feel very depressed, lethargic or agitated, and has a strong craving for cocaine. This is followed by an increase in appetite, feelings of exhaustion and a need to sleep. Over the succeeding weeks, sleep patterns begin to normalise, and fatigue and emotional disturbance start to abate, but craving for the drug often returns. Cocaine craving can return months or years after the last cocaine use.

The management of cocaine withdrawal is mainly directed towards controlling the intense dysphoria and craving. Drug treatment (e.g. antidepressants) may be tried, although supportive therapy and counselling are also needed.

Designer drugs

The term 'designer drug' was originally used to describe any substance deliberately synthesised in order to evade the legal restrictions on the sale and supply of drugs of abuse. In the USA, for example, the law is quite specific about which individual chemical entities are prohibited, so very minor changes to chemical structure might be used to create a drug which has the desired psychoactive effects, but which is not illegal. However, this original definition has been somewhat obscured by the fact that the term 'designer drug' is now usually used rather more loosely to describe any newly synthesised version of an existing drug intended for recreational use.

Most, if not all, designer drugs originate in the USA and are subsequently introduced into the UK. However, not all designer drugs that are established in the USA gain popularity in the UK. The designer drugs most commonly encountered are:

- phenylethylamines (e.g. Ecstasy, eve, MDA, DOM and related drugs) (*see* Amphetamines, 'Ecstasy' and related stimulants *above*)
- fentanyl derivatives (e.g. alpha-methylfentanyl)
- pethidine derivatives (e.g. MPPP)
- arylhexylamines (e.g. phencyclidine analogues).

Gamma hydroxybutyrate

Gamma hydroxybutyrate is a naturally occurring compound in the human brain, where it may function as a neurotransmitter. It has been employed medicinally in the treatment of alcoholism and in anaesthetics. It is not scheduled under the UK Misuse of Drugs Act, but is a prescription-only medicine.

Identification and street names

This drug is known by a variety of technical names, including sodium oxybate and 4-hydroxybutyrate. On the street it is usually supplied as a white powder or solution, and is known as 'GBH' or 'liquid X'.

Methods of administration

Usually the drug is taken orally, dissolved in water or a cold drink.

Actions

Gamma hydroxybutyrate has two distinct types of action. Firstly, it is reputed to build up human skeletal muscle and reduce body fat, and has been used by athletes and fitness enthusiasts as a substitute for anabolic steroids (*see* Chapter 8). Secondly, the drug has psychotropic properties which cause sedation, relaxation and euphoria, which can last up to 24 hours.

Side-effects

These include drowsiness, confusion and various other manifestations of CNS depression, including coma. Ataxia, vertigo and gastro-intestinal upset are well-known, but bradycardia, hypotension and various disorders of blood biochemistry have also been described.

Dependence and management

Withdrawal reactions have been described in a very small number of chronic users. Symptoms have included insomnia, tremor and anxiety.

Hallucinogenic fungi

Both species of mushrooms have a long history of abuse, but have quite different effects. Liberty cap contains two hallucinogenic alkaloids: psilocybin and psilocin. It is harvested between September and November. Fly agaric also has two psychoactive constituents: ibotenic acid and muscimol. It is usually picked in September.

Identification and street names

In the UK, two main species of fungi are abused because they contain psychoactive substances: together, they are termed 'magic mushrooms'. *Psilocybe semilanceata* (liberty cap) and *Amanita muscaria* (fly agaric) are both native to the UK. Liberty cap is a small, yellow or buff-coloured mushroom, about 10 cm high. Fly agaric is much larger and has a red cap flecked with white.

Methods of administration

Hallucinogenic mushrooms may be eaten raw, cooked or made into a drink; they may also be dried or frozen to preserve them for later use. In the UK, it is not necessarily an offence to possess these mushrooms in their raw state, although it is an offence to prepare them for consumption.

Actions

The effects of liberty cap range from mild excitement and euphoria in small doses, to hallucinations and perceptual disorders at larger doses. The consumption of about 30 mushrooms produces an effect similar to LSD. Hallucinogenic effects are often heralded by sympathomimetic effects (e.g. tachycardia, mydriasis and flushing). The hallucinations themselves are commonly visual, although they may also be auditory or tactile.

Fly agaric has a more depressant action on the CNS and often produces sleepiness, confusion, sensory illusions, euphoria and vivid dreams.

Side-effects

Both species may produce dysphoria or other unpleasant psychotropic effects (a 'bad trip'). Liberty cap may also cause ataxia, drowsiness, nausea and abdominal pain. Fly agaric has been reported to cause confusion, lack of co-ordination, headaches, vomiting and convulsions.

One important aspect of hallucinogenic mushroom abuse is the accidental ingestion of poisonous mushrooms picked in error.

Dependence and management

Mild to moderate psychological dependence may occur with hallucinogenic mushroom use; physical dependence and withdrawal symptoms have not been reported. Tolerance to the effects of hallucinogenic mushrooms develops rapidly; cross-tolerance may be exhibited between liberty cap and LSD.

Khat

Khat is cultivated from Yemen to Afghanistan and neighbouring regions, and the native populations chew the leaves for their stimulant effects. Khat use in other countries is rare, although immigrant communities may continue khat use in their country of settlement after importing the leaves by air. Traditionally, khat leaves are transported moistened and wrapped in banana leaves to keep them fresh; drying results in loss of active constituents, and the leaves are therefore stored in domestic deep freezers to reduce deterioration. The leaves contain the stimulant alkaloids, cathinone and cathine.

Identification and street names

Khat is the leaves of the shrub *Catha edulis*; the name is also spelled as 'qat' or 'kat'. The leaves are small and tear shaped, being less than 5 cm long. They must be fresh when used, not dried.

Methods of administration

Khat leaves are chewed into a large mass (quid), which is held inside the cheek. Generally, chewing lasts only a few hours, but may continue for days. Occasionally, the leaves are smoked or made into a drink.

Actions

The active constituents of khat resemble amphetamine in their actions, and the alkaloids may actually be metabolised into amphetamine derivatives within the body. The stimulant actions of khat are mediated by increased noradrenaline release and inhibition of its uptake. Initially, feelings of well-being, talkativeness and excitement are the predominant effects.

Side-effects

Dry mouth frequently occurs, necessitating the consumption of large quantities of water; constipation is common. Further chewing can result in side-effects similar to those seen with amphetamines (e.g. diminished appetite, dilated pupils, tachycardia and tachypnoea). Prolonged chewing of khat may cause mania, insomnia, hypertension, arrhythmias and hyperactivity. Khat psychosis has also been described following prolonged use.

Dependence and management

Tolerance to the effects of khat may develop as a result of depletion of noradrenaline stores, and reduced sensitivity and number of noradrenaline receptors. Withdrawal symptoms include lethargy and nightmares. Possession or consumption of khat is not illegal, but attempting to isolate the psychoactive ingredients is an offence.

LSD

LSD is a synthetic compound derived from the alkaloids found in ergot (*Claviceps purpurea*). It was first synthesised in 1938 by Albert Hoffman in his search to find stimulant drugs related to lysergic acid. LSD was subsequently marketed and became widely used by psychiatrists in the 1950s and early 1960s, particularly for the treatment of drug and alcohol dependence. It was used in the belief that it could release repressed thoughts from the subconscious. Other uses included treatment of personality disorders, sexual disorders, autism and terminal illness. However, well-controlled studies failed to demonstrate any therapeutic benefit.

The abuse of LSD achieved increasing popularity, which peaked in the 1960s and early 1970s. As a medicinal agent, LSD was withdrawn from the market in 1966 following increasing concern about its abuse.

Identification and street names

LSD is also known as lysergide or lysergic acid diethylamide. It is usually referred to on the street as 'acid' or 'trips'. LSD is illicitly synthesised in home laboratories and is distributed in a range of forms. In solution, it can be absorbed onto any suitable material (e.g. sugar cubes, blotting paper or small flakes of gelatin). Small pieces of absorbent paper, smaller than postage stamps, are impregnated with one dose of LSD; they are commonly decorated with a motif such as a cartoon character. A variety of tablets and capsules may also be produced. Very small tablets called 'microdots' or 'dots' containing a single dose are quite common.

Methods of administration

LSD is almost invariably taken by mouth, as it is well absorbed orally, although it can be injected or administered by the intranasal route. It is commonly used on an intermittent basis; users rarely resort to lengthy 'binges'. Peak effects are seen between 30 and 90 minutes following ingestion. The duration of effect is in the order of eight to 12 hours, although the intensity diminishes after four to six hours.

Actions

The LSD molecule resembles both serotonin and the catecholamines, and has some actions characteristic of each. It is the activation of serotonin pathways that are thought to be responsible for the psychedelic, or 'mind-altering', effects of LSD.

The psychedelic effects of LSD (commonly described as a 'trip') are not predictable and depend on numerous factors, including the environment and the user's emotional state, expectation, personality and previous experiences. Although traditionally classed as a hallucinogen, LSD actually tends to distort perception and cause illusions, rather than evoke true hallucinations (which by definition are not based upon a true sensory stimulus). Thus, there can be disturbances of perception relating to body image: body parts (or the whole body) may appear to enlarge or contract. Almost all sensory faculties are heightened. Synaesthesia may also occur, which is a distortion of sensory perception characterised by one sensory stimulus evoking a response in another (e.g. sounds are visual and colours are heard). Another common distortion is that time is passing very slowly or that the user or others are ageing rapidly.

Mood changes can be intense, variable and unstable, and thought control is disturbed, producing loss of short-term memory and emergence of the memory of events in the distant past. As a result of the effects of LSD, especially disturbance of cognition, users may believe they are having a mystical experience and may relate it to death and reincarnation. Bizarre thoughts and ideas may manifest.

Side-effects

Sympathomimetic effects often announce the beginning of a 'trip'; these include dilated pupils, a slight increase in blood pressure, tachycardia, tremor and pilo-erection. Muscle weakness, nausea and hyperthermia may also occur.

LSD can induce 'unwanted' psychotropic effects (commonly described as a 'bad trip'), although it is not known why they occur. Characteristic features include dysphoria, paranoia, acute panic reactions, delusions and distressing hallucinations; confusion and loss of contact with reality are also prominent. The effects of bad trips appear to diminish with time. Bad trips are more common with higher doses, although the dose is not thought to be the sole cause, as some individuals appear to have an increased susceptibility. Bad trips may occur in experienced persons who have previously enjoyed using LSD. Bad trips may also lead to accidental fatalities, although suicide is rare. Impulsive and irrational behaviour, which can be sudden and dangerous, may occur in a few cases.

'Flashbacks' are usually visual distortions that occur in the absence of recent drug intake. Users do not experience a full 'trip', but typically notice persistent visual aberrations (e.g. haloes or coloured patterns). They can occur months or years later and are more common in those who have used LSD several times. The cause is not known, although there may be precipitating factors (e.g. exposure to other drugs, sudden changes in light levels or stress).

Severe depression, sometimes accompanied by anxiety and panic, may occur following LSD use, but this is usually self-limiting. Psychosis may also occur, and can be a brief or prolonged episode. The condition usually resolves completely in time.

Dependence and management

Physical dependence is thought not to occur, but, as with all psychoactive substances, an element of psychological dependence may arise. Tolerance to the effects of LSD occurs after only a few regular doses. The development of rapid tolerance may be the reason for the intermittent pattern of LSD use. Tolerance is lost after four to six days. There are no withdrawal symptoms associated with discontinuation.

Opioids

Opioids are compounds that possess morphine-like activity; the term 'opiates' was previously used to describe naturally-occurring alkaloids from the opium plant *Papaver somniferum*. Opioids are used primarily for their analgesic, cough suppressant and antidiarrhoeal properties. Opium is now rarely seen in the UK, but it does continue to be used in other countries. The opium poppy grows in many countries (e.g. Afghanistan, Pakistan, Thailand, China and Indonesia) and is used to prepare raw opium, which may be smoked, eaten or drunk as an infusion.

Morphine is the principal alkaloid present in opium and is the standard opioid to which the activity of other opioids is related. Morphine was isolated from raw opium in 1803, and became established as an analgesic. In 1874, diamorphine, then called diacetylmorphine, was synthesised from morphine. Heroin dominates as the opioid obtained on the black market from illicit, imported sources, reflected by the large increase in heroin seizures, although a black market also exists for diverted medical supplies of most opioids.

Identification and street names

Diamorphine is universally known as heroin, but has various street names including 'dragon', 'skag', 'smack', 'H', 'hard stuff', 'horse' and 'junk'. Illicit heroin comes in a variety of forms; it is usually in powder form and off-white in colour, but can be anything from white to dark brown. Street heroin is commonly bought in small amounts (often called 'wraps').

Methadone is abused at street level, often when legitimate supplies for maintenance or detoxification are sold, or traded for other drugs. All other prescription opioids are also potentially abusable (e.g. morphine, buprenorphine and pethidine). Diconal has been very popular when it has reached street level because it also contains cyclizine (*see* OTC medicines *below*).

'Designer' opioids based on fentanyl are rarely seen in the UK (*see* Designer drugs *above*), but OTC opioids are probably abused quite widely (*see* OTC medicines *below*).

When the desired opioid is not available, users will commonly resort to others.

Methods of administration

Most opioids can be administered intranasally, smoked, by injection or by mouth. The preferred route depends on the particular opioid and the prevailing fashion. The oral route is not popular at street level because it does not produce a 'rush'. Liquid preparations or solutions made from crushed tablets may be injected.

Heroin is commonly administered by intravenous injection ('mainlining', 'shooting up' or 'making a hit'). It may also be injected just below the skin surface ('skin popping'), but this is only used when venous access is impossible. Heroin powder is mixed with a small quantity of tap water and heated, commonly in a teaspoon. A syringe is used to draw up the solution. An attempt is often made to remove impurities and undissolved material by using a makeshift filter (e.g. a piece of cotton wool or the filter-tip from a cigarette). Heroin base is relatively insoluble, and an acid is often added to increase solubility (e.g. citric acid or lemon juice).

Heroin can be mixed with cigarette tobacco and smoked; more commonly, it can be heated on a piece of aluminium foil and the vapour inhaled ('chasing the dragon'). Heroin may also be inhaled nasally as a powder ('snorting'). Abuse of buprenorphine by this route has also been reported. These non-intravenous methods may appear relatively harmless to some individuals in comparison with injection and can therefore lead to experimentation.

Heroin may be mixed with other drugs: a 'speedball' is a mixture of heroin with cocaine (or sometimes amphetamine). Such mixtures may enhance the psychoactive effects and prevent the severe depression that often follows stimulant use. Antihistamines (e.g. cyclizine) are sometimes used to enhance the effects of opioids, and benzodiazepines are commonly combined with opioids.

Actions

Different opioids vary in their onset and duration of action, rate of absorption, distribution, metabolism and excretion. These properties are generally conferred by the fat solubility and basicity of each compound. Heroin crosses the blood-brain barrier rapidly compared with other opioids and, consequently, has a shorter onset of action. It is hydrolysed to morphine in brain tissue, and it is probably morphine and its metabolites that account for the majority of its actions.

The euphoria following injection or smoking of opioids is intense (commonly described as a 'rush' or 'buzz'). It provides relief from anxiety or stress and produces intense pleasure. Euphoria is followed by relaxation, somnolence and lassitude, commonly described as being 'on the nod'.

Methadone is the second most commonly abused opioid. It has a longer duration of action than morphine. Buprenorphine also has a longer half-life than heroin. Pethidine has a shorter duration of action than morphine, but may cause more excitatory effects. The intense euphoria experienced with pethidine compared with other opioids is commonly described as 'edgy', 'jangly' or 'rough'.

Side-effects

Effects of opioids include nausea and vomiting, constipation, drowsiness, confusion, dry mouth, sweating, facial flushing, vertigo, bradycardia, palpitations, hypothermia, restlessness, mood changes and miosis. Difficulty in micturition, and biliary or ureteric spasm, may also occur. At higher doses, respiratory depression and hypotension are seen. Pethidine may produce excitatory effects, including hallucinations, muscle twitches, agitation and convulsions. Sexual dysfunction associated with opioid abuse includes loss of libido, and is common in users suffering from prolonged dependence. Women may experience amenorrhoea.

Dependence on opioids may be associated with general self-neglect and loss of appetite, which can result in nutritional deficiency.

Overdose is commonly inadvertent. It may be caused by lack of awareness of the degree of purity of the drug. Street samples of heroin differ in their purity, and overdose can result from using a product with a higher than expected concentration of heroin. Loss of tolerance following withdrawal can also result in overdose if the user returns to the same dose used before withdrawal. Initial use of a dose similar to that used by a friend who has developed substantial tolerance can also result in overdose. Signs of overdose include stupor, respiratory depression, coma, pulmonary oedema and respiratory arrest.

Dependence and management

Physical dependence develops gradually; users often believe that they are in control of the situation. The use of smokable forms of heroin does carry a risk of dependence, despite users often relating dependence to injection. As a result, the dangers can go unrealised.

Tolerance develops to all the psychotropic effects of opioids. It develops to such an extent that users often take doses which would be fatal to those who have not developed tolerance. The euphoric and pleasurable effects, which diminish in duration and intensity as tolerance develops, eventually become non-existent or brief. Tolerance is lost to a large extent following withdrawal from the opioid. There is substantial cross-dependence and cross-tolerance between different opioids.

Withdrawal symptoms associated with abrupt withdrawal of opioids in dependent users are variable in intensity, duration and onset, and also depend on the opioid used; other factors include total daily dose, interval between doses, duration of use, health status and personality characteristics. Generally, withdrawal symptoms in heroin-dependent subjects begin within a few hours, reach a peak within 36 to 72 hours, and then gradually subside; withdrawal symptoms associated with methadone dependence develop more slowly and may be less intense, but they are also more prolonged.

Common withdrawal symptoms include anxiety, craving, depression, restlessness, disturbed sleep or insomnia, and lassitude; other features include yawning, mydriasis, lachrymation, rhinorrhoea, sneezing, muscle tremor, sweating, irritability, anorexia, nausea, vomiting, dehydration, diarrhoea, bone pain, muscle cramps, abdominal pain, tachycardia, increased respiratory rate, hypertension and an increased body temperature. Alternate feelings of hot and cold in combination with pilo-erection may occur. Craving for opioids may last for several months, and sleep disturbances often take longer than other withdrawal symptoms to resolve.

The management of opioid withdrawal depends on the degree of dependence. Young heroin users with a short history of use, and who have used relatively small amounts daily, can often stop using heroin abruptly without pharmacological assistance. The intensity of withdrawal symptoms may be similar to an episode of influenza, and general supportive care may be all that is required. This form of opioid withdrawal is commonly referred to as 'cold turkey'. Some symptomatic treatment may be necessary.

Cross-tolerance between the opioids enables the administration of methadone to stave off withdrawal in those dependent upon heroin. Other opioids used in this way include buprenorphine and dihydrocodeine, although the latter is not licensed for this indication. Methadone, or other prescribed opioids, are given to achieve one of two basic objectives: some patients require a period of stabilisation on an assured supply of opioid before attempting withdrawal; other patients, depending on a variety of factors, will require life-long stabilisation on methadone to enable them to function as normal members of society. The first of these objectives is often called detoxification or supervised withdrawal; the second is methadone maintenance.

Methadone substitution is the commonest therapy used for opioid withdrawal and dependence. Methadone has a long half-life, which allows supervised, once-daily administration; it also has the same basic pharmacological effects as heroin, but does not cause the initial 'buzz' that an injection may cause. Doses that suppress withdrawal signs are administered in place of the opioid that the individual is dependent upon. If appropriate, a reducing regimen is agreed with the user. The rate of reduction depends on the opioid used, length of use, and whether the treatment is on an in-patient or out-patient basis. Where methadone maintenance is used, it is important to realise that this does not mean that the substitution has failed. Maintenance is a goal in itself, which removes the patient from the drug scene and prevents further injection. Maintenance is a long-term measure to stabilise and improve the lifestyle of the user. Users suitable for methadone maintenance include those with a long history of opioid dependence, and those who have had several unsuccessful attempts at withdrawal.

Buprenorphine has recently been licensed for facilitating opioid withdrawal or for maintenance. As a partial agonist at opioid receptors, it has potential advantages compared with methadone. Buprenorphine is much less likely to cause death by respiratory depression at high dose; it should oppose the action of any heroin administered simultaneously; and withdrawal may be more mild and, therefore, better tolerated. Two potential disadvantages are that being a tablet formulation, it can be ground up and injected, and, since it must be administered sublingually, supervising self-administration may be more difficult.

Lofexidine and clonidine are alpha-2-adrenergic receptor agonists that are used for the symptomatic treatment of opioid withdrawal. Hypotension is a troublesome side-effect for some patients taking clonidine, which is also not licensed for this indication. This led to the development of the less hypotensive lofexidine. Both drugs inhibit the release of noradrenaline, which is thought to be responsible for causing many of the withdrawal symptoms. It is important to realise that neither drug prevents withdrawal: they make it more bearable for the patient and may shorten its duration.

The opioid antagonist naltrexone is occasionally used. It can be used for the maintenance of detoxified, formerly opioid-dependent patients. It blocks the euphoric actions of opioids, and is given to former users to prevent recidivism. Treatment should be initiated in a drug dependency unit or other specialist centre. Naltrexone should not be given alone to patients currently dependent on opioids, since an acute withdrawal reaction will be precipitated. However, it can be given with clonidine or lofexidine to precipitate withdrawal in currently dependent opioid users, since the alpha-2 agonists will reduce the withdrawal symptoms. Despite this, oral sedatives are often needed when this regimen is employed, to help patients cope with the unpleasantness of the experience.

Relatively recently, a procedure known as 'rapid opiate detoxification under anaesthesia' (RODA) or 'ultra-rapid opiate detoxification' (UROD) has become more widely practised. This involves giving naltrexone to patients who are currently dependent on opioids to precipitate an acute withdrawal reaction, but the antagonist is given whilst the patient is receiving a general anaesthetic. Having emerged from six to eight hours of anaesthesia, patients are reported to be then relatively free of withdrawal effects. They are typically maintained on naltrexone thereafter.

Over-the-counter (OTC) medicines

The extent of the abuse of OTC medicines is not known; this is primarily because of lack of reporting and lack of research in this area. It is useful to distinguish between deliberate abuse (for a psychotropic effect) and inappropriate use in the mistaken belief that there is a medical need for the medicine. Laxatives and OTC analgesics usually fall into the latter category. The Council of the Royal Pharmaceutical Society of Great Britain states that:

> Every pharmacist must be aware of any problems in his area, whether or not they are general, or known to the Society. He or she should be aware of any products which are sold in excessive quantities or with abnormal frequency. Almost any substance can be abused . . .

Identification

The abuse potential of a large number of OTC medicines is recognised, and some of the common preparations involved are listed below:

- sympathomimetics (e.g. ephedrine, pseudoephedrine, phenylpropanolamine, phenylephrine)
- antihistamines (e.g. cyclizine, diphenhydramine, dimenhydrinate)
- laxatives (especially stimulant laxatives)
- analgesics (e.g. aspirin- or paracetamol-based preparations with or without codeine)
- opioids (e.g. codeine linctus, kaolin and morphine, Gee's linctus)
- dextromethorphan.

Methods of administration

When abused, most OTC products are taken by mouth. However, antihistamine tablets may be crushed for injection, and some oral sympathomimetic preparations are occasionally used in this way.

Actions and side-effects

Sympathomimetics (e.g. ephedrine, pseudoephedrine, phenylephrine and phenylpropanolamine) are included in a range of OTC products, particularly cold and influenza remedies. They are abused for a variety of reasons: to produce euphoria, to combat fatigue or to aid weight loss. Sometimes they may be purchased as a cheap and more readily available alternative to street amphetamines to relieve craving or withdrawal effects. Abuse of OTC sympathomimetics carries the same risks as abuse of other amphetamines to which they are chemically related (*see above*). Similar serious side-effects have been reported (e.g. paranoid psychosis, cardiac arrhythmias and hypertension). The abuse of stimulants such as ephedrine and pseudoephedrine has been associated with the development of tolerance and dependence.

Certain antihistamines can be abused, either individually or, more often, in combination with other drugs of abuse, especially opioids. Antihistamines which have been abused tend to be the older, more sedative drugs, which often have antimuscarinic actions (e.g. cyclizine, diphenhydramine and dimenhydrinate). They commonly cause sedation, dizziness and a lack of co-ordination. The use of antihistamines in combination with other depressant drugs may lead to more serious CNS depression. There has been much concern over the abuse of cyclizine which, when used in large doses, may cause euphoria. Doses used have sometimes been as high as 800 mg. Existing injection drug users are likely to crush tablets to form a solution to inject. Cyclizine potentiates the euphoric effects of opioids and has also been used with other drugs. Psychotic reactions may develop following abuse of cyclizine and dependence may occur. The Council of the Royal Pharmaceutical Society of Great Britain recommends that medicines containing cyclizine should be sold personally by the pharmacist.

Laxatives are commonly abused by patients suffering from eating disorders, in the belief that they will reduce gastro-intestinal transit time and impair the absorption of food. Some patients also have an obsession with regular bowel habit and take regular laxatives unnecessarily. Stimulant laxatives are abused most commonly. Abuse of laxatives can produce weight loss, dehydration and disturbance of electrolyte balance. Hypokalaemia can occur, producing symptoms that include fatigue, muscle weakness or cramps, headache, palpitations and abdominal pain. Long-term use is likely to cause an atonic colon, such that the peristaltic movements of the large bowel cease permanently.

OTC analgesics are sometimes taken indiscriminately. Unfortunately, when taken chronically, they can actually cause headache. Patients suffering from this drug-induced headache then continue to self-medicate with analgesics in the hope that this will alleviate the pain, which, of course, does not occur. This sets up a self-perpetuating cycle of analgesic administration that can be an under-recognised cause of chronic daily headache.

Opioids (e.g. codeine and morphine) are included in many non-prescription medicines for their analgesic, cough suppressant and anti-diarrhoeal properties. These preparations may be abused in their own right, or may act as substitutes for heroin when individual users cannot obtain a street supply. The OTC opioid of choice in this situation is codeine linctus, used to stave off symptoms of withdrawal. Pharmacists found guilty of supplying codeine linctus with the knowledge that it would be abused have been struck from the register by the Royal Pharmaceutical Society.

Dextromethorphan was developed as an opioid derivative, but it does not have typical opioid actions. It is used as a cough suppressant, but when abused in high doses it can cause euphoria, hallucinations, illusions and other perceptual distortions. Side-effects from these large doses include ataxia, confusion, tachycardia, hypertension, nausea, irritability and psychosis. A withdrawal syndrome has also been described.

Dependence and management

There are no published guidelines on how to deal with abuse of OTC drugs, or withdrawal reactions to them. The management of withdrawal from stimulants should be similar to that described under amphetamines (*see above*). Similarly, OTC opioid dependence should be managed, as for street opioids, by a local drug dependency unit or psychiatrist (*see above*); this may also be the best place to refer abusers of antihistamines or dextromethorphan. Laxative abusers are frequently referred to a gastro-enterologist, but a psychiatrist might also be of assistance. Those suffering from chronic daily headache should preferably be referred to a pain clinic.

Volatile substance abuse

Volatile substance abuse (VSA) refers to the intentional inhalation of volatile substances to achieve a state of altered mood, perception and behaviour. Many other terms are used to describe this activity including solvent abuse, 'glue sniffing' and inhalant abuse. However, the term VSA is the most appropriate as it encompasses glues, solvents and other volatile substances (e.g. aerosol propellants). The Royal Pharmaceutical Society of Great Britain has issued brief guidance to pharmacists concerning VSA (*see* Box 7.1).

Box 7.1 Advice to pharmacists on supply of solvents (from the Royal Pharmaceutical Society's guidance on the Code of Ethics and Professional Standards (RPSGB, 2000))

A pharmacist should be alert to the possibility of misuse of products containing organic solvents which can be used to cause intoxication and should not sell solvents or any product which the pharmacist believes may be purchased for this purpose. The products include adhesive plaster remover, collodions, dry cleaning fluids, organic solvents, certain glues and shoe cleaning fluids, and aerosols (which are misused because of their propellant content). Pharmacists are advised to prohibit the sale of such products by self-selection, to question regular purchasers, to investigate demands for large quantities, and to be particularly vigilant if the demand is from teenagers.

In the UK, VSA came to public attention in the 1970s, and began to cause great public concern in the 1980s. In the UK, VSA has been associated with 1477 deaths between 1983 and 1997; the annual figure rose steadily from 17 deaths in 1978 to a peak of 152 deaths in 1990. Since 1990, there has been a gradual trend towards fewer deaths per year; in 1997, for example, there were 73 deaths.

VSA is almost invariably associated with young people between ten and 16 years of age, although adult cases have been reported; the majority of users are male. In the UK, up to 10% of young people have experimented with VSA, and perhaps 1% are regular users. VSA occurs across all sections of the community.

Those who engage in VSA can be divided into two broad groups:

- Experimental users: young people may become involved in VSA through curiosity, excitement, experiment or as a result of peer pressure. Those involved are generally male and in their early teenage years, and usually practise VSA in groups and generally stop after a short period of time.
- Regular users: these users may have underlying social, behavioural or psychological problems, and regular VSA may provide an escape from reality. These subjects tend to be older than experimental users; they are also more likely to resort to VSA on their own.

In England, Wales and Northern Ireland, the Intoxicating Substances Supply Act 1985 controls the supply of potential products involved in VSA. It makes it illegal to sell a substance to a person under 18 years of age if the vendor knows, or has reasonable grounds for believing, that it is likely to be used for VSA. It is not an offence to indulge in VSA, but other legislation may be contravened during the process (e.g. breach of the peace or local byelaws). In Scotland, the Solvent Abuse (Scotland) Act 1983 permits prosecutions where supply to children is involved, although VSA itself is not an offence.

Identification and street names

All of the volatile substances listed in Table 7.2 are potentially subject to abuse. Many of the products are readily available, cheap and easily concealed.

Table 7.2 Preparations that are subject to misuse and their common volatile constituent(s)

Preparation	Volatile constituent(s)
Acrylic paints	Toluene
Adhesives	Acetone
	Ethyl acetate
	n-Hexane
	Methyl ethyl ketone
	Methylene chloride
	Toluene
	1,1,1-Trichloroethane
	Xylene
Aerosol propellants	Chlorodifluoromethane (Halon 22)
	Dichlorodifluoromethane (Halon 12)
	Dichlorotetrafluoroethane (Halon 114)
	Trichlorofluoromethane (Halon 11)
Anaesthetics	Enflurane
	Halothane
	Isoflurane
	Nitrous oxide
Anti-freeze products	Isopropanol
Bottled fuel gases, cigarette lighters	n-Butane
	Isobutane
	Propane
Car paints and thinners	n-Hexane
	Toluene
	Xylene
Chewing-gum remover	Trichloroethylene
De-greasing fluids	Tetrachloroethylene
	1,1,1-Trichloroethane
	Trichloroethylene
Dry-cleaning fluids	Tetrachloroethylene
	1,1,1-Trichloroethane
	Trichloroethylene
Fire extinguishers	Bromochlorodifluoromethane (BCF) propellants
Lacquers	Methylene chloride
	Toluene
	1,1,1-Trichloroethane
Nail polish remover	Acetone
Paint strippers	Dichloromethane
	Toluene
Petrol	Aliphatic hydrocarbons
Refrigerants	Dichlorodifluoromethane (Halon 12)
	Trichlorofluoromethane (Halon 11)
Shoe dyes	n-Hexane
	Methylene chloride
	Toluene
	1,1,1-Trichloroethane

Table 7.2 continued

Preparation	Volatile constituent(s)
Solvents	Acetone Carbon tetrachloride Chloroform Diethyl ether n-Hexane Methyl ethyl ketone Methyl isobutyl ketone
Spot removers	Carbon tetrachloride Tetrachloroethylene
Woodwork adhesives	Xylene
Typewriter correcting fluid and thinners	1,1,1-Trichloroethane
White spirit	Aliphatic hydrocarbons

Methods of administration

The method used to inhale volatile substances depends on the product. Adhesives, cleaning fluids and petrol may be poured onto a piece of cloth (e.g. a handkerchief or coat sleeve) and the vapour inhaled. More viscous substances may be poured into a plastic bag or an empty crisp packet, and the vapour inhaled by placing the bag over the mouth and squeezing the bag gently to force the vapour into the mouth or nose, or both ('huffing'). This method may also be used for other non-viscous volatile substances to maximise inhalation.

Aerosol propellants and bottled fuel gases are abused in a variety of ways, including spraying the contents into a large plastic bag and inhaling the contents. A particularly dangerous method of inhaling bottled fuel gas, aerosol propellants and fire extinguisher contents is to spray the contents directly into the mouth or nostril. Large body bags may also be used; these enable the body and volatile substance to be totally enclosed within the bag.

Actions

The range and magnitude of the effects of VSA are dependent on the circumstances of use. Important factors include the state of mind of the individual, the environment, the presence of other people and the relationship with other users in a group situation.

The characteristic feature of VSA is the rapid onset of action (the 'high'), which is followed by an equally quick recovery; the high can be maintained for several hours by repeated use. The initial effects following inhalation include euphoria, a sense of well-being, disinhibition, blurred vision and a feeling of invulnerability; visual or auditory hallucinations may also occur. After the euphoria has passed, the user may fall asleep for several hours.

Side-effects

During intoxication, solvents may cause various undesirable effects, including nausea and vomiting, dizziness, flushing, cough, sneezing, excessive salivation, lack of muscle co-ordination, slurred speech and convulsions.

VSA also carries a risk of sudden death. Solvents seem to sensitise the myocardium to the actions of catecholamines, and when stressed by exercise, for example, it is thought that fatal arrhythmias can develop. Other possible causes of death due to the direct effects of volatile substances include vagal inhibition and respiratory depression. Indirect causes of death associated with VSA include accidents, asphyxiation and inhalation of vomit.

Toluene seems to have particular toxic potential; it is also one of the solvents most slowly eliminated from the body. Physical damage associated with toluene abuse includes reduced lung function, as a result of damage to the alveoli and the vascular network of the lungs. Aplastic anaemia has been reported to occur following exposure and, rarely, liver and kidney failure. Neurological consequences of toluene abuse include the development of a cerebellar syndrome, with ataxia affecting the gait and arms. These symptoms may persist in some cases, especially following severe and prolonged use. Toluene can also cause mild peripheral neuropathy, although it is rare and only thought to occur with very prolonged use. Cognitive impairment may occur with chronic, long-term toluene use, although its severity is not related to the duration of use.

The local effects of VSA may become chronic, and include recurrent epistaxis, rhinitis, conjunctivitis, nasal and mouth ulceration, and perioral eczema ('glue sniffer's rash'). Systemic effects may include anorexia, weight loss, loss of concentration, depression, irritability, paranoia and fatigue.

Dependence and management

Psychological dependence may occur with VSA, especially in individuals who are regular users. Tolerance develops to the effects of volatile substances. Withdrawal symptoms may rarely occur, and include craving and a general feeling of dysphoria.

No treatment for withdrawal symptoms that may be associated with VSA is usually necessary, but where indicated, symptomatic relief may be appropriate.

The role of the pharmacist

Pharmacists are in an ideal position to help both those abusing drugs and the healthcare professionals that care for them. As detailed later, pharmacists can initiate needle exchange schemes and supervise the supply and self-administration of prescribed methadone or other agents used for drug dependency. Another important role is the detection of forged prescriptions.

However, there are many other opportunities for pharmacists to assist in this area of healthcare. All pharmacists should obtain a copy of *Drug Misuse and Dependence – Guidelines on Clinical Management*, published in 1999 by the Departments of Health for England, Scotland and Northern Ireland together with the Welsh Office (DoH *et al.*, 1999). This 'Orange Guide' provides a wealth of information on patient management which pharmacists will find of value for personal education. The Guide will also assist pharmacists in advising other healthcare professionals and, because this book is seen as the 'gold standard', pharmacists have an important role to play in enforcing the guidelines contained within it. The current edition states: 'community pharmacists provide a significant point of contact as part of the primary health care services and have regular (often daily) contact with the patient. Hence their role in the care of drug abusers is crucial, and communication in both directions between pharmacists and other healthcare professionals should be encouraged'.

Pharmacists have always been well placed to provide information to other professionals and the public. In the field of drug abuse and dependency, pharmacists can advise professionals on a range of clinical or technical matters, including choice of formulation, interactions, availability of products, side-effects and choice of therapy. Similarly, pharmacists can provide information and advice to the public. A sensitive and sympathetic attitude towards drug users is needed by pharmacists; research shows that some pharmacists still take the view that they are undesirable customers who are unpleasant, dishonest and a nuisance. The needs of drug users, and their relatives and friends, are essential considerations for pharmacists who are involved with drug abuse. A range of patient information leaflets is available, including a series of general, free leaflets from the Departments of Health. However, pharmacists should seek out local drug dependency services and stock leaflets advertising their services. Other local and national groups with an interest in drug abuse also provide leaflets and posters, although some organisations may charge for these.

Apart from leaflets, pharmacists can provide general healthcare information, and advice on symptomatic relief of minor ailments to drug abusers. Relatives and friends of abusers may be ignorant of the effects and consequences of abuse and dependency, and parents often feel helpless and frightened following the discovery of drug abuse by their child. Pharmacists are in a position to advise them and direct them to local, more specialised services. Patients receiving benzodiazepines should be made aware of their dependence potential, and whilst patient information leaflets may explain this, pharmacists may wish to stress the problem to particular patients, offer advice on how to minimise the risk of dependency or answer any queries that patients may have.

Pharmacists should liaise with local drug dependency teams, and be aware of the services available and the methods of referral. Making contact opens the door to co-operation, and pharmacists can help with the construction and implementation of local guidelines and protocols for a wide range of topics (e.g. methadone maintenance programmes, harm minimisation strategies and benzodiazepine prescribing). The 'Orange Guide' advocates the involvement of pharmacists in constructing multidisciplinary, shared care guidelines. In addition, the Advisory Council on the Misuse of Drugs has identified the need for pharmacists to be involved in regional and district plans for the reduction of harm from problem drug use, especially in the reduction in the spread of HIV infection.

Many of the drugs prescribed for drugs abusers are Controlled Drugs, so pharmacists' role in monitoring prescription legality is needed. As with other prescriptions, errors and drug interactions must also be investigated. The 'Orange Guide' provides an appendix listing the known interactions of methadone. Pharmacists should challenge inappropriate prescriptions, in the same way that they would in any other type of medicine. Examples of prescribing that should be challenged include: initiation of new long-term benzodiazepine prescriptions; prescribing potential drugs of abuse to known users of street drugs; patients trying to obtain potential drugs of abuse by deception; suspected abuse of prescription-only medicines; and inappropriately high doses of psychoactive drugs. The 'Orange Guide' can be an invaluable support when dealing with some of these situations.

Finally, it must be recognised that in the case of OTC medicine abuse or dependency, pharmacists are the suppliers of the abused substances. It is a tribute to pharmacists' existing vigilance that many abusers have to go to enormous lengths to conceal their regular habit from local pharmacists, perhaps by visiting many different pharmacies and travelling great distances in order to avoid suspicion. However, pharmacists must understand which products in the pharmacy can be abused, and make sure that their staff are aware. Solvent based products should not be forgotten. The Code of Ethics makes it clear that pharmacists should not sell a product which they suspect will be abused, and the Royal Pharmaceutical Society has a history of being strict with pharmacists who breach this. The pharmacist should attempt to challenge suspected abusers; often a discrete discussion is most appropriate. Whilst an offer of professional assistance may not always be welcome, the challenge may deter the patient from buying further supplies. Information on local patterns of OTC abuse and methods of dealing with it should be shared with neighbouring pharmacists, perhaps at local branch meetings.

Pharmacists should also work together nationally. The Pharmacy Misuse Advisory Group (PharMAG) is open to all pharmacists with an interest in substance abuse. It provides a national network of specialists who can support and advise each other, and has input into the activities of a large number of national bodies. At the time of writing, membership is free and includes a regular newsletter. The address to write to for membership is given below.

Needle exchange schemes

The role of pharmacists in preventing complications associated with drug abuse is clearly highlighted by the need to discourage the sharing of injection equipment. Participation in syringe and needle exchange schemes is considered to be an important role for community pharmacists in the prevention of the spread of

HIV infection, hepatitis B and C, and other infections. Providing free equipment may reduce sharing and use of contaminated equipment. Any continued sharing of injection equipment cannot be attributed solely to ignorance of the associated risks of infection, especially HIV infection. The most common reason for sharing may be that new equipment is not immediately to hand. The need to use drugs to avoid withdrawal symptoms may mean that sharing is the only means of obtaining the drug. There also may be a social acceptance of sharing injection equipment among friends and sexual partners; users might feel that friends will be insulted if they refuse to share. Some users may also believe that their previous injection habits have already increased their risks of infection and may continue sharing because they assume that any damage has already been done.

The Royal Pharmaceutical Society of Great Britain provides guidance on needle exchange schemes. The guidance states that pharmacists can, at their discretion, provide injection equipment to drug abusers, although it is also important to collect used equipment and dispose of it safely; a sharps container is suitable for the collection of used equipment brought in by users. Many community pharmacies participate in free syringe and needle exchange schemes in order to reduce the sharing of contaminated injection equipment. Such schemes are usually operated in collaboration with the Health Authority or Health Board. Pharmacists who decide to become involved in needle exchange schemes should follow the practice advice and professional standards provided by the Royal Pharmaceutical Society of Great Britain (Box 7.2).

An argument against needle exchange schemes is that the incidence of users choosing to inject drugs may rise as a result of increased availability. This may be true in those cases where users may have refrained from injecting because of the risks associated with using shared injecting equipment. However, measures aimed to control the spread of HIV infection should take precedence over the reduction of intravenous drug abuse.

Needle exchange schemes should not be instituted in a form that is threatening to users; in this respect, pharmacies are ideally placed to provide easy access, and are not associated with authority (e.g. compared with hospital-based needle exchange schemes). Pharmacies should be seen by users as being free of the stigma associated with specialist services and, in addition, allow for anonymity.

Pharmacists may express some concerns about becoming involved with needle exchange schemes. These include the need for:

- education and training for all pharmacy staff, which many pharmacists feel is necessary to alleviate the apprehension associated with dealing with users
- liaison with specialist services to provide support, and a place to which pharmacists can refer users for further advice
- pharmacy involvement in any given area to be wide, with a reasonable number of pharmacies taking part
- adequate arrangements for the supply of sharps containers, and their collection and disposal
- remuneration issues to be resolved.

These issues should be resolved locally in order to obtain the fullest support from all pharmacists. The most important aspect of the involvement of pharmacists in the prevention of complications associated with drug abuse by injection is their ability to reach those users in the high-risk groups. In addition, by providing advice and information, pharmacists are able to influence the user's practice of injection, and those who do not inject may be influenced never to attempt it.

Dispensing for drug users

A special prescription form, FP10(HP)Ad (in Scotland, HBP(A)), is available to doctors in NHS drug treatment centres for prescribing cocaine, dextromoramide, diamorphine, dipipanone, methadone, morphine or pethidine by instalments for addicts. In England and Wales, form FP10(MDA) is available to general practitioners for prescribing any Schedule 2 Controlled Drug to patients with drug dependency. In Scotland, general practitioners can prescribe by instalments on form GP10. It is important to be aware that all doctors who specifically want to prescribe diamorphine, cocaine or dipipanone to

Box 7.2 Practice advice for pharmacists providing needle and syringe exchange schemes

Provision of service

The aim of the service is to minimise the spread of HIV, hepatitis B and C and other blood-borne diseases which can occur as a consequence of injecting drug users sharing needles and syringes.

A protocol should be available in the pharmacy and should include procedures for:

- Minimising the risk to staff and members of the public
- Ensuring security of stock and premises
- Seeking to avoid, and action in the event of, needlestick injuries
- Dealing with spillage or contamination with potentially infected blood or body fluids.

Staff should be aware of the perceived health risks involved in providing services to drug misusers and be offered supportive prophylaxis.

The pharmacist is advised to liaise with, bearing in mind patient confidentiality:

- The local scheme co-ordinator
- The local health authority or health board
- Drug addiction clinics and drug teams.

The pharmacist is advised to work in collaboration with the police on general issues.

Service delivery

Supplies of syringes and needles should be accompanied by advice and encouragement to make use of any local drugs advisory service.

All clients should be encouraged to dispose of contaminated equipment safely, in properly designed sharps disposal containers which should be returned to the pharmacy.

Wherever possible, the person wishing to dispose of used needles and syringes should place the returns in the disposal container within the pharmacy.

The disposal container should be sited in a designated area of the pharmacy, where staff will not have inadvertent contact with contaminated waste material.

Approved health care information leaflets should be displayed if available.

Evaluation

Pharmacists are advised to keep the following records:

- Number of clients using the scheme
- Number of needles and syringes issued (preferably to each client)
- Number of used needles and syringes returned (preferably for each client)
- Dates of removal of sharps containers.

Training

Pharmacists and staff involved in the scheme should:

- Undertake any training required by Health Authority or Health Board
- Be instructed about the risk of needlestick injuries, infection and surface contamination
- Be trained to treat clients with respect and courtesy.

Standard of Good Professional Practice No. 17: Standards for Pharmacists Providing Needle and Syringe Exchange Schemes

Definition: Needle and syringe exchange schemes involve provision of clean syringes and needles and the collection of contaminated equipment used by injecting substance and drug misusers.

17.1 The pharmacist must be aware of local facilities for drug misusers and have established contacts with other health care professionals involved in the care of drug misusers.

17.2 All staff must be made aware that the pharmacy provides a needle and syringe exchange service and must be informed of the risk of infection, and precautionary measures to be taken.

17.3 Only appropriately trained staff should be permitted to be involved in a needle and syringe exchange scheme.

17.4 Supplies of needles and syringes must be made by the pharmacist or appropriately trained staff.

17.5 Clients must be encouraged to return used contaminated equipment but clean equipment must not be refused if they omit to do so.

17.6 Used equipment must be disposed of, normally by the client, in a properly designed sharps container available in the pharmacy.

17.7 Suitable arrangements must be made for the disposal of full sharps containers.

treat drug dependency require a special licence to do so.

Pharmacists have an important role in dispensing relevant medications and in ensuring their safe use. Many pharmacists undertake to monitor self-administration of methadone, or other substitution therapies, to ensure that the recipient does consume the prescribed dose on the premises. This prevents users taking the liquid home to inject, or to sell at street level. When non-compliance occurs or is suspected, the Department of Health advises pharmacists that they should agree with local drug dependency services when they can disclose this information to prescribers without the patient's consent. Patients should be made aware that pharmacists can perform this duty.

Forged prescriptions

Pharmacists should be aware that some drug users may attempt to forge prescriptions. It can be extremely difficult to detect a forged prescription, but all pharmacists should be alert to the possibility that any prescription calling for a potential substance of abuse could be a forgery.

The forger may make a fundamental error in writing the prescription, or pharmacists may get an instinctive feeling that the prescription is not genuine because of the way the patient behaves. If the prescriber's signature is known, but the patient has not previously visited the pharmacy, or is not known to be suffering from a condition that requires the drug prescribed, the signature should be scrutinised and, if possible, checked against an example on another prescription known to be genuine. Large doses or quantities should be checked with the prescriber in order to detect alterations to previously valid prescriptions.

If the prescriber's signature is not known, the prescriber must be contacted and asked to confirm that the prescription is genuine. The prescriber's telephone number must be obtained from the telephone directory, or from directory enquiries, not from the headed notepaper, as a forger may use false letter headings.

The dispensing of a forged prescription for a Controlled Drug or prescription-only medicine can constitute a criminal offence.

References

Department of Health, *et al.* (1999). *Drug Misuse and Dependence – Guidelines on Clinical Management.* London: HMSO.

Royal Pharmaceutical Society of Great Britain (2000). *Medicines, Ethics and Practice: A Guide for Pharmacists.* London: RPSGB.

Further reading

General

Centre for Pharmacy Postgradutae Education (1998). *Drug Use and Misuse – A Distance Learning Package.*

Rudgley R (1993). *The Alchemy of Culture.* London: British Museum Press.

Schuckit M A (1995). *Drug and Alcohol Abuse – A Clinical Guide to Diagnosis and Treatment.* New York: Plenum Book Company.

Wills S (1997). *Drugs of Abuse.* London: Pharmaceutical Press.

Specific subjects

Anonymous (1996). Managing abuse of anticholinergic medication in patients with psychotic disorders. *Drugs Ther Perspect* 8: 11–13.

Anonymous (1999). Few kick the cocaine habit for good. *Drugs Ther Perspect* 13: 5–8.

Brewer C (1997). The case for rapid detoxification under anaesthesia (RODA): a reply to Gossop and Strang. *Br J Intensive Care* July/August: 137–143.

Brown D T (1998) *Cannabis – the Genus Cannabis.* Amsterdam: Harwood Academic Publishers.

Galloway G P, Frederick S L, Staggers F E, *et al.* (1997). Gamma-hydroxybutyrate: an emerging drug of abuse that causes physical dependence. *Addiction* 92: 89–96.

Gossop M, Strang J (1997). Rapid anaesthetic-antagonist detoxification of heroin addicts: what origins, evidence base and clinical justification? *Br J Intensive Care* March/April: 66–69.

Hibbs J, Perper J, Winek C L (1991). An outbreak of designer drug-related deaths in Pennsylvania. *JAMA* 254: 1011–1013.

Home Office (1995). *Volatile Substance Abuse – A Report by the Advisory Council on the Misuse of Drugs*. London: HMSO.

Kalix P (1988). Khat: a plant with amphetamine effects. *J Subst Abuse Treat* 5: 163–169.

Klee H, Wright S, Rothwell J (1998). *Amphetamine Use and Treatment*. London: DoH. 13793 HP 4k IP Sep 98 SA (CLO).

Marsch L A (1998). The efficacy of methadone maintenance interventions in reducing illicit opiate use, HIV risk behaviour and criminality: a meta-analysis. *Addiction* 93: 515–532.

Monzon M J, Lainez J M (1998). Chronic daily headache: long-term prognosis following inpatient treatment. *Headache Q* 9: 326–330.

Paxton R, Chapple P (1996). Misuse of over-the-counter medicines: a survey in one English county. *Pharm J* 256: 313–315.

Preston A (1996). *The Methadone Briefing*. London: Island Press.

Schwartz R H (1995). LSD – its rise, fall and renewed popularity among high school students. *Ped Clinics N Am* 42: 403–413.

Ward J, Hall W, Mattick R P (1999). Role of maintenance treatment in opioid dependence. *Lancet* 353: 221–226.

Useful addresses

Pharmacy Misuse Advisory Group (PharMAG)
Dr Trish Shorrock
Needle Exchange Co-ordinator
Leicester Community Drug Team
Paget House
2 West Street
Leicester LE1 6XP
Tel: 0116 225 6400

Families Anonymous
Unit 37, The Doddington and Rollo Community Association
Charlotte Despard Avenue
London SW11 5JE
Tel: 020 7498 4680

Institute for the Study of Drug Dependence (ISDD)
Waterbridge House
32–36 Loman Street
London SE1 0EE
Tel: 020 7928 1211

National Association for Mental Health (MIND)
15–19 Broadway
London E15 4BQ
Tel: 0345 666163

Narcotics Anonymous
202 City Road
London EC1V 2PH
Tel: 020 7251 4007

Release
388 Old Street
London EC1V 9LT
Tel: 020 7729 9904

Re-Solv
30a High Street
Stone
Staffordshire ST15 8AW
Tel: 01785 817885

Standing Conference on Drug Abuse
Waterbridge House
32–36 Loman Street
London SE1 0EE
Tel: 020 7928 9500

TACADE
1 Hulme Place
The Crescent
Salford
Manchester M5 4QA
Tel: 0161 745 8925

Terence Higgins Trust
52–54 Grays Inn Road
London WC1X 8JU
Tel: 020 7831 0330

Turning Point
New Loom House
101 Backchurch Lane
London E1 1LU
Tel: 020 7702 2300

8

Sport and exercise

Steven Kayne

Promotion of sport and exercise for health

The apparent benefits of physical activity were recognised in some of the earliest civilisations, yet it is only relatively recently that the important and complex interaction between physical activity, physical fitness and mental and physical health has been acknowledged. It is now widely recognised that regular physical activity induces a variety of physiological changes (*see* The physiology of exercise *below*) that promote good health, whereas lack of activity can have a deleterious effect. For example, the relative risk of coronary heart disease associated with physical inactivity may be doubled. Although exercise does not necessarily guarantee an increased life expectancy, it can certainly improve the quality of daily life and delay deterioration in fitness due to age and inactivity.

During the 1960s, the Council of Europe put forward a charter, 'Sport for All', which included a wider range of activities than traditional competitive sports. This was followed in the UK by the creation of a Minister for Sport (a junior minister in the Department of Environment) and a national Sports Council, with responsibility for non-competitive activities (e.g. keep fit and yoga).

The 'Sport for All' campaign in the UK was officially launched in 1972. The Sports Council was subsequently replaced by four regional Councils in Belfast, Cardiff, Edinburgh and London. These bodies now work together with health agencies and local authorities in their own regions, undertaking projects and campaigns that seek to maintain current levels of participation and encourage, wherever possible, new participants to take up sport. The government also promotes physical activity as a means of improving public health through the Health Education Authority (HEA). The latter also deals with a range of other health aspects as detailed in Chapter 1. Despite the improvements made in the facilities available (e.g. a steady increase in the number of indoor sports facilities, swimming pools and golf courses), the ultimate aim of 'Sport for All' is still some way off. Participation in physical activity is clearly age-related, with a steady decline in activity amongst older groups. Only a third of people in the 55 and over age group participate in some form of exercise, typically walking, dancing, aerobics or golf. This rate is less than half that of the 16 to 24 age group. Surprisingly, the rate of decline in interest for indoor activities with age is even greater.

In some instances, physical activity may be a regular part of a person's normal working life (e.g. building or mining) or home life (e.g. gardening). However, increasing automation and the use of labour-saving devices significantly reduces the amount of activity required in some occupations, and many involve no physical work at all. It is, therefore, essential that anyone involved in sedentary occupations should reserve some of their leisure time for recreational physical activity.

Physical activity is a generic term that involves three elements:

- movement of the body produced by the skeletal muscle
- resultant energy expenditure that varies in its intensity
- a positive correlation with physical fitness.

Physical activity is sometimes called 'habitual sports activity' (HSA), particularly when it forms an important part of people's leisure activities. Sport and exercise, both structured activities, are often considered as two subcategories of HSA, and are ideal for those who are otherwise unable to achieve the desired levels of activity in their working life. Department of Employment surveys have shown that the average annual holiday entitlement for most full-time employees has doubled over the last 25 years from two to four or more weeks, and the average number of hours in a basic working week has dropped from 43 to around 35 hours. There is, therefore, more leisure time available for a greater number of people than ever before. More campaigns are required to bring to the attention of individuals the need to devote some of this time to regular physical activity.

It is not necessary to exercise at the level of elite athletes to attain health benefits: fitness may be improved at any age. Many people are not prepared to make time or do not have the inclination to take up a sport; they should be encouraged to seek alternative methods of exercise (*see* Participation in sports and exercise *below*), either in the privacy of their own homes, or just by walking briskly at every available opportunity. In fact, the annual General Household Surveys in Great Britain have shown that walking two or more miles is the most popular exercise activity. Learning the rules and skill for a sport and participating in organised events may provide additional benefits for improving self-esteem and self-confidence. Belonging to a sports club may also improve social skills as a result of interaction with other people.

Pharmacists can play a valuable part in promoting an increase in physical activity by being readily available to answer questions and offer advice to members of the public who wish to take up sport or exercise. Those suffering with chronic conditions or disabilities that preclude intensive exercise, but who nevertheless wish to partake in some form of physical activity will, in particular, require careful counselling. Advice may also be sought about the management of minor sports injuries or about drugs and dressings needed for sports club medical bags. The opportunity to impress on youngsters the dangers and futility of attempting to improve performance by taking drugs should not be missed.

Why people participate in sport

Considering the reason for individuals taking part in sports activities can often help with an assessment of the likely severity of an injury and the urgency with which an individual will seek treatment.

Competitive sport

Individuals whose sole aim is to improve their overall fitness should be advised to approach competitive sport with extreme caution. The additional psychological pressures of competition can significantly alter one's attitude. Most problems in this sector are dealt with by club medical staff or sports injury clinics.

Health

Appropriate regular exercise will help an individual enjoy enhanced well-being and encourage recovery from a medical condition. The exercise prescription will emphasise the necessary elements of activity. Accidents due to over-exuberance will usually be referred to a general practitioner, but clients may present in the pharmacy with simple sprains and strains or allergies.

Recreational sport

This is the enjoyment of sport for social aspects or for some gentle exercise to fill leisure time. People in this group are most likely to consult pharmacists for advice on injuries and illnesses.

The physiology of exercise

To appreciate the reasons for the benefits of sport and exercise (*see* The benefits of sport and exercise *below*), it is necessary to understand the physiology of exercise. Sports and exercise are not without their own health-risks (*see* The risks of sport and exercise *below*), and a knowledge of physiology will also enable an assessment to be made of an individual's capacity for activity, and whether or not medical referral is essential before taking part.

Energy is necessary to enable all functions of the body to be carried out, and is derived from the oxidation of glucose. Glucose is obtained from the metabolism of carbohydrates, fats and proteins, and undergoes oxidation in all cells of the body (cellular respiration) to produce carbon dioxide, water and energy. The energy is used to convert adenosine diphosphate (ADP) to adenosine triphosphate (ATP); the phosphate bonds of ATP store energy, which is yielded when required by hydrolysis of the terminal bond, forming ADP in the process. Complete oxidation of glucose proceeds through three stages (*see* Figure 8.1): glycolysis to produce pyruvic acid; the Krebs' cycle; and the electron transport chain. Oxygen is required for the latter two stages, and this process is therefore termed aerobic respiration. Oxygen is taken into the body during respiration at the same time that carbon dioxide is expelled. The heart pumps oxygenated blood received from the pulmonary circulation to the rest of the body, and deoxygenated blood to the lungs for oxygenation. Oxygen binds with haemoglobin in erythrocytes for transportation in the systemic circulation to the tissues. It therefore follows that during exercise, which increases the overall energy demand, all these processes must increase in efficiency to provide the extra oxygen required.

Anaerobic respiration occurs during sustained muscle activity, when there is insufficient oxygen to meet the requirements of aerobic respiration. The pyruvic acid produced by the oxidation of glucose cannot be completely oxidised and is converted to lactic acid (*see* Figure 8.1). Approximately 80% of the lactic acid is transported to the liver for conversion to glucose or glycogen, and the remainder accumulates in the muscles.

Most forms of exercise utilise both aerobic and anaerobic respiration.

Aerobic exercise

Exercise involving aerobic respiration requires that the oxygen demands of the active muscle must be fully met once the initial period of adjustment is over. To achieve this, there must be increases in respiration rate and depth, cardiac output and blood-flow to the muscles. Regular aerobic exercise induces adaptive changes so that future exercising becomes comparatively easier. However, this is not a long-term effect, and previous levels of unfitness will return if exercise sessions are discontinued. Aerobic exercise is of relatively low intensity, but can be of fairly long duration. It involves the movement of large muscle groups and causes participants to breathe more deeply, adding to the workload of the heart and lungs and raising the heart rate. Such exercise performed regularly will improve the cardiovascular and respiratory systems. Examples include walking, jogging, dancing and swimming. The capacity to follow these activities reflects an ability to take in and use oxygen and depends on three factors:

- effective external respiration
- effective oxygen transport from the lungs to cells
- effective use of oxygen within the cells.

Aerobic capacity is usually referred to as VO_2 max, the maximum rate of utilisation of atmospheric oxygen during continuous activity. It is expressed as mL/min/kg body weight. The scale for a man in his twenties might range from 38 (very poor) to 60 (excellent); for a man in his sixties the range would be from 20 to 40. A person's VO_2 max may be determined under laboratory conditions using a treadmill and apparatus to collect expired air. Inactivity decreases VO_2 max, whereas aerobic training for a few weeks can improve it substantially. VO_2 max improves as the maximum cardiac output increases (*see below*). VO_2 max starts to decline after 20 years of age, but the rate of decline can be decreased by regular exercise.

Anaerobic exercise

Exercise involving anaerobic respiration does not rely on a supply of oxygen to the muscles from the circulation, but can only be sustained for one to two minutes, as opposed to aerobic exercise, which in a fit subject, can be sustained for hours.

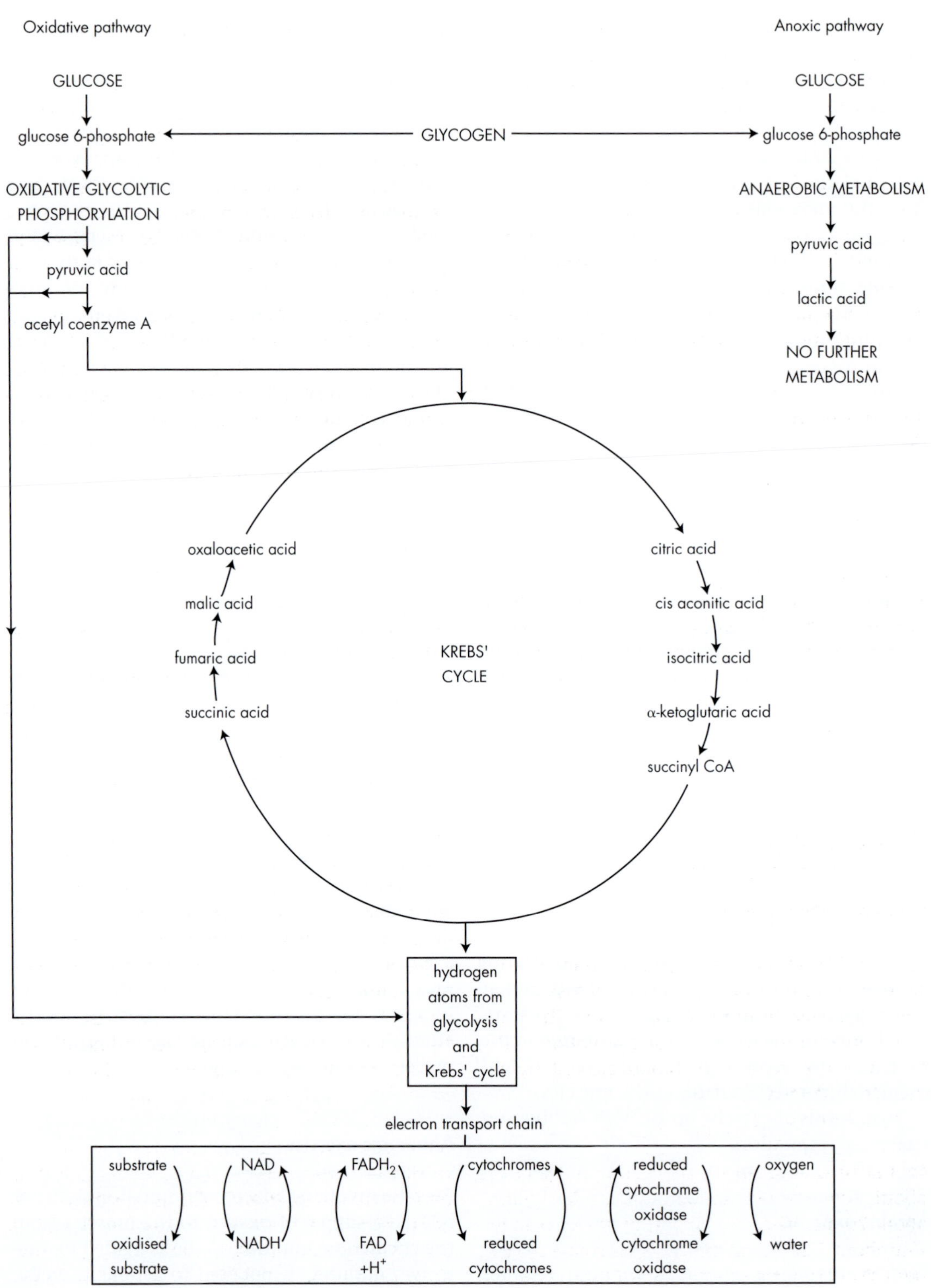

Figure 8.1 Outline pathways of glucose metabolism.

Anaerobic respiration occurs during short bursts of extremely strenuous activity (e.g. 100 metres sprint), when the supply of oxygen is insufficient to keep up with the exercising muscles (*see below*).

Isotonic exercise

Isotonic (endurance or dynamic) exercise involves muscle work during movement (e.g. cycling, running or swimming), and is of value in improving stamina and endurance. Isotonic exercise is dependent mainly on aerobic respiration.

Isometric exercise

Isometric (power or static) exercise (e.g. handgrip or weight lifting) involves a sustained increase in contraction of antagonistic muscles without movement. It is primarily employed to increase muscle strength. As a result, those that train regularly using isometric exercises are likely to be heavier than endurance athletes. They also tend to have more deposits of body fat. Isometric exercise is dependent mainly on anaerobic respiration.

Most forms of exercise employ both isometric and isotonic techniques.

Effects on physiological systems

Cardiovascular system

The cardiac output (CO) is the volume of blood pumped into the aorta from the left ventricle of the heart every minute. It is equal to the pulse rate (PR) multiplied by the stroke volume (SV), which is the volume of blood ejected by the ventricles at each heartbeat:

$$CO = PR \times SV$$

In a normal adult heart, the resting pulse rate is about 70 beats/minute, and the stroke volume about 70 mL. The cardiac output at rest is therefore about 5.25 litres/minute. To increase oxygen perfusion of the tissues to cope with the increased demand created by exercise, the cardiac output must be increased by raising the stroke volume or the pulse rate, or, as in response to exercise at altitude, both.

The pulse rate is controlled in part by the autonomic nervous system: the sympathetic division increases the rate; and the parasympathetic division lowers it. In people who have not been used to regular vigorous exercise, the cardiac output is mainly raised by an increase in the pulse rate. Physical training, however, increases the parasympathetic tone of the vagus nerve, and there is a much smaller rise in pulse rate for a given workload. Trained subjects, therefore, feel more comfortable than untrained individuals. In order to achieve the desired increase in cardiac output, trained individuals show a greater rise in stroke volume, which is produced by an increased ventricular capacity of up to 30%. This causes the heart to enlarge, but must be distinguished from enlargement caused by cardiac disease, in which the increased size is a result of muscular hypertrophy. The increase in size of the ventricular chamber reduces the pressure developed during systole. The resting pulse rate of highly trained individuals also falls, and may be as low as 40 beats/minute in elite athletes.

The cardiac reserve is the maximum that the cardiac output can be increased above normal during vigorous activity, and is expressed as a percentage. In the average adult, this reserve may be 400%, but trained athletes may achieve a 600% cardiac reserve. The actual cardiac output in trained athletes may reach 30 litres/minute or more during exercise. These cardiac changes reduce the work that the heart has to perform for a given workload and makes exercising progressively easier. These effects occur as a result of long-term isotonic exercise and may be apparent after a few weeks.

The optimum level of aerobic exercise needed by individuals varies with age, general health and fitness, and how active one has been in the past. In order to make appreciable gains in aerobic fitness, the heart rate during exercise must be raised above the resting heart rate by about 60% of the difference between an individual's resting and maximum heart rate. This is called the critical threshold, and above this, exercise is said to have a significant effect. In most subjects, movement should be sufficiently robust to raise the pulse to between 140 and 160 beats/minute in order to exceed the critical threshold. In isometric exercise, the arterial pressure rises, which increases the tension on the wall of the left ventricle. The cardiac output changes little and isometric exercise does not greatly improve stamina. Cardiac output increases linearly with increases in the intensity of aerobic exercise up to exhaustion. This is the result of increases in heart rate and stroke volume. The latter increases because the heart muscle contracts more forcefully, facilitating a more complete emptying of the ventricles with each heartbeat. Harmful effects are unlikely, provided that exercise levels increase slowly over a period of weeks, particularly if people have been following a sedentary life style.

The occurrence of occasional sudden and premature death in both amateur and professional athletes who appear to exhibit all the attributes of cardiorespiratory health and fitness has raised awareness of the underlying causes. Concern has been expressed as to the correct evaluation of conditioned athletes. The 'Athletes' heart' represents a gradual enlargement of the ventricles, but without a corresponding thickening of the walls. The heart beats more slowly but with greater force to eject a larger volume of blood in its stroke volume. Healthy, asymptomatic athletes are likely to alarm their physicians because of seemingly dangerous disturbances of heart rate and/or conduction. Arrhymias in highly trained athletes are, in fact, common.

Of all the cardiovascular measurements carried out on patients in hospital, the electrocardiogram (ECG) is considered to be one of the most important. Interpretation of the trace allows causal identification of an abnormal heart rhythm or an evolving heart attack. Physiological adaptations of the heart to prolonged, intense physical exercise produce a range of changes in the ECG. These changes are of interest because of their frequency and close resemblance to pathological changes occurring in certain organic heart diseases. The heart reacts to acute physical stress with a rapid increase in heart rate and a resulting increase in contractility. Regular physical training results in a permanent adaptation process in the heart that is not immediately reversible. The amount of training necessary to obtain adaptations in the ECG is unclear. An athlete who has ceased involvement in a moderate level of training within the past few months will still exhibit ECG changes associated with physical exercise. This should be borne in mind if evacuation to hospital and testing subsequent to an event is necessary as a result of either collapse or injury.

One way of differentiating between a 'normal' athletic heart and an athletic patient is to instruct the individual to stop training for some months. If the ECG abnormalities persist, they are more likely to be the result of pathological processes than of physical conditioning. However, such action is unlikely to meet with an athlete's immediate co-operation!

The heart, brain and skeletal muscles have increased oxygen demands during exercise, and blood must be redirected to these organs away from other parts of the body (e.g. gastro-intestinal tract). In vigorous activity, the blood supply to the heart tissue is increased by up to four or five times. The need for diversion of the systemic blood-flow decreases with training because the oxygen-extracting ability of the muscles improves (*see below*). The result is that the individual feels more comfortable during exercise as a result of fewer gastro-intestinal symptoms.

Regular exercising increases the network of blood capillaries supplying the muscles and improves the overall efficiency of the circulation. This has the added effect of lowering peripheral resistance, which has a beneficial effect on blood pressure.

The principal function of haemoglobin, which is contained in erythrocytes, is to transport oxygen in the blood. The normal blood-haemoglobin concentration is 14–18 g/100 mL of blood for males, and 12–16 g/100 mL of blood for females. A constant enhanced demand for oxygen by the tissues (e.g. as a result of physical training) increases the number of erythrocytes and, consequently, the amount of haemoglobin. Plasma volume may also rise, with the result that the haemoglobin concentration remains constant or may even drop, suggesting anaemia ('sports anaemia'). However, the actual oxygen-carrying capacity is higher because the total amount of haemoglobin present is greater. These rises in highly trained individuals may approach 40% above average values. Carbon monoxide, present in tobacco smoke and exhaust fumes from motor vehicles, binds with haemoglobin much more strongly than oxygen and, therefore, substantially reduces the oxygen-carrying capacity of the blood. Exercise can aid the removal of carbon monoxide from haemoglobin.

The core temperature, which is the deep body temperature measured by the oral or rectal method, may rise up to 41°C during intensive exercise. In order for this heat to be lost by conduction, convection and radiation from the skin, the volume of blood perfusing the skin increases during strenuous activity. Heat is also lost by evaporation of sweat. If any of these mechanisms are blocked, or the individual is unfit, heat stroke (*see* The risks of sport and exercise *below*) or even sudden death may occur.

Muscles

With regular training, local adaptive changes enable the muscles to increase the quantity of oxygen extracted from blood and improve its utilisation. There is an increase in the number of muscle capillaries, and the number and size of muscle mitochondria. In the average person at rest, about 15% of the cardiac output is used by the muscles. This percentage increases with exercise, and in trained athletes at maximal exercise may approach 90%. Muscles are also able to adapt to use greater amounts of lipids as an energy source. Training increases the bulk, strength and stamina of muscles, which are able to function longer aerobically (*see above*) as a result of improved oxygenation. The increase in muscle size is more likely to be a result of an increase in fibre size rather than number of fibres. Training also improves the strength of tendons and ligaments.

The energy required for muscular activity is produced from anaerobic and aerobic respiration. The mechanisms have been explained above and are summarised in Figure 8.2.

Creatine (Cr), or methylguanidine-acetic acid, is a physiologically active substance indispensable to muscle contraction. The normal daily intake of Cr is less than 1 g, obtained mainly from meat, fish and other animal products. However, the estimated daily requirement for the average individual is double that amount. The balance is produced in the body, mainly by the kidneys, together with smaller amounts from the liver and pancreas. The intake of exogenous Cr in the diet appears to play a role in the control of endogenous Cr synthesis by means of a feedback mechanism. Cr is formed from three amino acids: arginine, glycine and methionine. It reaches the muscle cells by an active membrane transport system.

There is a store of 120–140 g of Cr in the body, of which 98% is stored in muscle. Approximately 30% of muscle Cr is free; the balance is bound as phosphorous creatine (PCr), which is replenished at a rate of 20 mg/kg/day following its irreversible degradation to Cr. PCr is present in resting muscle in a concentration three to four times that of ATP, the immediate energy source for muscle contraction. If cellular ATP concentration falls too far, fatigue occurs.

The rate of ATP hydrolysis to ADP and free phosphorus (P) is set by the power output of the muscles (i.e. the intensity of the exercise). Regeneration of ATP at a rate close to that of its hydrolysis is vital if fatigue is to be delayed. Indeed, a decline in the rate of resynthesis of ATP as a result of depletion of PCr is recognised as a

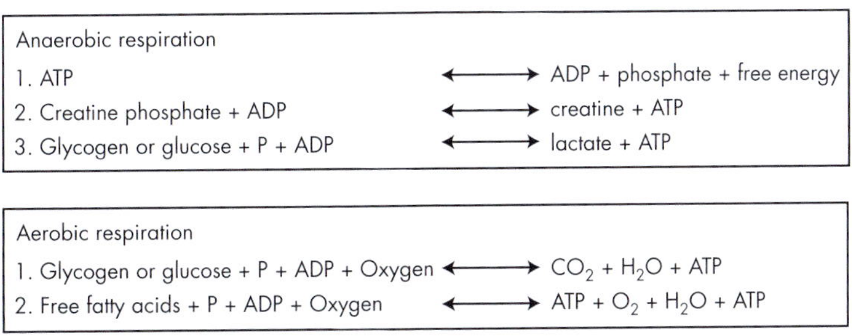

Figure 8.2 Energy for muscular contraction.

possible cause of reduction in muscle power in maximal intensity exercise.

In the regeneration of ATP, transfer of the phosphate group from PCr is catalysed by the enzyme creatine kinase (Cr kinase), resulting in the restoration of ATP and the release of free Cr. The creatine kinase reaction is extremely rapid. As the muscle PCr concentration can fall to almost zero, it is likely to contribute significantly to the energy supply required for short bursts of high intensity exercise. During the recovery stage following exercise, the Cr kinase reaction is reversed using oxygen resulting from a metabolic process in the mitochondria.

The lactic acid that accumulates as a result of anaerobic metabolism (*see* Figure 8.2) during sustained muscle activity must eventually be catabolised, and the extra oxygen required for this process is termed the 'oxygen debt'. The additional oxygen is 'repaid' at the end of the activity by a continued increase in the depth and rate of respiration.

Muscle fatigue and pain is caused by a combination of factors, including the build up of lactic acid and carbon dioxide in the tissues and a reduced supply of oxygen. To avoid fatigue, adequate levels of ATP must be maintained in the tissues to supply the energy required. As fatigue develops, levels of ATP, phosphocreatine and high energy phosphates decrease, and levels of lactate, ADP, inorganic phosphates and hydrogen ions increase. In high intensity exercise, glycolysis will result in the formation of pyruvate at a rate higher than that at which it can be removed by oxidative metabolism. This leads to a build up of lactate within the muscle. Muscle pH falls as a result of the glycolysis, and is thought to be involved in the development of fatigue. The breakdown of PCr acts as a buffer mechanism within the cells, delaying the point at which a critically low pH is reached. An increased availability of PCr for breakdown may increase the buffering capacity in the muscles (*see* Ergogenic aids *below*).

All these biochemical changes may cause symptoms of fatigue. The response of the muscle filaments becomes progressively weaker in the face of sustained contraction, and activity must either cease or switch to the slower aerobic pace. Proponents of the 'burn' as the goal to be attained in 'aerobics' (aerobic exercises) are, in fact, promoting an anaerobic activity.

Sprinting is a particular athletic event in which a short distance (e.g. 60 to 100 metres) is run at high speed. However, sprinting may also be employed in everyday life (e.g. in running for a bus or, at its most extreme, to escape from danger). Sprinting requires anaerobic metabolism in the muscles, and for unfit individuals, any increase in activity above their normal level may be comparable to a 'sprint' in terms of muscle metabolism and fatigue. If oxygen were provided at a sufficient rate to keep pace with oxidative processes to produce enough energy for a sprint, the blood supply to the muscles would have to increase to such an extent that there would be no room in the muscles for sufficient myofibrils to sustain the contraction, or enough mitochondria to cope with the oxidative processes. Anaerobic metabolism, therefore, is a means of allowing short periods of sustained muscle contraction. Longer periods require aerobic metabolism and the activity must therefore continue at a slower pace (e.g. marathon running). Regular aerobic training will, however, increase the capacity for sprinting by increasing the number of capillaries in the muscles.

There are two types of fibre present in skeletal muscles: fast fibres, which contract quickly and with great strength, and are suitable for anaerobic exercise; and slow fibres, which are more suitable for aerobic exercise. The proportion of each type of fibre present in the muscles of an individual is genetically determined, and a born sprinter is unlikely to become an elite marathon runner or vice versa. However, training does improve performance above baseline in both types.

Respiratory system

The total lung capacity (TLC) in adult males is approximately six litres, but at rest only 10% of this is used. The tidal volume is the amount of air that moves into and out of the lungs with each breath, and at rest is 500 mL. Of this, 150 mL occupies the dead space (i.e. those parts of the airway not involved in gaseous exchange), which means that only 350 mL reaches the alveoli. The tidal volume increases during exercise: at maximal breathing, when the largest proportion of the TLC is used, it is referred to as the vital capacity (VC). This may be between 3 and 5 litres in adult males, which still leaves a residual volume of 1 to 1.5 litres. The VC of males is 50% greater than that of females. The effort required for respiration is minimal at rest, but obviously increases as activity increases, and additional muscles are employed.

The average respiration rate at rest is 12 respirations/minute. Since the tidal volume is 500 mL, the average volume of air inspired every minute is six litres. The maximum breathing capacity (maximum ventilation volume) in adult males in a normal atmosphere is 125 litres/minute. The volume of air taken in during a deep inspiration may be as much as 3.6 litres. Exercise increases the rate of respiration and the volume of air inspired per minute.

Respiration rate is controlled primarily by the concentration of carbon dioxide in the blood. Thus, if the concentration falls, respiration rate decreases until the blood-carbon dioxide concentration rises to normal levels. Oxygen only acts as a stimulus if there is a severe reduction in blood-oxygen concentration, because haemoglobin remains at least 85% saturated until quite low oxygen concentrations are approached. However, with further reductions in oxygen concentrations to extremely low levels, anoxia of the inspiratory area in the medulla results in a diminished response to impulses received from chemoreceptors, and breathing may stop altogether.

Overbreathing immediately before an event is thought by some athletes to improve performance because a few vital seconds may be gained by temporarily removing the desire to breathe. Carbon dioxide is flushed out from the lungs, reducing the blood concentration to such an extent that respiration temporarily stops. The oxygen remaining in the lungs diffuses slowly into the blood, but eventually a very low blood-oxygen concentration stimulates breathing. At about the same time, or shortly afterwards, the blood-carbon dioxide concentration rises sufficiently to act as a further stimulus. The interaction of both stimuli are required to maintain respiration. It is possible to hold one's breath for up to one minute after a deep inspiration, and this too may be used to gain time, especially in swimming. Eventually, respiration is stimulated by rising blood-carbon dioxide concentrations. Athletes may combine breath-holding with overbreathing in an effort to further increase the time of non-breathing. However, this practice should not be encouraged as it may produce anoxia severe enough to cause syncope, which is particularly dangerous for swimmers.

Alveolar diffusion capacity, which is a measure of the gaseous exchange efficiency of the alveoli, varies even among healthy subjects, and training cannot increase this function above an individual's inherent maximum. Thus, the oxygen saturation of blood will be different among highly trained athletes. However, through intensive training, the muscles can adapt to a certain amount of oxygen lack (*see above*).

The main consequence of sport and exercise at high altitude results from the lower availability of oxygen in the air. Lower oxygen pressure in the inspired air gives a lower oxygen pressure in the alveoli; this in turn leads to less oxygen in the blood. At sea level, blood haemoglobin is 96% saturated; at an altitude of 2300 metres, saturation falls to 90%. Below about 1500 metres, there is little appreciable fall in VO_2max, but thereafter there is a 10% drop per 1000 metres gain in height. Physiological adaptation results in increased pulmonary ventilation. Simultaneously, the heart increases its output by up to a third, raising both pulse rate and stroke volume. With time, the body produces new erythrocytes and the blood oxygen carrying capacity rises. Muscle enzymes also adapt and become more efficient.

The benefits of sport and exercise

Exercise and the maintenance of good health

Some benefits of regular exercise to the participant are shown in Table 8.1.

The functioning of muscles and the respiratory and cardiovascular systems is improved by regular exercise (*see* The physiology of exercise *above*), and many studies have shown that this is a major contributory factor to the reduced risk for

Table 8.1 Benefits of exercise

Benefit	Examples of typical outcomes
Decreases incidence of disease	Reduced hypertension
	Decreased risk of diabetes
	Less discomfort during pregnancy
	Reduced incidence of osteoporosis
	Less respiratory disease
Improved cardiovascular and respiratory systems	Decreased risk of heart attack
	Relief from cardiac disease
	Increased capacity for work
	Faster recovery after strenuous activity
Reduced stress	Reduced anxiety, tension
	Enhanced quality of sleep
	Easier to relax
	Improved reactivity to stress
Improved appearance	Reduced body weight
	Enhanced self-esteem
	Decrease in amount of food eaten
Increased flexibility	Decreased incidence of low back pain
	Joints, tendons and ligaments more flexible
	Relief in arthritis

ischaemic heart disease. Generally, the forms of exercise of most benefit to the heart are those that involve the movement of large muscles and an increase in blood-flow to the tissues (i.e. aerobic exercises). Exercise is also of value in maintaining ideal body-weight, which is itself of benefit in reducing the risk for ischaemic heart disease. Exercise cannot replace cardiac tissue that is already damaged, but may aid in the improvement of residual performance (*see* Exercise in the management of disease *below*). Other studies have shown reduced risks for cancer, hypertension, and stroke, and improved glucose tolerance.

Inactivity is associated with loss of bone mass; conversely, exercise has been shown to increase bone mass and may aid in the prevention of osteoporosis. This effect may occur at any age, and in the elderly, the increase in bone mass is greater than the amount of bone lost. Similarly, exercise can prevent the muscle atrophy that occurs with inactivity, as well as reducing the stiffness associated with arthritis or other conditions that limit joint movement. However, exercise is contra-indicated during the acute stages of inflammation in osteoarthritis or rheumatoid arthritis.

Exercise has psychological benefits that are particularly marked in depressed or anxious patients. Some workers have claimed that this is caused by the release in the brain of endorphins, although the evidence is still inconclusive. Others have postulated that exercise may promote feelings of increased self-confidence or reverse the feelings of apathy commonly experienced by depressed individuals. Whatever the mechanism, it is generally agreed that regular exercise is of benefit in the prevention and management of depressive disorders.

Some studies have shown that exercise is of value in stress management and prevention, although the evidence is inconclusive and the mechanism unclear. The effect may be mediated through the same pathways that improve anxiety and depression. Alternatively, it may simply be that exercise represents an active form of relaxation (i.e. by concentrating on something different for a short time, allowing individuals to clear the day's problems from their minds). It may also be a positive way of relieving frustrations. However, it is important that the chosen form of exercise does not represent additional stress, and it is suggested that for those with stressful lifestyles, aggressive competitive sports should be avoided unless the subject finds them particularly enjoyable and rewarding.

Exercise during pregnancy is of benefit to delivery, and has been associated with a reduced incidence of abortion and prematurity; it does not appear to adversely affect the well-being of the newborn. However, careful consideration of the type of activity undertaken is necessary: anaerobic exercises, contact sports, horse riding, skiing, water-skiing, SCUBA diving or any activity involving extreme environmental changes are not recommended. Any other form of physical activity that may have been carried out before pregnancy may be continued in moderation, avoiding vigorous exercise, particularly during the third trimester. The intensity and duration of exercise should be reduced as pregnancy proceeds. For those who previously did not undertake regular exercise but who wish to start a programme during pregnancy, walking and swimming are the best options. It has been suggested that three sessions a week lasting no more than 30 minutes each is adequate and should not be exceeded. The risks of exercise during pregnancy are discussed in The risks in medical conditions *below*.

Exercise only produces long-term benefits if it is carried out regularly. Protection against disease stops when regular activity ceases; cardiovascular disease is not prevented in old age because of a high level of fitness when young, unless fitness is maintained during the intervening years.

Exercise in the management of disease

The following conditions have been shown to respond positively to exercise. Activities may involve both aerobic and anaerobic phases of exercise.

Arthritis

Exercise for patients with arthritis remains the subject of considerable debate, as it has long been known to exacerbate both inflammatory and degenerative arthritis. However, anaerobic exercise has been found to be beneficial in the treatment of chronic arthritis amongst carefully chosen patients. The aim here is to make muscles work as hard as they can without causing extra pain. This is achieved by lifting weights of differing amounts according to individual requirements. There are two different approaches: isotonic exercise makes the muscles move the joint through the maximum range available; the aim of isometric exercise is to use weights to tense the muscles without actually moving the joint. Exercise is contra-indicated during the acute inflammatory stages of osteoarthritis, and in rheumatoid arthritis, when it is limited by pain. During rehabilitation, physiotherapy and regulated exercise programmes contribute to the restoration and maintenance of full muscle functions so as to give maximal support to the inflamed joints.

Asthma

A supervised and controlled programme of exercises has been shown to be beneficial in those with obstructive airways diseases (e.g. asthma or chronic bronchitis) in reducing dyspnoea and improving exercise tolerance. The most suitable exercises are those that can be performed at home (e.g. stair-climbing), with regular assessments at out-patient clinics.

Atherosclerosis

Exercise increases the plasma-HDL concentration, which has a beneficial effect on cholesterol levels, and reduces the concentration of the more harmful LDLs (*see* Chapter 2, Fats and cholesterol). It also increases fibrinolysis and, therefore, aids in the dissolution of blood clots. These properties may help to explain the epidemiological evidence linking sustained regular exercise with the prevention or slowing of atherosclerosis.

Coronary disease

Exercise may be of benefit after myocardial infarction in reducing the oxygen requirements of the residual heart muscle for a given work-load. Patients are, therefore, more able to cope comfortably with everyday activities and meet the demands imposed by occasional increased effort. It is not recommended that cardiac patients undertake isometric exercise (*see* The physiology of exercise *above*), because the increase in blood pressure during exercise may place too great a strain on the heart. Patients should not attempt to design their own exercise programmes, but should be trained under medical supervision.

Regular exercise has a beneficial effect in hypertension as it eventually brings about a reduction in blood pressure. The decrease is of the order of 13/12 mmHg, although the fall is not so substantial in normotensive subjects. Regular exercise also reduces the blood pressure response to a given work-load. Hypertensive patients should avoid severe, prolonged isometric exercises (*see* The physiology of exercise *above*) because of the association with a rapid increase in blood pressure. Moderate isotonic exercises are permissible once blood pressure is under control with antihypertensive drugs. However, the response of patients must first be determined.

Diabetes

In insulin-dependent (Type I) diabetes, activities help lower the blood glucose level. Specific recommendations vary according to the patient's degree of metabolic control and any associated conditions. Hypoglycaemia is a complication that must be carefully watched. In non-insulin-dependent (Type II) diabetes, aerobic exercise is also the exercise of choice. It should involve the large muscle groups of the legs and upper body and should be performed frequently. Because the majority of these patients are obese and are often sedentary, the development of an exercise programme can present a considerable challenge. Concordance may be low.

The recommendation to use exercise training therapeutically to lower glucose and lipid levels stems from the pronounced effects of acute exercise on the metabolism of glucose, insulin and lipids. A single exercise session improves and partially normalises both insulin responsiveness and sensitivity for glucose utilisation. Exercise training has been shown to improve insulin sensitivity in those with Type II diabetes, probably as a result of enhanced insulin action in skeletal muscle. Because of the limited duration of benefit, exercise must be performed routinely to be effective (i.e. at least every second day). The possible therapeutic benefits of exercise training for people with Type II diabetes include the following:

- reduced blood glucose and insulin levels
- improved oral glucose tolerance
- improved insulin secretion response to oral glucose stimulus
- improved peripheral and hepatic insulin sensitivity
- improved blood lipid and lipoprotein concentration
- decreased hypertension
- reduced risk of cardiovascular disease
- increased physical fitness
- increased energy expenditure and resulting weight reduction
- enhanced quality of life and feeling of well-being.

Precautions need to be taken by diabetics during exercise. With proliferative retinopathy, a common complication of the disease, exercise may result in retinal or vitreous haemorrhage. Strenuous exercise can lead to soft tissue or joint injuries in persons with peripheral neuropathy.

Obesity

Obesity has been linked with adverse effects on health (*see* Chapter 2, Diet and related diseases), and is generally associated with lack of exercise. However, inactivity cannot really be considered a sole aetiological factor of obesity, but rather a consequence, as once obesity is established, the level of exercise tends to fall. Regular endurance exercise training can favourably modify the abdominal fat distribution profile that is typical in older men and women and can reduce obesity, especially if combined with a suitable weight-reducing diet (*see* Chapter 2, Dietary needs of specific groups). This is particularly important for those individuals whose rate of weight-reduction appears to be slowing despite a drastic reduction in dietary energy intake. The American College of Sports Medicine recommends that people should engage in regular physical activity that promotes a daily energy expenditure of at least 300 calories. As the fat-free mass (FFM) decreases with reducing weight, so too does the basal metabolic rate (BMR), which means that slimmers have to further reduce their energy intake to continue losing weight. This may be offset to some extent by increasing the level of physical activity, which increases the overall energy expenditure. Exercise does not, however, increase the BMR and the increase in energy expenditure as a result of physical activity is not sufficient to be used as a means of reducing weight alone; it is only of benefit as an adjunct to dietary measures.

Osteoporosis

Osteoporosis is the most common metabolic bone disease; it literally means 'porous bones'. It may be defined as 'a reduction in bone mass leading to fracture upon minimal trauma'. In women, there is often a period of rapid bone loss beginning at the menopause and lasting for about ten years. The condition is often the underlying cause of fractures of the vertebral column, wrist and hip suffered by post-menopausal women. Several studies have demonstrated a retardation of the rate of bone loss in post-menopausal women with aerobic exercise, compared with non-exercising controls. An increase in bone density has also been reported. In one trial, spinal bone density increased with 45 minutes of light aerobic training twice weekly for eight months in women aged from 50 to 73. Total body calcium has also been shown to increase in a group performing aerobic exercise three times per week over a period of one year. Exactly how this is achieved is the subject of considerable debate. Some suggestions are that exercise places physical stress on bones, which respond by becoming bigger, and by increases in blood flow, circulating nutrients to the bones. In addition to exercise, the most efficient way of protecting bone density is by administering hormone replacement therapy.

The exercise prescription

In designing exercise prescriptions, the best programme for an individual is chosen, with lifestyle, social circumstances and preferences being considered. Exercisers fall into three groups: those who are unwell, those who will be unwell if they do not exercise and those who are comparatively well and fit, but want to be even fitter. The motivational processes in each group are likely to be different. Knowledge of, and belief in, the health benefits of physical activity may motivate initial involvement. However, subsequently a significant proportion of drop-outs from medically supervised group exercise programmes occurs within the first six months of commencement, reaching as high as 50% of participants, albeit followed by a slower rate thereafter. Patient adherence with unsupervised exercise appears to be subject to the same early drop-out as supervised exercise. The factors affecting adherence to an exercise prescription are rather different to those governing concordance with a drug prescription. The main considerations are time to carry out the exercises and enjoyment or ability to complete the tasks set.

The risks of sport and exercise

General adverse effects

The ultimate adverse effect that may occur during exercise is sudden death, which is usually the result of heart failure. The occurrence of occasional sudden and premature death in both amateur and professional athletes who appear to exhibit all the attributes of cardiorespiratory health and fitness has raised the consciousness of the underlying causes. Concern has been expressed as to the correct evaluation of conditioned athletes. The implication is clear: some or all of these sudden deaths could (and perhaps should) have been avoided with an appropriate screening programme. However, identifying all athletes at risk for exercise related sudden death is difficult, particularly if they are asymptomatic. Mass screening is expensive, and in many cases is claimed to be unreliable. The problem of interpreting athletes' ECG traces has already been highlighted (*see* The physiology of exercise *above*).

However, this is not a common event; the risk of sudden cardiac death during strenuous activity is generally greatest in those who do not regularly exercise (e.g. less than 20 minutes per week). The risk may be reduced by establishing a programme of exercise of gradually increasing intensity.

In some instances, particularly in elite athletes, chronic intense exercise training may interfere with hormonal mechanisms, causing changes in endocrine regulation as a result of altered physiology. Gonadal dysfunction in women is one example of this. At the extreme, regular physical exercise that becomes compulsive can be viewed as a form of dependence, or addiction, that is similar to drug abuse in its intensity. Some researchers have found that male runners deprived of participation in their sport for two weeks suffered from withdrawal symptoms, although in a form milder than drug withdrawal.

Other adverse effects that may arise are generally as a result of attempting to do too much exercise while still unfit, poor preparation for a sports event, failure to take into account prevailing environmental conditions or over-exercising when suffering from certain diseases. Small injuries often become exacerbated by keen exercisers returning to activity before healing is complete.

Exercise to music in groups provides an enjoyable activity for many people, both men and women, and they join aerobic classes. Good aerobics classes feature qualified instructors who are able to devise exercise programmes for separate groups, noting individual abilities. Poor instructors do not attempt to individualise exercises and use the same activities for all, regardless of age or fitness. This is unacceptable at best, and positively dangerous at worst. For those who are unwilling or unable to join an aerobics class, a whole library of exercise videos exists, from the ultimate fitness package to concentration on one body part. Unfortunately, the stimulus of constant encouragement from an instructor and support from fellow exercisers is missing. Further, there is the possibility of injury through attempting activities which are too ambitious.

Specific problems

Anaemia

Anaemia may often be diagnosed in athletes on the basis of a reduced blood-haemoglobin concentration (*see* The physiology of exercise *above*). Medical investigation of anaemia is necessary, particularly in men, to exclude serious pathology (e.g. peptic ulceration). In women, anaemia may be a true diagnosis if pregnant or experiencing regular heavy menstrual losses, and requires treatment with iron supplements. Diets deficient in iron may also be a contributory factor. Haematuria is associated with long-distance running, although the underlying reason is not clear. All patients with haematuria should be referred for medical investigation, but reassured that 'exercise haematuria' is not necessarily serious.

Haemoglobinuria, which also produces a reddish-coloured urine, may occur in long-distance runners or karate players. It is caused by repeated severe jarring, resulting in local haemolysis, and is more common in men than women. The oxygen-carrying capacity of the blood does not fall below normal and treatment is not required. Prevention may be effected by the use of some means of protection (e.g. springy insoles in running shoes or changing from road running to cross-country running).

Asthma and breathing difficulties

Exercise-induced asthma can be provoked by inhaling irritant substances, sometimes in very small quantities, and is recognisable by identifying a fall in peak expiratory flow. Irritation of the nose provokes rhinitis; irritation of the bronchi leads to difficulties in breathing, especially in exhalation, and wheezing. Running, particularly in a cold environment, is the most likely to provoke such an attack, swimming the least. Medical investigation should be considered to exclude a serious disorder (e.g. bronchiectasis or tuberculosis).

Chest pain

Chest pain may occur for a variety of reasons (e.g. angina pectoris, indigestion, musculoskeletal injury within the chest, oesophagitis or referred spinal pain) and should always be investigated before continuing further exercise. Exercise is not contra-indicated in controlled angina pectoris, provided that the exertion is not too vigorous. Regular attacks of palpitations should always be referred for investigation, although they are not uncommon in athletes, either during recovery from intensive exercise or at rest, and do not necessarily represent any serious pathology.

Circulatory problems

Syncope may occur at the end of a period of intense physical exercise (e.g. a marathon run), and is usually the result of a dramatic fall in blood pressure caused by the abrupt cessation of activity. The pumping action of the muscles on the blood circulation is suddenly stopped, and a large volume of blood pools in the dilated vessels of the lower legs. Falling from the vertical to the horizontal position will restore the blood-flow, and there is no cause for alarm, provided that no injury is sustained in the fall. Occasionally, collapse may be caused by cardiac arrest, which should always be excluded. Syncope during physical activity should always be thoroughly investigated and all forms of exercise discontinued until the cause has been elicited.

Environmental dangers

A number of problems resulting from activities in extreme environmental conditions may be identified (e.g. heat stroke in marathon runners, hypothermia in hillwalkers and long-distance swimmers or altitude sickness and frost-bite in mountain climbers). They generally affect the homoeostatic mechanisms of the body and, if severe, may endanger life.

High temperatures

Exercising in conditions of high air temperature and relative humidity for extended periods of time can be dangerous, especially for the unfit, and may result in heat stroke (sunstroke). The core temperature rises, and relies on various mechanisms to lower it (*see* The physiology of exercise *above*). Anything that acts to block these mechanisms (e.g. heavy clothing, a still or humid atmosphere, or dehydration) causes the core temperature to rise further, and eventually brain cells may be destroyed. Severe cases may result in some degree of permanent brain damage on recovery.

Some drugs (e.g. antimuscarinics, barbiturates and phenothiazines) or diseases (e.g. diabetes mellitus) may also impair heat regulatory mechanisms. Heat stroke is characterised by a core temperature around 41°C or more, confusion, headache, irritability and a hot dry skin. Blood pressure is usually normal to start with, but eventually falls during the final stages. Immediate treatment is necessary, and the patient should be sponged with tepid water and fanned with cool air to lower the core temperature to about 38°C. Further decreases by these means should be avoided, to prevent the risk of precipitating hypothermia. It is preferable not to use cold water for sponging or cold air for fanning because the resultant cutaneous vasoconstriction may impair the mechanism of heat transfer from the centre of the body to the surface. Administration of fluids and electrolytes may also be necessary.

Vigorous activity in hot conditions causes profuse perspiration and results in excessive loss of salt and water from the body. The average loss of sweat during light work is two to three litres/day, but during heavy physical activity in hot weather, the maximum rate of production may reach two to four litres/hour. The rate does, however, fall off as perspiration continues and may be as little as 0.5 litres/hour after 24 hours of sustained sweating. Sweat contains salt, and large salt losses may occur at maximal sweating rates. If these losses of salt and water are not replaced, salt-depletion heat exhaustion or water-depletion heat exhaustion or both may occur.

Salt-depletion heat exhaustion occurs if there are excessive salt losses during intense activity, and is characterised by painful contractions in exercised muscles during the post-exercise phase (heat cramps). Additionally, there may be fatigue, headache, nausea and vomiting, postural hypotension and weakness. Treatment involves the oral or parenteral administration of sodium chloride. Water-depletion heat exhaustion is characterised by dehydration and thirst. The face and eyes may have a sunken appearance, and the skin feels cool and clammy; the condition may be complicated by heat stroke. The concentration of electrolytes in the body fluids rises and death occurs when the amount of fluid lost approaches 15 to 25% of the initial body-weight. Treatment requires rehydration by the oral administration of water or, in more severe cases, the administration of glucose 5% intravenous infusion. Losses of body fluid during a marathon run may approach three to four litres (or more in hot weather), and hypovolaemic shock may occur if inadequate fluid is taken during a race. Runners should ensure that they have taken plenty of fluid before the start of a race, and take advantage of all drinks available during the event. Shock may not become apparent until as long as 20 minutes after completion of the race.

Heat exhaustion may be prevented by drinking plenty of fluids before, during and after prolonged sessions of intensive physical activity, particularly if undertaken in hot conditions. Salt supplementation may also be necessary in some individuals although, for many, the daily intake of dietary sodium is far in excess of requirements. Salt cannot be absorbed from the gastro-intestinal tract during exercise and should be taken before or after an event. Replacement salt solutions must be hypotonic, and a sodium chloride 0.5% solution is generally considered adequate. Sodium Chloride Tablets BP are available and should be dissolved in water before administration. It is essential that plenty of fluid should be taken with salt supplements, and if this is not available, salt supplementation is not recommended. Salt solutions may cause nausea and vomiting, and sustained-release formulations are available to minimise gastro-intestinal side-effects. There is no advantage to be gained by excessive salt supplementation, which in the short term causes fluid retention, and in the long term has been linked with the development of hypertension. Regular training or acclimatisation in a hot climate causes an increase in overall sweat production and a decrease in sodium concentration of sweat. Highly trained athletes may not, therefore, require as great a salt supplementation as might be expected.

Low temperatures

Hypothermia may develop during a marathon race in the presence of cool weather, wind or rain, particularly if the athlete is ill-clad or running slowly. The runner should avoid early fatigue caused by starting the race at too fast a pace, because fatigue lowers the rate of heat production. If necessary, a lightweight garment that is both waterproof and windproof should be carried. Hillwalkers, climbers and skiers may also be at risk of hypothermia if inadequately dressed or injured in ambient temperatures close to 0°C. As the air temperature drops below freezing point, there is the additional hazard of frost-bite.

Mild hypothermia occurs with a core temperature below 35°C, and is characterised by shivering and an intense feeling of cold. However, the subject is usually still alert and, unless injured, should be self-motivated to take action to keep warm. A core temperature of below 32°C results in severe hypothermia, which causes apathy, impaired judgement, coma and, eventually, fatal ventricular fibrillations. Treatment is required when the core temperature falls below 34°C; recovery is unlikely if the core temperature falls below 26°C. The patient should be thoroughly dried and re-clothed in warm, dry clothing, and then wrapped in a foil blanket, if available. Rapid re-warming (e.g. by immersion in hot water) can be dangerous in some situations and should be avoided. Warm drinks, preferably containing sugar, should also be given once the core temperature has risen above 31°C.

Alcohol should never be given to hypothermic patients or ingested following exercise in cold conditions, because this can accentuate or precipitate hypothermia. After a period of vigorous exercise, the subject will almost certainly have used up most of the carbohydrate reserves and be reliant on the formation of glucose from amino acids (gluconeogenesis) as an energy source. This reaction involves pyruvic acid as an intermediate product. However, alcohol metabolism also utilises pyruvic acid, which is then unavailable for conversion to glucose. There is consequently insufficient pyruvate to replace the glucose used during the period of exercise. The result is hypoglycaemia, which adversely affects the homoeostatic mechanisms controlling core temperature, and hypothermia may develop. Hypoglycaemia also contributes to the patient's mental confusion.

Frost-bite is marked by areas of hard white skin, usually on the extremities, although severe cases may extensively involve the limbs. Small areas may be treated by immersion in hand-hot water to induce thawing, but more severe frostbite requires evacuation of the patient to an intensive care unit in hospital and should not be treated by rapid re-warming.

Exercise at altitude
The increased respiration that occurs at high altitude (*see* The physiology of exercise *above*) removes more carbon dioxide than usual, causing periodic irregular breathing and insomnia. This adds to fatigue and impairs sporting activity. Other symptoms include irritability, headache, dry throat, gastro-intestinal upsets, visual disturbances and vertigo. People who are resident or train at high altitude often claim an advantage over low-altitude colleagues. Although it is certainly necessary for athletes to train at altitude if they intend to compete in such an environment, there is little evidence to support its widespread worth in normal sea-level activities.

Gastro-intestinal symptoms

Exercise is characterised by a flow of blood away from the gastro-intestinal tract towards the muscles and lungs. Changes in endocrine secretions lead to variations in gastro-intestinal motility, blood-flow and absorption, but the exact mechanism is unclear. It may be an indicator of poor fitness, as some people appear to be more susceptible than others.

Gastro-intestinal disturbances are more often associated with running than cycling or swimming. 'Runner's diarrhoea' is related to the severity of the exercise. Incontinence and rectal bleeding are not uncommon. In endurance events (e.g. marathon and long-distance cycling events), 30 to 50% of participants may develop stomachache, vomiting and heartburn. There are also reports of gastro-intestinal bleeding (melaena or haematemesis). Again, the mechanism is unclear, and it is essential to exclude serious pathology (e.g. peptic ulceration or colorectal cancer) before attributing this symptom to the stresses of the exercise. For those who appear to be susceptible, training programmes should be rescheduled to be less intense, increasing gradually to the required level. Non-steroidal anti-inflammatory drugs should be avoided, particularly during the few days before a race.

Dehydration because of insufficient fluid replacement has been shown to increase the frequency of gastro-intestinal symptoms.

Hormonal problems in women

Amenorrhoea and oligomenorrhoea may occur in women who regularly undertake intensive endurance exercising (e.g. long-distance running) and may be caused by impairment of cyclical secretion of luteinising hormone, although there are insufficient data to support this conclusively. Women with low body-weight and low body-fat are particularly prone; emotional disturbances caused by intensive training schedules and competition may also be a contributory factor. Amenorrhoeic athletes should be referred for medical investigation, although menses generally resume on reduction of exercise and fertility is not usually impaired.

The risks in medical conditions

General conditions

Anyone suffering from anaemia, chronic disorders of the cardiovascular, renal, or respiratory systems, metabolic disorders or thyroid disorders must consult their doctor and have a full medical examination before undertaking any exercise programme. It is generally considered that exercise is contra-indicated in such disorders until the condition has been brought under control. Medical assessment is also advised for patients recovering from acute conditions, and in those with hypertension or musculoskeletal disorders.

Cardiac disease

Sport and exercise may uncover underlying cardiac defects or disease (e.g. when a person collapses while running or playing sports). Cardiac disorders (e.g. ischaemic heart disease, myocardial disease and valvular heart disease) reduce the cardiac reserve of the heart. Faulty valves (either as a result of incompetence or stenosis) increase the workload of the heart muscle under normal conditions; exercising causes further increases. A person with valvular heart disease is, therefore, unable to cope with the same level of physical activity as someone with a normal heart.

Chronic myocarditis may lead to cardiomyopathy and possibly cause sudden death during exercise. However, a controlled and supervised exercise programme may be of benefit in preventing further cardiac damage following myocardial infarction (*see* The benefits of sport and exercise *above*).

Diabetes mellitus

Exercise may precipitate hypoglycaemia in Type I diabetes mellitus, and it can occur up to several hours after physical activity unless preventive measures are taken. A patient should be medically assessed before undertaking a programme of sport or exercise. It may be necessary to reduce the insulin dose before anticipated exercise and to inject at a site not being exercised (to minimise the increase in absorption that occurs from exercising muscles, presumably as a result of increased blood-flow). Doses should not be administered less than one hour before exercise. Some diabetics, especially the lean, may need to ingest carbohydrate before exercising and during prolonged sessions, and a meal should always be taken within three hours of completing the activity. It may be helpful for those who wish to undertake vigorous exercise regularly to monitor their blood-glucose concentrations before, during and after exercise, in order to assess their personal response to physical activity and to allow reasonably accurate predictions of future requirements to be made.

Type II diabetics on diet therapy alone do not generally experience problems related to altered blood-glucose concentrations, and need only observe the same precautions related to taking up exercise as the general population. However, those on oral antidiabetic agents may experience hypoglycaemia during prolonged physical activity, and should first seek medical advice. Exercise has, however, been shown to be beneficial in both types of diabetes mellitus and should be encouraged. Vertigo during exercise may simply be related to stress or it may be indicative of a serious disorder (e.g. iron-deficiency anaemia or cardiac disease), particularly if it occurs on changes in posture. Exercise is contra-indicated until medical investigations have been carried out.

Infections

Exercising is contra-indicated during infections, particularly viral infections, because there is often an associated risk of myocarditis. The extra workload placed on the inflamed heart results in reduced exercise tolerance, which is characterised by breathlessness and fatigue, and can be responsible for sudden death during exercise. Exercise may also prolong convalescence and increase the incidence of postviral depression (e.g. following influenza or Epstein-Barr virus infection). Patients should not, therefore, resume exercising until fully recovered.

Respiratory disease

Exercise tolerance is reduced in those with obstructive airways disease because more work is required to force air through constricted passages. Also, any disorder that increases the dead space of the lungs reduces the efficiency of respiration. Fluid accumulates in the air spaces of the lungs in pulmonary infections, reducing the efficiency of gaseous exchange. Emphysema results in reduced elasticity of the alveoli, which lowers the amount of air expelled. Some diseases (e.g. asthma, bronchitis and emphysema) influence the distribution of blood to different parts of the lungs, which reduces exercise tolerance because alveolar gaseous exchange is dependent on adequate perfusion. Similarly, exchange can only take place across healthy alveolar walls, and any disease that affects the lining (e.g. emphysema, pulmonary fibrosis or viral infections) reduces the efficiency of respiration. Carbon dioxide diffuses into the alveoli faster than oxygen diffuses into the blood, so the primary effect of impaired gaseous exchange is reduced oxygenation of the blood rather than an increase in the blood-carbon dioxide concentration. Exercises may, however, be beneficial in the management of obstructive airways disease, but full medical supervision is necessary (*see* The benefits of sport and exercise *above*).

Exercise may cause attacks of asthma in susceptible individuals, and for some asthmatics this is the only provocative factor. Breathlessness and wheezing characteristically occur after exercise, or may arise after a few minutes into continuous exercise. Exercise-induced asthma (EIA) usually peaks about five to ten minutes after exercise and abates after 30 to 60 minutes. The severity of the attack is related to the intensity of exercise, but further exercise two to four hours later (the refractory period) fails to elicit the same intensity of response. This property is made use of by some asthmatic athletes who induce asthma some time before an event. EIA does not necessarily occur every time a susceptible individual exercises, but may be precipitated by specific factors. Cold, dry conditions are more likely to induce an attack than a warm, moist atmosphere, and it is noteworthy that swimming is less likely to induce asthma than running. EIA may also be related to stress or the presence of certain allergens (e.g. pollens) in the air. Known precipitating factors should be avoided and prophylactic therapy administered (but *see* Table 8.4 on page 224 for a list of drugs banned in sports competitions).

Effects of medication

It may be necessary to consider the effects of any medication on performance or ability to partake in sports or strenuous exercise programmes. Some drugs (e.g. morphine) depress the rate of respiration, which ultimately slows down the rate of gaseous exchange between the alveoli and the blood. Alterations in fluid and electrolyte balance affect the plasma concentrations of some drugs (e.g. lithium), and toxic effects may arise if the patient becomes dehydrated during intense exercise. Studies have shown increased absorption of medication from transdermal delivery systems (e.g. glyceryl trinitrate patches) during strenuous physical activity, which may be related to an increase in cutaneous blood-flow and increased skin temperature. For the performance-enhancing effects of drugs in sport, *see* Participation in sports and exercise *below*.

In the past, patients suffering from diabetes or epilepsy were advised against certain forms of exercise. With sensible precautions, it is now acknowledged that these individuals can exercise effectively and become involved in sport. Pharmacists can provide a useful source of information in this respect.

AIDS and sport

According to the World Health Organization consensus statement on AIDS and sport, no evidence exists for a risk of transmission of HIV virus when any affected persons do not have bleeding wounds or other skin lesions, and there is no documentary evidence of HIV being acquired through participation in sport. However, if a lesion is observed or a bleeding wound occurs in any participant, it is prudent for medical attention to be given immediately. The area should be cleansed with disinfectant and securely covered. HIV is not believed to be transmitted through sweat, urine, respiratory droplets, swimming bath water or toilets. The possibility of injecting steroid abusers acquiring HIV through injecting practices has given cause for concern. This has implications for pharmacists through needle exchange schemes, which were set up for opiate abusers, but are now being expanded to include all drug abusers. Sports injectors generally use short, narrow gauge needles.

Pregnancy

Exercise during pregnancy may pose some risks for the mother or foetus, although if carried out sensibly and in moderation, it has been shown to be of benefit (*see above*). A pregnant woman should seek medical advice to assess whether or not it is safe for her to exercise. Absolute contraindications include any factors that predispose to prematurity (e.g. incompetent cervix, more than one foetus or a history of premature labour), or any factors that cause decreased oxygenation of the uterus or placenta (e.g. pregnancy-induced hypertension or smoking). Relative contraindications should be assessed on an individual basis taking into account all other factors present, and include anaemia, arrhythmias, diabetes mellitus, essential hypertension, thyroid disorders or extremes of weight. Vigorous exercise by pregnant women has been seen to produce foetal bradycardia and should therefore be avoided. Hyperthermia may have an adverse effect on the foetus, and pregnant women should avoid exercising to such a level or in conditions that significantly raise the core temperature. For the same reason, post-exercise saunas or hot baths are not recommended.

Sports medicine

Sports medicine may be defined as:

> the medical and paramedical supervision of people involved in sport and exercise and the treatment of their injuries and illnesses whether sustained in training or competition, to facilitate a return to their own particular level of activity as soon as possible.

Sports persons are like any other member of the community; they suffer from a whole range of common injuries and diseases. Because of their participation in sport, they are subject to a greater risk illness and injury in certain circumstances. Pharmacists, as health advisers, are ideally placed to respond to requests for advice on treatment.

Injuries are more prevalent in the unfit; the risks may be significantly reduced by improving strength, stamina, suppleness, playing skill and by using good quality equipment.

The general principles of treating sports injuries

The different reasons for injuries arising during sports or exercise are:

- Trauma
  - abrasions and lacerations
  - bruises
  - dislocation
  - fractures
  - ligament injuries (sprains)
  - muscle injuries (strains)
  - tendon injuries.
- Overuse syndromes
  - bursae injuries
  - inflammation of muscles
  - inflammation of tendon and attachments
  - joint problems
  - stress fractures.
- Miscellaneous
  - blisters
  - burns/friction
  - cramp
  - delayed onset muscle soreness (DOMS).

Risk factors for injuries resulting from sports or exercise activity may be intrinsic (resulting from personal actions) or extrinsic (resulting from environmental influences) (Table 8.2).

Attention to many of these factors will reduce the risk of injuries to a large extent. The type of injury occurring during sports and exercise generally varies with the type of activity being undertaken. Trauma is more likely to occur during combat or contact sports (e.g. boxing, judo or rugby); overuse injuries are more commonly a feature of sports involving repetitive movements (e.g. golf or tennis). Traumatic and overuse injuries mainly involve bone and soft tissue, with soft-tissue injuries accounting for over 80% of all sports injuries. There are more injuries involving the limbs than head and trunk, and the incidence in the lower limbs is greater than in the upper. Overuse injuries occur most commonly in the tendons of the ankle, hip, knee, shoulders and wrist.

In treating an injury the main aims are as follows:

- decrease the amount of damage from the initial injury
- decrease pain and inflammation, and restrict any collateral damage in areas away from main site
- decrease the possibility of secondary damage through infection
- increase the healing ability of the damaged tissue
- increase the flexibility and strength of muscles
- increase the aerobic and anaerobic fitness appropriate to sports activity being followed
- allow skills to be re-attuned
- attempt to correct any causal factors (e.g. muscle imbalance).

Injury to soft tissues causes the release of prostaglandins (especially prostaglandin E_2) and other inflammatory mediators (e.g. bradykinin, histamine and serotonin), which cause swelling, pain and bruising. Applying the principles of treatment to soft-tissue injuries involves reducing the risk of infection where the skin has been

Table 8.2 Examples of risk factors for sports and exercise injuries

Risk factor	Example
Intrinsic or personal risks	
Age	Affects ability to pursue exercise to varying intensity
Anatomy	Body shape and size. Misalignment of feet and/or legs or other parts of the body
Disabilities	Presence of debilitating disease (e.g. diabetes) or handicap
Existing weaknesses	Insufficient rehabilitation from previous injury (sprains and strains), arthritis, old fracture
Fitness	Insufficient aerobic capacity, and strength and flexibility
Extrinsic or environmental risks	
Climatic conditions	Temperature and altitude
Equipment	Inappropriate for surface (e.g. grass, synthetic or wood) ill fitting, poor quality or poorly maintained
Training programme	Inappropriate duration, frequency and intensity
Training surface	Hard, irregular contours and sloping

broken, minimising initial swelling and pain, and promoting rapid healing. It is also important to reduce the risks of secondary damage. The injured area should be examined periodically for signs of inflammation, which is characterised by erythema, swelling and tenderness. There may be decreased mobility and pain. More ominous findings that warrant referral include fever, severe pain on movement and persistent pain at rest.

The four essential elements in the early management of soft-tissue injuries can be remembered by the acronym RICE:

- Rest
- Ice
- Compression
- Elevation.

The RICE regimen may then be followed by other measures (e.g. heat treatment and drug treatment) and rehabilitation.

Rest

Immobilisation is recommended for the first 24 hours to avoid aggravating the injury, prevent further bleeding and minimise inflammation and swelling. It may be necessary to avoid bearing weight on an affected limb. If longer-term immobilisation of an area is indicated, it is essential to ensure that this does not prevent long-term movement in unaffected joints, as this will promote atrophy of tissues and loss of co-ordination. Soft-tissue injuries should not be massaged or manipulated at this stage, as this could aggravate the lesion. Prolonged rest for muscle injuries is usually discouraged because the collagen scar tissue formed is unable to contract, and repair is associated with some loss of flexibility.

Ice

Cooling the injured area (cryotherapy) reduces the local blood-flow and decreases the metabolic rate in peripheral cells, thus limiting the extent of inflammation and degree of pain. Commercial ice-packs or home-made packs containing crushed ice may be used, or, if nothing else is to hand, cold water will help. Cooling sachets are available, and contain two separated chemicals that undergo an endothermic reaction when brought into contact with each other. However, these are not as efficient in cooling the body and do not last long enough to be effective. Cold treatment should be administered for up to 30 minutes and repeated every two hours over the first 24 hours. For severe injuries, it may be necessary to continue the applications for 48 hours. Ice and ice-packs should always be wrapped in damp cloths to prevent skin burns, and should not be left on for longer than the recommended time. Cooling aerosol sprays are also available, but their effect is likely to last for less time than ice-packs. Injuries should not be cooled if the patient suffers with atherosclerosis or a peripheral vascular disease (e.g. Raynaud's syndrome).

Compression

Compression involves the application of pressure over the injured area, and is employed to decrease bleeding and the flow of inflammatory exudate, and therefore reduce swelling. A compression bandage should be applied after the ice has been removed. It is necessary to extend the bandage 20 centimetres above and below the injured area, but it is vital that the bandage is not applied so tightly that blood-flow is totally impeded. Compression should be applied for at least 24 hours, although large lesions may require compression for longer.

Elevation

The injured area should be raised above the level of the heart to aid drainage of fluid and reduce swelling.

Other measures

Heat treatment (thermotherapy) is the application of heat for 20 to 30 minutes by means of an infra-red lamp, hot-water bottle or heat-pad. Heat causes vasodilatation, which increases the flow of blood to the injured area, and is of benefit to relieve the pain produced by muscle spasm. Heat also promotes relaxation of muscles before exercising, and therefore reduces the risk of further injury. If applied to joints, heat improves mobility by reducing the viscosity of synovial fluid. However, heat should not be used during the first 48 hours following a soft-tissue injury because of the risk of re-bleeding. Heat treatment should not be used for open wounds or on patients with reduced skin sensation, who would be unable to detect a burn.

Alcohol is a vasodilator and should be avoided for up to 72 hours following an injury, in order to minimise bleeding into the damaged area. Ideally, it should also be avoided before or during exercise. Hot baths should also be avoided initially in favour of showers or tepid baths, to avoid the risk of re-bleeding.

Ultrasound treatment and laser therapy may increase blood-flow and reduce inflammation. Non-steroidal anti-inflammatory drugs may be of benefit, but to be effective should be administered for up to three to five days, starting as soon as possible after the injury. Prolonged administration in most cases is unnecessary. Topical counter-irritant products, which produce a sensation of warmth, are widely available, but are of limited value and should never be used under a dressing or on open wounds.

Rehabilitation

Prolonged rest leads to loss of suppleness, strength and stamina. Gentle exercise, dictated by the extent of pain, should commence after 24 hours (or longer where indicated, *see below*) to restore the full range of movement of a part and minimise the permanent loss of strength associated with the formation of scar tissue. Controlled isometric exercises (*see* The physiology of exercise *above*) of increasing intensity are beneficial in aligning the randomly orientated collagen fibres of new scar tissue. Injured areas may require support (which does not involve compression) during rehabilitation by means of suitable bandages.

Prevention

The frequency of sports injuries may be reduced by warming-up properly before the event, to increase the blood-flow to the tissues, and by gentle cooling-down exercises afterwards. The latter may be difficult if you have been soundly beaten! Warming-up has the effect of raising the temperature of the tissues, making them more elastic and, therefore, less susceptible to tearing. Suitable warm-up exercises include muscle stretches, running on-the-spot and loosely shaking all joints.

Protective equipment is essential for those activities where direct contact with playing equipment or other players is associated with a high risk of injury. Correct footwear is also important, including the use of cushioned insoles to act as shock-absorbers and reduce the stress on joints. Different sports (and different playing surfaces) require different designs of footwear, and sports shoes should not be used interchangeably. The UK Amateur Athletic Association has ruled that children should not participate in running events longer than five kilometres on the basis that severe injury to rapidly growing tissue may result in permanent deformity.

Table 8.3 lists suggestions of items that may be included in a sports medical bag to cover the basic requirements of first aid in the event of sports injury. However, there may be more specific requirements for a particular sport, and some governing bodies actually lay down rules dictating the contents of sports club medical bags.

The management of specific injuries

Blister

A blister is the common name for a vesicle or, if large, a bulla. It is a fluid-filled sac on the surface of the skin, and may be formed during sports and exercise as a result of repeated friction between the skin and a hard object (e.g. ill-fitting shoes). Intact blisters are best left untreated, and further damage prevented, if necessary, by a non-adherent protective covering. If aspiration is undertaken, all equipment used should be sterile and the covering flap of skin left, in order to reduce further the risk of infection. Friction burns may be treated by cooling the affected area and the oral administration of an analgesic. Broken skin may require cleansing and covering with a non-adherent dressing to prevent infection. If extensive areas are involved, hospital treatment may be required.

Bursitis

This inflammation of a bursa (a sac-like fluid-filled cavity surrounding soft tissues and protecting them from friction) may be caused by trauma or overuse. Treatment comprises the administration of non-steroidal anti-inflammatory drugs or local corticosteroid injections. Surgical aspiration may be necessary in chronic cases.

Capsulitis

This is inflammation of a joint capsule and may be caused by trauma or overuse. General methods of treatment may be sufficient (i.e. rest and the application of heat or cold), with administration of non-steroidal anti-inflammatory drugs or local corticosteroid injections. Gentle exercises should be started once the pain and inflammation have subsided. Severe cases may require manipulation under anaesthetic.

Delayed onset muscle soreness (DOMS)

Muscle pain and stiffness are not uncommon in muscles that have been subjected to unaccustomed intense physical activity, and characteristically appear 24 to 48 hours after the exercise. The mechanisms responsible are unknown, although it has been established that there is damage to the muscle fibres and membranes. Greater damage is caused by exercises that involve an increase in muscle length than those that rely on muscle shortening. Exposure of the muscle to similar exercise at a later date does not produce pain. There is some risk of further injury if already damaged muscles are exercised vigorously, and the pain and discomfort experienced as a result may impair performance. It is, therefore, advisable to prevent DOMS by gradually working up to a particular intensity of exercise.

Haematomas

As muscle fibres rupture, blood seeps into the interstitial spaces to form haematomas, which cause pain and loss of function. Haematomas should be treated by the RICE regimen. Large haematomas may require immobilisation of the injured area for 24 to 48 hours. They are eventually resorbed, although this may not happen and surgical aspiration may be necessary.

A haematoma may be invaded by osteoblasts (possibly derived from the periosteum) and these initiate ossification in the soft tissue. This condition is termed myositis ossificans and is characterised by pain, stiffness and reduction in movement. Massaging thigh injuries may predispose to this condition and should therefore be avoided. Ossification may be further encouraged

Table 8.3 Suggestions of items to include in a medical sports bag to administer basic first aid in the event of sports injury

Item	Purpose	Examples	Comments
Wound cleansing			
Disinfectants and cleansers	to cleanse and disinfect skin and wounds	Cetrimide Chlorhexidine Povidone-iodine Sodium chloride 0.9% (sterile solutions may also be used for eye irrigation)	Chlorinated solutions (e.g. dilute sodium hypochlorite solution) are no longer recommended for wound cleansing as they are considered too irritant
Swabs	to apply the disinfectants and cleansers	Gauze Swab BP Absorbent Cotton BP Absorbent Cotton Gauze BP	Absorbent cotton hospital quality should not be used for wound cleansing
Wound dressing			
Absorbents	to absorb wound exudate and provide protection	Absorbent Cotton BP Absorbent Lint BPC Calcium Alginate Dressings (Drug Tariff) Gauze and Cotton Tissue BP Perforated Film Absorbent Dressing BP	
Haemostatic dressings	to stop bleeding	Calcium Alginate Dressings (Drug Tariff)	
Tulle dressings	to apply to abrasions, burns and other skin injuries, usually beneath an absorbent dressing	Paraffin Gauze Dressing BP Chlorhexidine Gauze Dressing BP	
Retention bandages	to hold dressings in place and to aid in the application of pressure to stop bleeding	Cotton Conforming Bandage BP Elastic Net Surgical Tubular Stockinette (Drug Tariff) Elasticated Tubular Bandage BP Open-wove Bandage BP	
Standard dressings	comprises an absorbent pad and retention bandage in one complete sterile dressing, used for wounds that are bleeding severely	Triangular Calico Bandage BP	May also be used as a sling A selection of sizes is recommended, including an eye pad

Table 8.3 continued

Item	Purpose	Examples	Comments
Adhesive dressings ('plasters')	an absorbent pad (which may be medicated) surrounded partly or completely by a piece of extension plaster, used to cover minor wounds	Elastic Adhesive Dressing BP Semipermeable Waterproof Plastic Wound Dressing BP	
Surgical adhesive tape	to secure dressings	Elastic Surgical Adhesive Tape BP Permeable Non-woven Surgical Synthetic Adhesive Tape BP Zinc Oxide Surgical Adhesive Tape BP	May also be used as a skin closure for small incision wounds May also be used to immobilise small areas
Management of soft-tissue injuries			
Cooling aids	to reduce the blood-flow in soft-tissue injuries and minimise further damage and swelling	Ice Ice-packs Cooling sachets	
Compression bandages	to provide pressure to reduce the flow of blood and inflammatory exudate	Cotton Crepe Bandage BP Crepe Bandage BP Elastic Adhesive Bandage BP	
Support bandages	to provide support for an injured area during active movement	Cotton Crepe Bandage BP Crepe Bandage BP Elasticated Tubular Bandage BP Open-wove Bandage BP	 Provides light support only.
Miscellaneous			
Wide-necked thermos flask or insulated bag	to carry ice or ice-packs		
Bucket, sponge and towel	for general cleaning purposes		
Scissors, safety pins and forceps	to cut up dressings and for general surgical use		

by exercise, and treatment of myositis ossificans includes immobilisation. Gentle exercising may commence when ossification appears to have stopped or is receding. Surgery is only indicated in the later stages to remove an old lesion.

Overuse injuries

As the name implies, an overuse injury is the result of carrying out the same activity for too long or too often. It may also be the result, in those unaccustomed to a particular activity, of doing too much too quickly. Muscle pain and stiffness, bursitis, capsulitis, tendinitis and tenosynovitis, and blisters and friction burns are all examples of overuse injuries. In general, initial treatment comprises the RICE regimen and the administration of non-steroidal anti-inflammatory drugs. A programme of exercise of gradually increasing intensity should be implemented, except for those conditions where complete rest is indicated (*see below*). Some modifications in action may be necessary to prevent further injuries: these may include changes in playing technique, exercise schedule, equipment (e.g. changing to padded running shoes) or modifications to the activity itself (e.g. cross-country running instead of road running).

Sprains

A sprain is an injury caused by overstretching or twisting a ligament, and may vary from damage of a few individual fibres to complete rupture. Symptoms include pain, swelling and tenderness. A complete rupture (which may be relatively painless) usually produces abnormal or excessive movements. Initial treatment of sprains comprises the RICE regimen and administration of non-steroidal anti-inflammatory drugs, followed by gentle exercise of gradually increasing intensity. Immobilisation may be necessary for severely damaged ligaments, and a complete rupture must be repaired surgically.

Strains

A strain is tearing apart of muscle fibres, and is characterised by pain and swelling. Muscle strains may be graded according to severity: grades 1 and 2 involve damage to the fibres only and the muscle sheath remains intact; grade 3 is partial rupture of the fibres and sheath; and grade 4 is complete rupture. Treatment of muscle strains involves the RICE regimen (*see above*) and an early encouragement back to activity. Grades 3 and 4 may require surgical repair.

Stress fractures

Stress fractures may result from the repeated application of stress to a bone without any evidence of direct trauma. Pain appears after exercise initially, but may progress to more severe and continuous pain. There is local tenderness and in some cases a lump. X-rays may appear clear, although eventually callus formation may be evident, indicating a healed stress fracture. It is essential to rest the affected bone for four to six weeks to prevent progression to complete fracture, but isometric exercises (*see* The physiology of exercise *above*) are recommended to prevent muscle atrophy.

Tendinitis and tenosynovitis

Injuries to tendons may involve complete or partial rupture, which produces pain and, if rupture is complete, loss of function. Partial ruptures may allow limited, albeit painful, movement. Tendon ruptures require immobilisation for one to two weeks, or longer. Inflammation of the tendon itself produces tendinitis, and of its outer covering, tenosynovitis. There is pain on movement and swelling may be visible. Treatment comprises rest, either cold or heat treatment, and the administration of non-steroidal anti-inflammatory drugs or local corticosteroid injections into the tendon sheath to control the inflammation; this should be followed by regular exercise of gradually increasing intensity. Chronic cases may require immobilisation or surgical decompression.

Specialist help for sports injuries is available from sports injury clinics (both in the NHS and on a private, fee-paying basis), and a list of addresses may be obtained from the UK Sports Council (*see* Useful addresses *below*).

The treatment of exercise and sports-related conditions

Anxiety and stress

Anxiety and excitement can affect performance in competitive sport, and the underlying mechanisms are complex. Methods of dealing with stresses surrounding sports performance are available, but pharmacists will undoubtedly be occasionally asked to recommend suitable medicines. Homoeopathic remedies (e.g. Argent. Nit., Aconite or gelsenium) might be considered.

Stress incontinence may be brought on in women during exercise, and is usually caused by a weakness of the urethral sphincter which prevents the urethra from closing tightly enough to withstand pressure on the bladder (*see also* Harman, 1989). Up to 33% of women may suffer from such leakage. A supporting device made from polyvinyl formyl sponge is available for insertion into the vagina.

Fungal infections

The most commonly occurring fungal infection is athlete's foot (Tinea pedis). Presentation is usually as itchy, flaking skin between the toes. A red, sore area is left as the scales peel off, and this lesion can become soggy, spreading to the whole foot. Secondary bacterial infection is possible, necessitating medical referral. Old-fashioned remedies (e.g. Whitfield's ointment and potassium permanganate) have been largely replaced by creams for dry infections, powders to keep the foot dry, sprays, solutions and paints. Ideally, treatment should be with a broad-spectrum antifungal which is effective against any yeasts that may be present as well as the mycoses: imidazoles (miconazole and econazole) are the most effective.

Other fungal infections include ringworm of the body (Tinea corporis), caught occasionally from people, but more usually as a zoonose from animals. Ringworm of the groin ('Jock itch') appears as an itchy red area around the genitals and upper thighs.

Headache

Headaches associated with a sports injury to the head should be referred immediately. In some sports in which intense concentration is necessary, headaches may be triggered by a visual problem, and referral to an optician should be considered. Occasional tension headaches may be treated with suitable OTC analgesics. A combination product may be helpful, and in some cases the athlete's preference for a particular brand has been shown to be significant.

Head lice (Pediculosis capitis)

These ectoparasites live on the scalp where they feed on blood. Infestation can be checked by combing the hair with a fine toothed comb over a piece of white paper and looking for live lice, which appear as brown specks. Head lice cause itching and irritation of the scalp and may provoke an eczema-like reaction. They can be spread by direct head-to-head contact (e.g. in a rugby scrum). However, in the warm damp environment occurring in most changing rooms, it is entirely possible that they can be spread by sharing combs, brushes and protective head gear. Various local insecticide policies exist for the eradication of head lice.

Scrumpox

In rugby, this troublesome rash is commonly caused by the Herpes simplex virus and is highly infectious, spreading by direct contact via clothing or towels, or by droplet spread. Other sources of infection are *Staphlococcus aureus* and *Streptococcus pyogenes* (causing impetigo and erysipelas respectively) and the fungus Tinea barbae. In all cases, patients should be referred to the general practitioner with advice to stop playing sport in the interim period.

Verrucae

Plantar warts (verruca plantaris) are caused by a virus that penetrates moist skin. They are most commonly found on the soles of the feet, having been caught from others by walking barefoot across the floor of a changing room or communal showers. Treatment involves gradual destruction of skin in the lesion while protecting the healthy surrounding area. Salicylic acid may be recommended in its various formulations, and there are numerous OTC products widely advertised for the removal of warts and veruccae.

Water-related conditions

Swimmers are susceptible to a number of illnesses, including conjunctivitis, otitis externa and skin and gastro-intestinal problems, together with various fungal infections and verruccae.

Sports nutrition and sports drinks

Athletes are always searching for nutritional supplements that will give them sufficient advantage over fellow competitors to ensure a position on the victory podium. To a great extent, this accounts for the reports of illegal drug taking in sport. The ideal for some professional athletes is to find a product that is effective in improving performance, but which is not on the International Olympic Committee's (IOC) Medical Committee banned list. Long-term safety would not seem to be a prime concern.

Energy requirements

Basic nutrition is as important in preparing athletes for events as physical training, and peak performance cannot be reached if there are nutritional deficiencies. Women may be at a disadvantage if suffering from iron-deficiency anaemia as a result of heavy menstrual losses.

The dietary energy requirements of an athlete, and in particular those participating in endurance events, are much greater than those of a sedentary individual. Adverse conditions (e.g. hot or humid weather) must also be taken into account and salt and fluid intake adjusted accordingly (*see above*). The daily dietary energy requirements (*see* Chapter 2, Energy requirements) of a young male athlete may be between 12.7 and 17.5 MJ (3024 and 4167 kcals), compared with about 10.6 MJ (2550 kcals) for a sedentary young man. The energy required for physical activity is provided by the oxidation of carbohydrates and fats. Excess dietary carbohydrate is stored as glycogen in muscles (about 350 g) and liver (about 100 g). Liver glycogen is broken down into glucose to maintain the optimum plasma-glucose concentration necessary for brain and nervous system functioning, and for use by muscles during exercise. Glycogen in muscles is converted when required to glucose-6-phosphate, which is metabolised to provide ATP. However, there is insufficient stored glycogen to last for more than about 90 to 120 minutes in trained individuals, and stores are only mobilised in those muscles actually in use. Fat stored in adipose tissue provides an additional source of energy for many hours of work, although it cannot be relied upon as the sole source because the oxidation of fat is only able to supply 50% of the energy required at any time.

Mineral and vitamin supplements

Many special diets have been put forward as being essential for peak athletic performance, some of which may be extremely faddist. However, generally, there is nothing to be gained by taking megadoses of vitamins and minerals (*see* Chapter 2, Vitamin and mineral supplements), or consumption of vast quantities of proteins. Excess protein is not laid down in muscle tissue, but is used as an energy source or stored as glycogen or fat. Carbohydrates are metabolised to glucose, which is used as a source of energy or stored as glycogen or fat. Fats are a highly concentrated source of energy able to supply twice as much energy weight for weight as carbohydrates and proteins, but are not metabolised fast enough to be of use in shorter athletic events. The recommendations for intake of dietary fats are the same in athletes as for other individuals (*see* Chapter 2, Fats and cholesterol) and should not be exceeded. There is no advantage to be gained by laying down deposits of fat in the body in anticipation of endurance events. This is harmful to health in the long term since obesity has been linked with many diseases, and merely increases the energy required by the athlete to move the extra body-weight.

It has been suggested that an increase in the intake of some vitamins is essential if physical activity is increased. This is only true for thiamine and niacin (nicotinic acid and nicotinamide), where the Reference Nutrient Intakes (RNIs) are related to dietary energy intake. The RNI for thiamine is 400 mg/4.2 MJ (1000 kcals) and for niacin is 6.6 mg/4.2 MJ (1000 kcals). The RNIs for other vitamins and minerals remain the same for all levels of activity (*see* Chapter 2, Table 2.1). Carnitine is a dietary supplement that has been claimed to increase endurance and thereby improve athletic performance. These claims have not been adequately proven, although carnitine does have a role in long-chain fatty acid metabolism.

The average diet contains salt far in excess of the daily requirement and, in most cases, will be sufficient to meet the additional demands created by profuse sweating during exercise. If evaporation of sweat is inhibited (e.g. by heavy clothing), sweating will be excessive and sodium losses even greater. Salt supplementation (*see above*) may be required in such instances, but is generally more efficient if taken prophylactically, rather than during exercise.

Anyone anticipating training sessions or exercise should not eat anything later than 2.5 to 3 hours beforehand, as doing so may cause gastrointestinal discomfort during the event. Food eaten at this stage should be rich in carbohydrates and low in fats and proteins, which take longer to digest. Carbohydrates ingested 0.5 to 1 hour before an event have the effect of stimulating a sudden increase in plasma-insulin concentration, which prevents mobilisation of fatty acids, and thus allows premature depletion of the glycogen reserves. However, glucose in solid form or solution may be taken immediately before exercise without adverse effect. Fluid replacement (*see above*) is necessary during long events (e.g. marathon runs). Minerals are not absorbed during exercise because of gastrointestinal stasis and should be taken with fluid before the event rather than during it. Marathon runners are only able to cope with small, but frequent, quantities of a dilute glucose solution (e.g. no more than 5 g/100 mL) during a race, and must rely on using body stores of glycogen and fat as a source of energy.

Ergogenic aids

Ergogenic agents are supplements that aim to maximise the efficiency of energy utilisation. They may be used at different times and different frequencies during training and competition. In the following examples, caffeine is used once, carbohydrate loading is used during training and competition, creatine is used principally during training, and sodium bicarbonate loading is used immediately prior to competition.

Caffeine

Caffeine enhances performance in endurance events by releasing free fatty acids and thus exerting a glycogen-sparing effect. It also reduces fatigue and is of most benefit to marathon runners. Its presence in urine is permitted up to a maximum concentration of 12 mg/mL. Above this level, caffeine is considered to be a stimulant and is banned by the IOC Medical Committee. Athletes taking caffeine need to be careful not to consume coffee, tea and certain soft drinks during competition. There is a strong possibility that the limit will be reduced to 8 mg/mL in the near future, representing a daily consumption of about three cups of coffee or four soft drinks.

Carbohydrate loading

Diets have been devised for endurance events to double or treble the glycogen stores in the muscle. About seven days before an event, the athlete totally depletes his muscles of glycogen by intensive activity. The diet over the next two to three days is rich in proteins and fats but low in carbohydrates, which is followed by three to four days of a diet rich in carbohydrates and low in proteins. Training should be reduced during this phase, particularly when little carbohydrate is being ingested. Response to such a technique is varied, and individuals should assess their personal response well in advance of an event. However, it is unlikely to work more than twice in a 12-month period. Some authorities feel that the low-carbohydrate phase is unnecessary. Elite marathon runners undergoing intensive training sessions will regularly deplete their stores of muscle glycogen, and all that may be required before the event is to reduce activity and adopt a high-carbohydrate, low-protein diet for two to four days.

Creatine (Cr)

The biggest ever survey of British sportsmen and women, organised by the *Independent* newspaper in 1998, revealed widespread use of Cr, which is claimed to have similar performance enhancing effects to steroids. The enthusiastic endorsement of Cr by high-profile professional athletes has raised its popularity among teenagers and amateurs. It has also prompted questions about the long-term safety of the supplement.

During brief intense anaerobic actions (e.g. sprinting, jumping or weightlifting), phosphate-creatine (PCr) regenerates ATP to provide the energy necessary to maintain muscle contractions (*see* Fig. 8.2). The aim of supplemental Cr is to increase the resting levels of PCr, so as to regenerate more ATP and maintain a high power output longer, delaying fatigue and improving performance. Cr is also thought to buffer the lactic acid that builds up during intense exercise.

Studies have shown the concentrations of PCr and free Cr in resting human skeletal muscle to vary widely. Several factors may be responsible, including dietary Cr uptake and relative amounts of slow-twitch and fast-twitch fibres. The fast-twitch fibres have a higher total Cr content than the slow-twitch fibres. For reasons not yet understood, females appear to have slightly higher resting levels of Cr than males. The starting point, therefore, is far from being fixed. Muscle Cr levels increase an average of 20% after six days of supplementation at 20 g per day ('rapid loading'). These higher muscle levels can then be maintained by ingesting 2 g per day thereafter. A similar, but slower, 20% rise in muscle Cr levels can be achieved in one month by ingesting 3 g per day ('no-load method').

The long-term effects and possibility of adverse reactions are beginning to cause considerable concern, particularly as the death of three American wrestlers was linked to its use. Substantial renal dysfunction has been reported in a patient who had taken a Cr supplement to augment his pre-season soccer-training regime. Cr supplementation may cause an electrolyte imbalance, leading to a predisposition to dehydration and heat-related illness. There are no reliable scientific data on possible adverse reactions at present.

Sodium bicarbonate loading

In high intensity exercise of between one and seven minutes duration, the main source of ATP is anaerobic glycolysis. A build up of lactic acid leads to a fall in pH, and this causes the muscle contractile mechanism to shut down, a decrease in the generation of muscle force, and onset of fatigue. The body's internal buffering system initially deals with this build-up of acid in the early stages, but when the pH falls below 6.3 (acidosis), glycolysis is inhibited.

The increased buffering capacity by raised ingestion of sodium bicarbonate is claimed to protect against acidosis. The resulting rise in extracellular pH establishes a gradient that causes movement of hydrogen and lactate ions out of the cell. Cellular pH rises, delaying the onset of fatigue and improving performance. The value of using bicarbonate loading depends on the type of exercise, its intensity and its duration, but many positive reports have appeared in the literature. The normal dose quoted for a 70 kg man is 0.3 g of sodium bicarbonate in one to two litres of fluid taken one to two hours prior to an event. It is necessary to drink plenty of water, because the sodium loading requires an influx to the intestine.

Sports drinks

There are three main types of drinks used in sport:

- The most common form of carbohydrate replacement is in the form of glucose high-energy drinks. Its use is permitted in events that require short sessions of inactivity between periods of activity (e.g. between heats in athletic events or at half-time in sports matches). Those involved in activities involving a high degree of skill require regular glucose supplementation in order to avoid hypoglycaemia, because the nervous system can only use blood-glucose as a source of fuel and is unable to utilise the body's fat stores.
- Isotonic drinks are used to replace fluid and electrolyte losses, and are generally low in carbohydrate. They are only of value in intermittent activity, when gastro-intestinal inhibition may be sufficiently reversed to allow absorption of minerals. They serve to replace sweat losses. Sweeter replacement fluids are less well tolerated than slightly sharper tasting drinks.

Cool drinks increase the chances of absorption by promoting peristalsis.

- There are various products on the market that can provide a balanced diet in a can of flavoured drink. Such an intake is more easily absorbed than solid food and is useful for those with tight schedules or insufficient time for eating and resting during competition.

The use and abuse of drugs in sport

Drugs to enhance performance

In high-level sports competitions, athletes are under enormous pressure to succeed, both for honour and for financial rewards. To win and break records is the all-consuming goal. In order to attain this, some athletes resort to the use of artificial means to increase performance, without considering the ethical issues or the personal risk: benefit ratio. Training for sports competition is not always synonymous with training for health. Abuse of drugs causes unwanted side-effects, and, in some cases, even death; some adverse effects may not become apparent until years later. Sports authorities have introduced measures to stop what is effectively cheating and to protect athletes from irreparable damage to their health.

Difficulty in obtaining some agents through legitimate channels may drive athletes to black-market sources of dubious origin, further increasing the risk to their health. Health education for athletes is necessary to first explain that, in many cases, the evidence supporting the claims of enhanced performance is lacking or contradictory; and second, that performance enhancement cannot be justified if, as a result, health is compromised.

History

In 1865, canal swimmers in Amsterdam, and many European cyclists, were charged with taking a mixture of heroin and cocaine; in the early years of the twentieth century, alcohol and strychnine were taken by boxers and marathon competitors. Thus, the use of performance-enhancing drugs in sport is certainly not a new problem. Drugs taken in this way undermine the foundation of fair competition, involve cheating and can be dangerous to health. Athletes have to be protected from themselves; they are often caught up with striving for better performance and fail to look beyond the next medal. They may resort to any method that has been passed on by word of mouth from other competitors (or ruthless coaches) that seems to bring their goal nearer.

Drug testing

Individual governing bodies of sports have drawn up lists of banned classes of drugs. There are absolutely no exceptions to the rules, and doctors cannot prescribe any of the drugs covered by the list; they must seek alternatives for patients wishing to participate in sports competitions. Subjecting sportsmen and women to tests to detect the presence of banned substances, and subsequent disciplinary action for those with positive results, may act as a deterrent to some. However, there are others whose determination is such that they devise ways and means of 'cheating' the test itself. Testing is usually carried out on a sample of urine because it is a non-invasive technique and therefore considered the most convenient and least obtrusive means of analysis. Urine also has the advantage that any drugs present are more concentrated than in blood, and there is less interference with the test from the normal constituents of urine than those of blood.

Laboratories undertaking drug-testing must be accredited by the IOC, which guarantees that samples are analysed in accordance with recognised procedures and to the highest standards. The level of 'doping' control in individual countries is variable, and the concern of many athletes is that urine analysis during the competition itself will not necessarily detect drugs that have been used during training (e.g. anabolic steroids). Many of those who abuse these substances have become knowledgeable about drug kinetics and can plan their dosage schedules ahead to minimise the risk of detection, or use masking agents when they know a test is likely to take place. As a result, some nations (including the UK) have introduced random drug testing during training for major competitions.

Banned drugs

The Medical Commission of the IOC has drawn up a list of banned substances, classifying them into five categories:

- Class A – Stimulants
- Class B – Narcotic analgesics
- Class C – Anabolic agents
- Class D – Diuretics
- Class E – Peptide and glycoprotein hormones and analogues.

Stimulants

Stimulants continue to be a big problem, constituting the greatest percentage of total positive samples detected by IOC-accredited laboratories (45% in 1994–96) (formerly, the biggest detected problem was with anabolic steroids). Stimulants have been shown to improve athletic performance in some studies, although others have shown conflicting results. They increase alertness and mood and mask fatigue, but do not prevent exhaustion. Judgement is impaired and eventually performance deteriorates. The effects of stimulants are not perceived by the subject, who continues the sporting activity with a significantly increased risk of injury. Sympathomimetics in high doses improve blood-flow and act as mental stimulants. However, adverse effects include anxiety, increased blood pressure, headache, palpitations and tremor. These compounds are often present in non-prescription medicines for coughs, colds and influenza.

Narcotic analgesics

Narcotic or opioid analgesics may be used to mask pain and permit activity in the face of injury, which is not to be recommended. However, they are more likely to be abused for their euphoric effects. These agents also produce respiratory depression, which is a serious adverse effect for anyone contemplating intensive physical activity. The major risk of these drugs is their dependence potential (*see* Chapter 7).

Anabolic agents

This class includes anabolic androgenic steroids and beta$_2$ agonists.

First used in 1954, anabolic steroids are synthetic derivatives of testosterone used to increase strength and lean body mass, and to decrease recovery time from exercise. These agents are used during training rather than the event itself, and are one of the most widely abused class of drugs in sport. Adverse effects are associated with the use of anabolic steroids: some are irreversible; others may be fatal. Adverse effects include acne, aggressiveness, depression, enlargement of the clitoris, fatigue, foetal damage, gallstones, gynaecomastia, hypertension, increased plasma-LDL concentrations and decreased plasma-HDL concentrations, infertility, jaundice, liver disorders, menstrual irregularities, oedema, premature closure of the epiphyses in adolescents, priapism, prostate enlargement and testicular atrophy. Delayed-onset adverse effects, sometimes appearing only some years later, include ischaemic heart disease, stroke and liver cancer. Irreversible masculinising effects in women include hirsutism, male-pattern baldness and deepening of the voice. Anabolic steroids enhance the development of muscles, but not tendons; this increases the risk of injuries.

Testosterone is used in the hope that, as it is naturally present in the body, its use will not be detected. The IOC has included it in the list of banned substances under anabolic steroids by requiring that the ratio in the urine of testosterone:epitestosterone should not exceed 6:1.

Beta$_2$ agonists may be used orally or by injection to increase altertness, reduce feelings of tiredness and increase competitiveness or aggression. They may also be administered systemically to increase muscle size, strength and power. Adverse effects include tremor, palpitations, muscle cramps, restlessness, insomnia, nausea, rapid heart rate, dilation of peripheral blood vessels, headaches and anxiety. These drugs are commonly used to treat asthma.

Diuretics

Diuretics may be used for one of two reasons: firstly, they produce a rapid loss in weight as a result of fluid loss and therefore may be taken immediately before a weigh-in (e.g. in boxing); secondly, they may also be used as masking agents to produce a dilute urine.

Peptide and glycoprotein hormones and analogues

Chorionic gonadotrophin (HCG or human chorionic gonadotrophin) administered to males causes an increase in the concentrations of endogenous androgenic steroids, and its use in sport is therefore banned.

Corticotrophin (ACTH or adrenocorticotrophic hormone) increases the concentrations of endogenous corticosteroids (which have a stimulant action) and its use in sport has consequently been banned.

Human growth hormone (HGH or somatotrophin) is used to increase size and strength, although the evidence for this effect in normal, healthy adults is lacking. Unlike anabolic steroids, the enlargement produced by growth hormone is non-specific and many organs may be involved. This is probably less likely to be a problem in adults, in whom most of the growth receptors will be inactive, than in children and adolescents. It is predicted that the long-term use of growth hormone could produce acromegaly, cardiomyopathy, diabetes mellitus, hypertension and hyperhidrosis. However, to date, there are only anecdotal reports available to confirm this. In some cases, other drugs (e.g. clonidine, propranolol and vasopressin) may be used to stimulate increased release of endogenous growth hormone from the pituitary gland.

Drugs with partial restrictions

Some drugs (e.g. corticosteroids and local anaesthetics) may be used under certain conditions, and notification to the relevant authorities may be required. Certain formulations, or only specific indications, may be permitted.

Beta-blockers (e.g. atenolol, propranolol, sotalol) reduce heart rate, anxiety and tremor, and are consequently used in precision sports. Their use is banned by the IOC in certain sports only, for example, in archery, shooting and freestyle skiing.

Alcohol is a source of calories that may be used as a fuel source; it also reduces anxiety. Its use is not banned by the IOC, although breath-alcohol or blood-alcohol concentrations may be determined at the request of an international sports federation. However, other sports authorities may have different rules: for example, the International Skiing Federation bans the use of alcohol by competitors because of its disinhibiting effect.

Cannabis is also not banned by the IOC Medical Commission for use in sport, although tests may be requested by an international sports federation. However, UK law prohibits its possession and use.

Table 8.4 lists examples of substances included in the above categories. Details of some of the drugs that may be taken by athletes without contravening these regulations are described below.

Banned procedures

'Blood doping' is a technique to improve blood-haemoglobin concentrations and consequently oxygen consumption. It involves taking up to 900 mL of blood from the competitor and freezing it some weeks before an event. It is then re-infused one to two days before the event. However, it can take months for some individuals to recover after blood has been taken. The alternative is to infuse donor blood before the event, but this method introduces risks of serum sickness and transmission of blood-borne diseases (e.g. AIDS and hepatitis). There is always an increase in viscosity following blood transfusion, which carries a risk of blood-vessel blockage. Blood doping is banned by the IOC, although there are, as yet, no means of detection.

Oxygen 100% is used in some sports because it is felt that increased oxygen in the muscles improves performance and reduces recovery time from exercise. However, studies carried out to assess its effectiveness have not been conclusive. Oxygen is also inconvenient because it can only be administered if the activity is temporarily stopped, and the effects are short-lived. However, it is often used in American football and has not been banned by the IOC.

Illicit drugs

The use of illicit drugs (e.g. amphetamines, heroin, cocaine and cannabis) is a problem in society as a whole rather than one specifically confined to athletes, and is discussed in Chapter 7.

Therapeutic drugs

It may be necessary for sportsmen and women to occasionally take medication to relieve the symptoms of minor illnesses or to treat more

Table 8.4 Examples of substances and methods banned by the Medical Commission of the International Olympic Committee (IOC)

Class A

Stimulants

Amfepramone
Amineptine
Amiphenazole
Amphetamine
Bambuterol
Bromantan
Caffeine[a]
Carphedon
Cocaine
Cropropamide
Crotethamide
Dimethylamphetamine
Ephedrines[b]
Etamivan
Ethylamphetamine
Etilfrine
Fencamfamin
Fenetylline
Fenfluramine
Formoterol
Heptaminol
Mefenorex
Mephentermine
Mesocarb
Methoxyphenamine
Methylamphetamine
Methylenedioxyamphetamine
Methylphenidate
Nikethamide
Norfenfluramine
Parahydroxyamphetamine
Pemoline
Pentetrazol
Pentylentertrazol
Phendimetrazine
Phentermine
Phenylephrine
Pholedrine
Pipradrol
Prolintane
Propylhexedrine
Pyrovalerone
Reproterol
Salbutamol[c]
Salmeterol[c]
Selegiline
Strychnine
Terbutaline[c]
and related compounds

[a] The definition of a positive is a concentration in urine in excess of 12 μg/mL.

[b] For cathine, the definition of a positive is a concentration in urine in excess of 5 μg/mL. For ephedrine and methylephedrine, the definition of a positive is a concentration in urine in excess of 10 μg/mL. For phenylpropanolamine and pseudoephedrine, the definition of a positive is a concentration in urine in excess of 25 μg/mL.

[c] Permitted by inhaler only to prevent and/or treat asthma and exercise-induced asthma. Written notification by a team doctor is necessary to the relevant medical authority.

Class B

Narcotic analgesics

Buprenorphine
Dextromoramide
Diamorphine (heroin)
Hydrocodone
Methadone
Morphine
Pentazocine
Pethidine
and related compounds

Class C

1 Anabolic androgenic steroids

Androstenediol
Androstenedione
Boldenone
Clostebol
Danazol
Dehydrochlormethyltestosterone
Dehydroepianrosterone (DHEA)
Dihydrotestosterone
Drostanolone
Fluoxymesterone
Formebolone

Table 8.4 continued

Class C	19-norandrostenediol
1 Anabolic androgenic steroids (contd)	19-norandrostenedione
Gestrinone	Norethandrolone
Mesterolone	Oxandrolone
Metandienone	Oxymesterone
Metenolone	Oxymetholone
Methandriol	Stanozolol
Methyltestosterone	Testosterone[a]
Mibolerone	Trenbolone
Nandrolone	and related compounds
[a] The definition of a positive is the administration of testosterone or the use of any other manipulation such that the ratio of testosterone:epitestosterone in the urine exceeds 6:1.	
2 Beta$_2$ antagonists	Reproterol
Bambuterol	Salbutamol[a]
Clenbuterol	Salmeterol[a]
Fenoterol	Terbutaline[a]
Formoterol	and related compounds
[a] Authorised by inhalation as described under Class A.	
Class D	
Diuretics	Hydrochlorothiazide
Acetazolamide	Indapamide
Bendroflumethiazide	Mannitol[a]
Bumetanide	Mersalyl
Canrenone	Spironolactone
Chlortalidone	Triamterene
Ethacrynic acid	and related compounds
Furosemide (frusemide)	
[a] Prohibited by intravenous injection.	
Class E *Peptide and glycoprotein hormones and analogues* Chorionic gonadotrophin (HCG or human chorionic gonadotrophin) Corticotrophin (ACTH or adrenocorticotrophic hormone) Growth hormone (HGH or somatotrophin) and all the respective releasing factors of the above-mentioned substances Erythropoietin (EPO)	*Pharmacological, chemical and physical manipulation* The IOC Medical Commission bans the use of substances and of methods which alter the integrity and validity of urine samples used in doping controls. Examples of banned methods are catheterisation, urine substitution and/or tampering, inhibition of renal excretion (e.g. by probenecid and related compounds), epitestosterone or bromantan administration.
Blood doping The practice of blood doping in sport is banned by the IOC Medical Commission.	*Alcohol and marijuana* Alcohol and marijuana are not prohibited, although tests may be carried out at the request of an International Federation.

Table 8.4 continued

Local anaesthetics
Injectable local anaesthetics are permitted under the following conditions:

- that bupivacaine, lidocaine, mepivacaine, procaine, etc. are used but not cocaine
- only local or intra-articular injections may be administered; intravascular injections are not permitted
- only when medically justified (i.e. the details including diagnosis, dose and route of administration must be submitted immediately in writing).

Glucocorticosteroids
The use of glucocorticosteroids is banned except for topical use (aural, ophthalmological or dermatological), inhalation therapy (for asthma or allergic rhinitis) and by local or intra-articular injections. Any team doctor wishing to administer corticosteroids intra-articularly or locally to a competitor must give written notification to the IOC Medical Commission.

Beta blockers
Beta blockers are banned in certain sports, including archery, bobsleigh, diving, curling, synchronised swimming, luge, modern pentathlon, shooting, ski jumping and freestyle skiing. Examples of banned beta blockers include acebutolol, alprenolol, atenolol, labetalol, metoprolol, nadolol, oxoprenolol, propranolol, sotalol, and related substances.

The presence in a urine sample of all listed substances (except those substances that are allowed up to a certain level) or their major metabolites, and substances belonging to the banned classes even if they are not listed, will constitute an offence.

The information contained in this table is taken from one of the booklets in the Doping Control Information series produced by the Sports Council. Copies of the booklets may be obtained from the Doping Control unit of the Sports Council (*see* Useful addresses).

Other governing bodies (both national and international) may produce their own lists of banned substances or there may be sport-specific restrictions. For example, the Modern Pentathlon bans the use of anxiolytic sedatives, hypnotics, neuroleptics and tricyclic antidepressants, and an up-to-date copy of the list specific for a competitor's particular sport and event should always be consulted.

serious acute disorders or injuries. Some competitors may have a chronic condition (e.g. asthma) that requires long-term administration of drugs. The side-effects of some drugs (e.g. nausea, drowsiness or fatigue) may impair athletic performance or may have adverse effects during physical activity (*see* The risks of sport and exercise *above*). The benefits of exercise must be weighed against the potential risks. Where possible, alternative means of treatment should be sought (e.g. homoeopathy could be a possibility) or, if none are available, a programme of physical activity should be designed to minimise the associated risks. Banned substances may be inadvertently taken, which is particularly likely to happen if non-prescription medicines are purchased or athletes do not tell prescribers that they intend to compete.

Many common non-prescription remedies for coughs and colds contain sympathomimetics that are banned. Now that drug testing may be carried out during both training and competition, and in the close season, it is prudent for pharmacists to enquire whether potential clients are involved in sport before making a suggestion. Some herbal products (e.g. ginseng) often contain substances that are not declared on the label and can give a positive dope test. Ma Huang (Chinese ephedra) contains ephedrine. At present, there is no legal requirement for ingredients to be listed on the labels of herbal products or dietary supplements. Competing athletes using such products may inadvertently ingest banned substances.

Participation in sports and exercise

The effects of training

The effects of training are to increase the maximum capacity for work so that less effort is required for the same work-load, and the maximum intensity and duration of work increases. Changes only occur in those muscles that are exercised, including heart and respiratory muscles. To be of benefit to health, physical activity must therefore be intense enough to significantly increase the heart rate and respiration rate. Regular physical activity can improve stamina, suppleness and strength.

In healthy subjects, the maximum heart rate at peak exercise is about 200 beats/minute at 20 years of age, and decreases with age. The minimum amount of physical activity required to induce a training effect is three sessions of 20 minutes each week of aerobic exercise, during which time the heart rate should be increased to between 60 and 70% of the maximum. There is marked individual variation in maximum heart rate. Those over 35 years of age, the obese, or anyone with a pre-existing medical condition may require a medical examination (including an ECG) before commencing (*see below*).

Exercising vigorously every day is neither necessary, nor is it recommended because the risk of injury is increased. A refractory period of 24 to 48 hours is essential to allow the worked muscles to recover. Overtraining is also likely to cause fatigue and a loss of interest. Some individuals, however, prefer not to rest on the days between exercise sessions, but alternate periods of light and hard exercise, or alternate sports that use different muscles. Those who are not used to vigorous activity should start exercising gently at first and increase the intensity in small stages at intervals of eight to ten weeks. Although the aim is to work the muscles and cardiovascular and respiratory systems, the individual should not feel unduly distressed.

Injuries during sport and exercise may be prevented by warming-up before and cooling-down afterwards. Participants should be realistic in their choice of activity and choose within their capabilities. Progress in a new venture or in returning to an old one after a period of inactivity should be gradual, and with appropriate intermediate objectives. It is important to remember that many vigorous activities require a certain level of fitness for safe participation, and although such activities are of enormous benefit in improving and maintaining fitness, they may not be suitable for getting fit. Thus, it may be necessary to first undertake a graded programme of suitable training exercises.

Training is a long-term commitment, and individuals who stop it completely will soon return to being unfit. They may also become obese if dietary adjustments are not made to meet the reduced level of physical activity.

Fitness tests

An initial routine medical examination to assess the safety of sport or exercise for an individual may include screening for, or testing of, the following:

- degree of obesity
- blood pressure
- heart and lung sounds
- ECG
- tendon reflexes
- enlargement of lymph nodes
- herniation in the groin.

Additional tests may be required if routine medical examination reveals abnormalities. Sport-specific tests (e.g. chest X-ray for SCUBA diving) may also be necessary.

Fitness tests are tests carried out under controlled conditions to assess an individual's fitness and, consequently, their capacity for exercise. Fitness may be assessed by measurement of various parameters, including cardiovascular fitness, muscular endurance and strength, flexibility and body composition (i.e. proportion of body fat).

The basis of all the different tests is to increase the workload on the subject by a known amount and measure the response either during the test or at the end of it. The easiest parameter to measure is the final pulse rate. There is some risk of cardiac arrest attached to the tests, but when compared with the risk in the general population, these tests are considered to be relatively safe, provided they are supervised by trained personnel and adequate means of resuscitation are available.

The simplest test is the step test, which involves stepping on and off a step of predetermined height for a given time, followed by measurement of pulse rate. The results are read against standard tables to give the fitness index. There are many variations of step height, length of test and intervals of final pulse measurement, but the most important point is that whatever parameters are chosen, they must remain constant to enable comparisons.

Bicycle ergometry involves the use of a modified bicycle with a variable-resistance drive wheel that can be adjusted to different work-loads. The subject pedals against the resistance for a given time, after which the pulse rate is measured and compared against standard tables. More sophisticated tests may involve the measurement of gases inhaled and exhaled to determine VO_2 max (*see* The physiology of exercise *above*).

Many different types of treadmill are available to suit medical purposes or for training athletes. They may be horizontal, or raised through successive gradients to increase the workload. Pulse rate is usually measured before and after the test; alternatively, experienced personnel can measure pulse rate and blood pressure during the test.

Exercise programmes

A distinction is usually drawn between weight-bearing and non-weight-bearing exercise. The former is a physical activity (e.g. walking or running) in which the legs support the weight of the body; examples of the latter are swimming and cycling. Another classification identifies high-impact movements that have an unsupported airborne phase (e.g. jumping) and low-impact movements, where one foot is in contact with the ground at all times (e.g. walking). It should be noted that a low-impact exercise may not necessarily be low intensity; similarly, a high-impact exercise may not be high intensity. Some activities may fall into both categories.

Table 8.5 provides an example of guidelines for an eight-week walking programme of anaerobic exercise.

The main features of an aerobic exercise programme are summarised in Table 8.6. The acronym is appropriately given the letters FITT.

Sport and exercise for special groups

The elderly

Physical activity naturally falls with advancing age, and with it there is a decline in fitness, stamina, strength, suppleness and co-ordination. Eventually, the deterioration may be such that everyday tasks cannot be carried out (e.g. carrying shopping or doing housework) and the individual loses independence. It has been estimated that 20% of the decline is as a result of inactivity. This degenerative process may be retarded by maintaining a reasonable level of activity to suit the ability of the individual. Movement of each joint through its full range each day maintains joint mobility; swimming or stair-climbing increases strength; and various activities (e.g. digging, swimming, walking or housework) carried out at least three times a week improve stamina. Elderly people who regularly undertake some form of exercise often show improved concentration and mood compared with more sedentary individuals. They may also be afforded some degree of protection against hypothermia

Table 8.5 Example of an anaerobic exercise programme

Weeks	Age up to 50	Age above 50	Times per week
1 to 2	12 mins	6 mins	2 to 3
3 to 4	15 mins	10 mins	2 to 3
5 to 6	17 mins	12 mins	3 to 4
6 to 8	20 mins	15 mins	3 to 4

Table 8.6 The features of an aerobic programme – FITT

Frequency	most authorities consider three to five days per week is optimal
Intensity	exercise at 50 to 85% of VO_2 max or 75% of maximum heart rate improves fitness
Time	a duration of about 20 min per session is recommended
Type	a continuous activity (e.g. jogging, swimming or walking)

during the winter because of the effect that physical activity has in raising body temperature. Additional social benefits may be gained through attending local exercise classes for the elderly.

Elderly people are not precluded from participating in many sporting activities, and are likely to gain benefits from the excitement and challenge of competition and joining in any social events organised by their particular club. It is recommended that anyone contemplating a programme of vigorous exercise should first seek medical advice to ensure that there is no underlying condition that first requires treatment, or which may contra-indicate intensive physical activity. Enquiry must also be made about any medication, as the effects of some drugs (e.g. antihypertensive drugs, beta-blockers, calcium-channel blockers, diuretics, some psychotropic drugs and insulin and oral antidiabetic drugs) may compromise the safety of exercise. Warming-up and cooling-down exercises are recommended for anyone exercising, but their importance must be particularly stressed for the elderly. It is also important to emphasise that elderly people should not exercise in extremes of environmental temperature, which may precipitate hypothermia or hyperthermia, because the homoeostatic control mechanisms may not function as efficiently as in younger adults.

Disabled athletes

Exercises can be tailored to meet the capacity and abilities of most subjects, and the disabled will benefit as much from physical activity as able-bodied people. It is a misconception that people with disabilities are fragile and are not able to do anything for themselves. This attitude is likely to lead to a worsening of the disability, with a concomitant reduction in the level of the individual's independence. In fact, for such individuals, exercise may have an even greater impact on improving the quality of life by increasing stamina, strength, dexterity and co-ordination, thereby maximising residual capacities. The effort required to carry out everyday tasks may be reduced, resulting in increased independence and self-confidence. It may also help prevent the emergence of a secondary disability.

Where possible, aerobic exercises involving the movement of large muscles to improve cardiopulmonary performance and exercises to work the joints should be carried out. Exercises in water are particularly advantageous as they are non-weight-bearing. However, there will be those with types of disability that make many exercises impractical or difficult, and exercises of sufficient intensity to significantly improve cardiovascular fitness are just not possible. This should not, however, preclude them from engaging in physical activities of low intensity, increasing the programme gradually to remain within their capabilities and comfort at each stage. It is now not uncommon for physically disabled people to learn a sport, and there are many organisations and clubs that can help. The added advantage of sports participation is that it brings people with disabilities together, and they can learn and benefit from each other's experiences in coping with the tasks of everyday life.

People with mental handicaps suffer impairment of learning processes, and there may also be associated physical disabilities (e.g. impaired co-ordination). However, there is no reason why they should not participate in sports or exercise, which in addition to improving physical fitness, may well have beneficial effects in improving learning ability, mood and self-confidence. They may also find it enjoyable, and, for the energetic young, it may prove a valuable means of 'releasing energy' and relieving frustrations that they are unable to channel in other directions. Skilled help is necessary for both physically and mentally handicapped people to participate in sports and exercise safely and effectively, particularly when starting. A medical assessment should be undertaken initially, to assess the most suitable form and appropriate intensity of sport or exercise to ensure that the individual is not put at risk of injury.

The British Sports Association for the Disabled (BSAD) is funded largely via the Sports Councils and is responsible for the development of disabled sport at non-elite level. It supports the full spectrum of sports played by disabled people, organising national championships where possible. As disabled people progress towards more elite level, they may compete under the organisational umbrella of organisations covering specific groups (e.g. wheelchair athletes, cerebral palsy, blind, amputees and the deaf).

The role of the pharmacist

To help meet the challenges that have emerged with regard to sport and exercise and the use of medication, a discipline called 'sports pharmacy' is emerging. It may be defined as:

> the science and practice of dispensing medication and medical equipment for individuals participating in exercise or sport, and the provision of information and advice on exercise programmes and the treatment and prevention of simple injuries.

For many people, participation in sport or exercise is a daunting prospect, even if they have already been convinced that it will be beneficial to their health. They may fear that exercising will be uncomfortable or painful, or they may worry about potential injuries. Many of those who have not played any sport since school are likely to be lacking in confidence or too embarrassed to learn (or re-learn) a new skill. Lack of time is an important factor in many people's lifestyles, and a reorganisation of other activities may be necessary. Pharmacists should, where necessary, emphasise that it is not necessary to run marathons to become fit, and explain the overload principle of training (i.e. it is only necessary regularly to increase physical activity above usual levels for a minimum of 20 minutes three times a week). Pharmacists can also suggest, for those who wish to learn a sport, that perhaps the best way is to join a beginner's class so that everyone will be at a similar level of playing skill, and possibly fitness. The social advantages of participating in a sport, particularly if it involves membership of a sports club, could also be stressed.

People's goals and capabilities vary enormously, and pharmacists' initial task is to assess what these are. There are many different ways of exercising, and pharmacists could find out what local facilities are available through the local council offices, adult education centres or private clubs, and pass the information on to those interested. However, not everyone has the time or the inclination to take up a sport, and some people may prefer solitary exercise rather than group exercising. One of the most popular, convenient and least obtrusive ways of exercising is walking. As long as the pace is brisk (i.e. faster than normal walking pace) and forms a regular part of an individual's normal routine, there will be a training effect. The most enjoyable way is to specifically 'go for a walk', particularly in areas of interesting scenery. However, for those truly pressed for time, there are ample opportunities throughout the course of a normal day's work to 'walk rather than ride'. Stair-climbing instead of using a lift, or walking short distances instead of taking a car, bus or train is of great benefit; the extra time taken is probably negligible compared with the time wasted in rush-hour traffic or waiting for public transport. There is the additional benefit of boosting the body's levels of vitamin D by carrying out physical activities outdoors (*see* Chapter 2, Vitamins). For those who may have difficulties in coping with sport and exercise (e.g. the elderly, or physically or mentally handicapped), specialist help is available from various organisations (*see* Useful addresses). Pharmacists can help by passing such information on and by displaying some of the many leaflets available from such organisations.

Pharmacists may become involved with amateur or professional sports clubs, and be asked for advice about items for a medical bag to enable first-aid to be carried out on-site at a sporting event. Team doctors and physiotherapists will have their own specialist requirements (e.g.

suturing equipment, drugs for emergency use, inflatable splint, infra-red lamp and strapping) in addition to the basic items needed to cleanse and dress wounds and carry out the RICE regimen (*see* Sports medicine *above*). Many low-key events will not have professional medical help available, and it will be the responsibility of the coach to administer first-aid, followed by medical referral where necessary. For suggestions of items that may be included in a sports medical bag to cover the basic requirements of sports injury first-aid, *see* Table 8.3.

Pharmacists presented with requests for advice by an athlete for the treatment of a minor ailment should first ascertain what the problem is and then check the relevant list of banned substances before counter-prescribing. The IOC produces one such list (*see* Table 8.4), but there may be further restrictions imposed by other national or international organisations, and there may be some sport-specific restrictions. A competitor should, therefore, make himself fully aware of all regulations governing his specific event and present the information to pharmacists before purchasing medicines or having a prescription dispensed. Athletes may be confused over nomenclature of substances on the banned list (e.g. trade or generic names, or metabolites), and seek guidance from pharmacists.

In general, coughs and colds cannot be treated with any product containing sympathomimetics (e.g. ephedrine, phenylpropanolamine or pseudoephedrine) or codeine. However, dextromethorphan and pholcodine are not banned, and antitussive preparations containing these agents may be recommended. Hayfever may be treated with antihistamines and sodium cromoglicate, but not sympathomimetics (however, some antihistamines are currently banned in the modern pentathlon). There is no ban on the use of non-steroidal anti-inflammatory products. Aspirin and paracetamol are permitted as analgesics, but codeine is not, which precludes the use of combination analgesic products. Products containing morphine or codeine may not be used to treat diarrhoea, although diphenoxylate and loperamide are permitted. Hyoscine may be used as a gastro-intestinal antispasmodic and an anti-emetic. Topical corticosteroids are permitted for the treatment of skin conditions, but there are partial restrictions imposed on the use of other corticosteroid formulations.

It is also necessary to be aware of prescription-only medicines that are banned, because there may be instances where patients have omitted to tell the prescriber that they intend to participate in a registered sporting event, and turn instead for advice to the pharmacist dispensing the prescription. Antibiotics and antihistamines are allowed, but care must be exercised when prescribing the latter when contained in multi-ingredient preparations. Oral contraceptives are usually allowed. The use of some sympathomimetics (e.g. orciprenaline, rimiterol, salbutamol and terbutaline) is allowed in aerosol formulations for the treatment of asthma. Fenoterol is banned because it is metabolised to a stimulant, parahydroxyamphetamine. Sodium cromoglicate and nedocromil are also allowed for the treatment of asthma, but isoprenaline is banned. Anticonvulsants may be used by epileptics, provided that a declaration has been made beforehand. A list of drugs that may be used when competing can be obtained from the four Sports Councils. The Sports Councils have produced a 'Doping Control in Sport' advice card. Supplies of the card may be obtained from the Doping Control Unit of the Sports Council (*see* Useful addresses *below*). Other national bodies (e.g. Sport New Zealand) produce similar cards.

References

Harman R J (1989). *Patient Care in Community Practice*. London: Pharmaceutical Press.

Further reading

Harries M (2000). *ABC of Sports Medicine*, 2nd edn. London: BMJ Books.

Kayne S B, Wadeson K, MacAdam A (2000). Is glucosamine an effective treatment for osteoarthritis? A meta-analysis. *Pharm J* (in press).

Lillegard W A, Butcher J D, Rucker K S (1999). *Handbook of Sports Medicine*. Oxford: Butterworth-Heinemann.

Marchand J (1990). *Sport for All in Europe*. London: HMSO.

Martin M, Yates W (1998). *Therapeutic Medications in Sports Medicine*. Baltimore, MD: Williams & Wilkins.

Mottram D R, ed. (1996). *Drugs in Sport*, 2nd edn. London: E & F N Spon.

Reilly T, Secher N, Snell P, *et al.*, eds (1990). *Physiology of Sports*. London: E & F N Spon.

St. John's Ambulance, St. Andrew's Ambulance Association, British Red Cross Society (1997). *First Aid Manual: The Authorised Manual of St. John Ambulance, St. Andrew's Ambulance Association, and the British Red Cross Society*, 7th edn. London: Dorling Kindersley.

Useful addresses

British Olympic Association
1 Wandsworth Plain
London SW18 1EH
Tel: 020 8871 2677

British Sports Association for the Disabled
The Mary Glen Haig Suite
34 Osnaburgh Street
London NW1 3ND
Tel: 020 7383 7277

Chartered Society of Physiotherapy
14 Bedford Row
London WC1R 4ED
Tel: 020 7242 1941

Disabled Living Foundation
380–384 Harrow Road
London W9 2HU
Tel: 020 7289 6111

Exercise Training for the Elderly and/or Disabled (EXTEND)
22 Maltings Drive
Wheathampstead
Hertfordshire AL4 8QJ
Tel: 01582 832760

Irish Sports Council
21 Fitzwilliam Square
Dublin 2
Ireland
Tel: +353 1240 7700

Keep Fit Association
Francis House
Francis Street
London SW1P 1DE
Tel: 020 7233 8898

The National Sports Medicine Institute of The United Kingdom
c/o Medical College of St Bartholomew's Hospital
Charterhouse Square
London EC1M 6BQ
Tel: 020 7251 0583

The Royal Association for Disability and Rehabilitation (RADAR)
Unit 12, City Forum
250 City Road
London EC1V 8AF
Tel: 020 7250 3222

Sport England
16 Upper Woburn Place
London WC1H 0QP
Tel: 020 7388 1277

Sport Scotland
Caledonia House
1 Redhews Rigg
Edinburgh EH12 9DQ
Tel: 0131 317 7200

Sports Council of Northern Ireland
House of Sport
Upper Malone Road
Belfast BT9 5AA
Tel: 0289 038 1222

Sports Nutrition Foundation
The National Sports Medicine Institute of the United Kingdom
c/o Medical College of St Bartholomew's Hospital
Charterhouse Square
London EC1M 6BQ
Tel: 020 7251 0583

Welsh Insitute of Sport
Sophia Gardens
Cardiff CF11 9SW
Tel: 02920 300 500

9

Health and travel

Larry Goodyer

The number of people travelling overseas for business or pleasure has risen steadily since the introduction of international air travel. Significant numbers also leave the UK for the continent. This steady increase has been reflected in an upsurge in requests to pharmacists for advice about health during travel. The range of destinations is varied and includes more tropical countries than ever before. The advice on prophylaxis against infectious diseases is constantly being updated, and it is essential that pharmacists keep abreast of all major developments in travel health. However, the problem of contracting infectious disease must be viewed within the context of the various other health hazards (Table 9.1). Although a very high percentage of travellers will experience a bout of diarrhoea, mortality from any infectious disease is below 1% of all deaths. The main causes of death are cardiovascular disease and accidents.

There are a variety of infectious diseases that may befall the unwary and unprepared traveller (*see* Prevention and management of conditions associated with travel *below*). The risk of contracting any of these diseases varies considerably, and depends upon the destination, activities while abroad, standard of foreign accommodation and numerous other factors (e.g. state of health and medical history).

Table 9.1 Travel health hazards

- Accidents
- Altitude/climate
- Chronic illness
- Dermatological, e.g. sunburn
- Iatrogenic
- Infections
- Travel sickness

This chapter deals with some of the precautions that need to be taken before and during travel to minimise illness and discomfort; the preventive measures that need to be taken to avoid contracting infections; management of some conditions associated with travel; and action that may be necessary on returning home. In the UK, information on recommendations for immunisation and all aspects of health abroad can be found in Department of Health (DoH) leaflets, which are updated regularly. Information is also published by the World Health Organization (WHO). Prominent display of available literature in the pharmacy helps to confirm pharmacists as a source of information on health and overseas travel. Also available are a number of computerised databases and on-line resources with which pharmacists should be familiar.

Action to be taken before travelling

Immunisation

Immunisation against infectious diseases is an important medical consideration before setting out overseas. Malaria chemoprophylaxis must also be considered in advance of travel (*see below*). Pharmacists have perhaps a lesser role to play in travel vaccination, as general practitioners will now stock a range of vaccines for use by the practice nurse. Pharmacists should still have a general overview of the current use of travel vaccines in order to deal with queries from the public. It should also be remembered that the planning of vaccination schedules is the subject initially bringing the traveller into contact with other health professionals, allowing for the opportunity to address a variety of health issues. Certainly, those pharmacists working more closely with general practitioners may become involved in the issues concerning travel vaccines.

A clear distinction must be drawn between mandatory immunisation requirements necessary for entry to a country and recommendations for immunisation because of the potential risks to the traveller. Some vaccines are administered as courses in which doses must be separated by specified time intervals; some vaccines may not be given at the same time as others. It is absolutely essential, therefore, that travellers start their vaccination programmes well in advance of the date of departure. It is recommended that travellers visit general practitioners at least two months before travel, and even longer if planning hepatitis B vaccination. There are a few rules that apply to the administration of live vaccines:

- it is important that the administration of live vaccines is postponed until at least three months after stopping oral corticosteroids and six months after stopping cancer chemotherapy
- in theory, live virus vaccines should be given at least three weeks before or three months after an injection of normal immunoglobulin, which may interfere with the immune response. This does not apply to yellow fever vaccine, since normal immunoglobulin does not contain antibody to the virus. Polio is another live vaccine, and for those about to travel, if there is insufficient time, the recommended interval may have to be ignored
- if two live vaccines are required, they should be administered at the same time or three weeks apart
- live vaccines are usually avoided in immunosuppressed individuals or those with human immunodeficiency virus (HIV).

In general terms, travel to Europe, North America, Australia and New Zealand does not warrant protection unless a stop-over is made outside these areas. The specific measures required vary according to stop-overs and final destinations. Information and details of addresses and telephone numbers of UK organisations that can be contacted for further information can be obtained from BNF 14.6; some useful addresses are also listed below (*see* Useful addresses *below*). Not all vaccines that may be required for travel are available at NHS expense: for example, yellow fever and Japanese B encephalitis vaccination must be purchased privately.

Diphtheria, measles, mumps, poliomyelitis, rubella, tuberculosis and tetanus are all given routinely as part of the UK childhood immunisation programme and only booster doses may be required for some of these. However, full courses may be required by those who did not receive vaccines during childhood, or if courses were not completed.

Cholera

Cholera is primarily a disease resulting from poor sanitation and hygiene, but is rarely a problem in travellers. Part of the reason for this is that certain strains of vibrio cholera have become less virulent over the years. Therefore, the symptoms of sudden massive and life-threatening diarrhoea are rarely seen in otherwise healthy individuals. Indeed, travellers who contract cholera may experience little worse than a severe bout of traveller's diarrhoea. It does remain a serious problem in the young and elderly, and in those who are malnourished or otherwise debilitated. In these individuals, the use of oral rehydration therapy may be life-saving. The cholera vaccine previously used has been found to provide an unacceptably low level of protection. Therefore, in recognition of the fact that vaccination against cholera cannot prevent the introduction of infection into a country, the World Health Assembly amended the International Health Regulations in 1973 so that cholera vaccination should no longer be required of any traveller. Unfortunately, travellers to some destinations in developing countries have reported that customs officials will occasionally demand a certificate in lieu of a bribe. A more effective oral cholera vaccine has been developed, but it is not yet (2000) licensed in the UK.

Hepatitis

Hepatitis A and hepatitis B occur throughout the world, particularly in warm climates where hygiene and sanitary conditions are poor. Hepatitis A is transmitted by the faecal-oral route and has no carrier state. Infection commonly arises as a result of eating raw seafood that has been contaminated by sewage, or by eating vegetables grown in soil fertilised with human faeces.

The risk of contracting hepatitis B is increased by the high prevalence of asymptomatic carriers in many parts of the world. Hepatitis B is transmitted predominantly in blood and blood products, although its presence in saliva, menstrual and vaginal fluids, and seminal fluid allows the possibility of additional modes of transmission.

Passive immunisation against hepatitis A for travellers to endemic regions can be carried out by administering human normal immunoglobulin injection, which protects for three to five months. This has largely been replaced by the more reliable active vaccination, prepared from inactivated hepatitis A virus. A first dose of the adult vaccine will provide protection for up to one year; if a booster is given within one year, ten years' protection will be achieved.

Active immunisation with hepatitis B vaccine is available for travellers considered at high risk (e.g. healthcare staff, patients with malignant diseases, immunocompromised patients and homosexual men). It is also worth considering for travellers on longer journeys (i.e. longer than three months) where medical facilities may be poor. It should, however, be borne in mind that the immunisation schedule takes up to six months to confer adequate immunity.

Japanese B encephalitis

Japanese B encephalitis is a rare, but serious, insect-borne infection that occurs in most of the Far-East and South-East Asia. It tends to be more prevalent during the monsoon season in certain rural pig-breeding areas. Travellers visiting such regions for extended periods may be advised to seek vaccination. At present, Japanese B encephalitis vaccine is only available on a named-patient basis. Also, some concerns have been raised regarding the safety of this vaccine; in rare cases, it is associated with serious delayed hypersensitivity reactions.

Meningitis

This vaccine is sometimes recommended to those travelling to certain destinations in Asia or Africa. In particular, the disease tends to cause seasonal epidemics across the 'meningitis belt' of Africa. A single vaccination against the A and C strains is required.

Poliomyelitis

Despite its disappearance from many developed countries of the western world, poliomyelitis is still prevalent in developing nations, especially in areas with poor healthcare facilities. Poliomyelitis is contracted via the faecal-oral route or nasopharyngeal secretions.

A large proportion of the UK population and that of other western countries is protected against poliomyelitis as a result of active immunisation programmes carried out during childhood since 1955. Nevertheless, travellers with no record of immunisation wishing to visit developing countries must be immunised before setting out. Single, oral booster doses are recommended every ten years for those who have been previously immunised.

Rabies

Apart for those working with animals, other travellers may also need to consider vaccination against rabies. This will mainly be for destinations where the incidence is very high and supplies of vaccine or antibodies unreliable. All travellers should be advised to seek medical help and vaccination if bitten by a mammal, whether or not pre-exposure vaccination has been given.

Tetanus

The risk of contracting tetanus is rare on holidays of limited physical exertion; the risk is somewhat increased when participating in holidays of greater activity (e.g. adventure holidays, trekking and safaris). Most people in the UK will have been vaccinated during childhood, but booster doses are necessary every ten years or following injury. The DoH particularly stresses the need for travellers to regions without medical facilities to be immunised before departure.

Tick-borne encephalitis

Tick-borne encephalitis occurs in the forested areas of Scandinavia and Central Europe, particularly Austria, Czechoslovakia, Germany and Yugoslavia. A vaccine is available from a limited number of centres in the UK on a named-patient basis.

Tuberculosis

This has become a growing worldwide problem in recent years, and presents a particular hazard to those with HIV infection. Those planning travel to certain developing countries for extended periods of time, especially if close contact with the local population is likely, should consider their immune status with regard to tuberculosis. Most children in the UK are immunised with BCG at the age of 12; resistance is retained through early adulthood. Older adults may therefore require testing (e.g. Tine test), but unfortunately the effectiveness of BCG in adults has not been established.

Typhoid fever

Typhoid fever is a disease resulting from poor sanitation and hygiene. Vaccination should be recommended to all travellers to endemic regions intending to stay for longer than two weeks, and especially for travellers to the Indian subcontinent, from where most of the 200 cases reported annually in England and Wales derive. However, it should be emphasised to all prospective travellers that vaccination is not a substitute for, but an adjunct to, basic hygienic measures (*see* Prevention and management of conditions associated with travel *below*). The older, whole cell typhoid vaccine was associated with a high incidence of minor reactions (e.g. local inflammation, fever and malaise). It has been largely superseded by a capsular polysaccharide vaccine, which requires a single dose to provide three years' protection. A live attenuated oral vaccine is also available but, owing to the somewhat complicated dosing schedule, may be less reliable.

Yellow fever

Travellers to some parts of Africa and South America are at risk of contracting yellow fever which, like malaria, is transmitted by mosquitoes. As there is no effective treatment for the infection, the importance of prevention cannot be overemphasised (*see* Prevention and management of conditions associated with travel *below*). A yellow fever vaccine is available from a number of centres in the UK and, after administration, patients are issued with an International Certificate of Vaccination. The certificate becomes valid after ten days and lasts for ten years following initial vaccination; it is immediately valid on revaccination within the ten-year period. Certificates are required for entry into many parts of Africa and South America. Some countries (e.g. in Asia) may require a certificate of vaccination if travellers have come from an endemic region.

Travel and diabetes mellitus

Travelling can be a source of worry to diabetics, and in particular insulin-dependent diabetics, but taking adequate precautionary measures can help allay fears.

Immunisation schedules and malaria prophylaxis are the same for diabetics as non-diabetics (*see above*). It is essential that diabetics ensure that they have sufficient supplies of insulin, syringes and urine/blood testing equipment in their luggage. Air travellers should carry insulin in hand luggage to prevent it freezing in the luggage hold at high altitudes; it is also then available for use in the event of unexpected delays before departure, while airborne or if luggage is lost. If insulin injections are required while airborne, only half as much air should be injected into the vial to take account of the differences between cabin pressure and ground pressure (*see* Air travel *below*). Travellers should be reassured that, although refrigeration of insulin is necessary for long term storage in high ambient temperatures, it is not essential for short periods during a journey or in temperate climates.

A means of identification (e.g. a doctor's letter or statement of current treatment, and the name and address of the doctor or clinic) is important for diabetic travellers. It can help to smooth passage through customs if luggage is searched and the presence of needles and syringes is queried. Identification can also help first-aiders attending a solo diabetic traveller who has lost consciousness as a result of hypoglycaemia.

If diabetics are known to experience motion sickness, it is important to prevent vomiting because of the risk of dehydration, hyperglycaemia and diabetic ketoacidosis. Drugs for motion sickness may be used by insulin-dependent diabetics. If vomiting occurs, carbohydrate intake should be maintained by sipping fluids containing glucose.

Long-distance travel across time zones can pose special problems for insulin-dependent diabetics in the timing of their injections. All insulin-dependent diabetics should be advised to consult their doctor or diabetic clinic well in advance of travelling and, if necessary, have a dosage adjustment schedule worked out for them. It should also be borne in mind that the level of physical activity during a holiday may be somewhat different from that at home, and further adjustments in insulin dose, carbohydrate intake, or both, may be required. Non-insulin-dependent diabetics taking oral hypoglycaemic agents do not need to adjust their dosage schedules on account of different time zones.

Regular dietary management may be a particular problem for diabetics. If normal eating times are delayed, additional snacks may be necessary to prevent hypoglycaemia. Diabetics should always carry a readily available form of glucose in case of insulin overdose or other cause of hypoglycaemia; this is particularly important while travelling.

Prolonged sitting in any form of transport may prevent adequate circulation in the toes and feet. This is a particular hazard for diabetics. Regular walking breaks, or determined efforts to move the toes and feet whilst otherwise immobile, will help to promote adequate bloodflow. Legs should not be crossed while sitting for prolonged periods.

Travel and HIV infection

There is no vaccine available to protect against HIV infection, and travellers must be aware of the mode of transmission of infection and means of prevention (*see* Prevention and management of conditions associated with travel *below*).

People who have already contracted HIV infection should consult their doctor for assessment of their fitness to travel and advice concerning any medication they may require. WHO has advised that no restrictions should be made on entry requirements into any country for people infected with HIV, because such measures are ineffective and impractical in the fight against spread of the disease. Nonetheless, many nations have taken it upon themselves to impose a variety of restrictions that travellers with HIV infection should be aware of.

Air travel

Flying can be a stressful experience, especially for those who do not fly regularly. Elements of travel that cause most stress include overcrowding, delays at airports, altered eating habits and travel across time zones; consequences of these include fatigue, indigestion, insomnia and nausea. The predominant reasons for requests for doctors during a flight include anxiety, convulsions, mental illness, stress, and cardiovascular and gastro-intestinal disorders. Recommendations on advice for people with pre-existing medical conditions are outlined in Table 9.2.

Some drugs (e.g. antiepileptics, insulin and oral contraceptives) require regular dosage intervals to be effective, and patients taking such medication may run into difficulties when crossing time zones. The recommendations are to remain on 'home-time' during a long journey, and to adjust carefully dosage intervals after arrival. It is also strongly recommended that all essential medication is kept in hand luggage. In addition, it is worth keeping some supplies in the main luggage in case either is lost in transit. Epileptics may need to increase their dose of antiepileptic drugs to avoid seizures induced by the stresses of flying and should consult their doctor well in advance of the flight.

The environment within an aircraft is pressurised to counteract the low atmospheric pressure and decreased temperature at high altitudes. At all altitudes, the conditions within the aircraft

Table 9.2 Advice for people with pre-existing medical conditions who may be contemplating air travel

Condition	Advice	Reason
Anaemia, severe	not fit to fly	impaired oxygenation of tissues exacerbated by hypoxia
Cerebrovascular accident	do not fly for at least three weeks	impaired oxygenation of tissues exacerbated by hypoxia
Diabetes mellitus	*see* Travel and diabetes mellitus	
Epilepsy	dose of antiepileptics may need to be increased; patient should consult doctor	risk of stress-induced seizures
Fractured skull	do not fly for at least seven days	expansion of gases may damage brain tissue
Gastro-intestinal haemorrhage, recent (e.g. as a result of peptic ulceration)	do not fly for at least 21 days	rebleeding may occur
Heart failure, uncontrolled	not fit to fly	impaired oxygenation of tissues exacerbated by hypoxia
Infectious diseases	do not fly	risk of contagion of other passengers
Myocardial infarction and severe angina	do not fly for at least two weeks, and preferably not before two months	impaired oxygenation of tissues exacerbated by hypoxia
Ostomies	carry extra bags and dressings	pressure changes may result in increased venting of gas and cause the bag to split
Otitis media, severe	do not fly	inability to vent the Eustachian tubes causes pain and discomfort, and may cause internal damage; patients with grommets may, however, be able to fly because grommets are not an airtight fit
Plaster casts	plaster may need to be split for long journeys	air trapped in the cast may expand and compress the limb
Pneumothorax (collapsed lung)	do not fly until lung has re-expanded	expansion of gases may impair lung function
Psychiatric disorders	trained escort and sedation may be required	stress and excitement of flying may exacerbate some psychiatric conditions
Respiratory disorders that cause breathlessness at rest	flying permissible if fit to walk 50 m and climb 10 to 12 steps	impaired oxygenation of tissues exacerbated by hypoxia
Sinusitis, severe	do not fly	inability to vent the Eustachian tubes causes pain and discomfort, and may cause internal damage
Skin diseases, repulsive	do not fly	carriers feel that offence may be caused to other passengers and air crew, who must handle food, and cannot provide nursing assistance
Surgery, recent		
– abdominal	do not fly for at least ten days	expansion of gas may weaken wound
– air introduced into a body cavity (e.g. laparoscopy)	do not fly until the condition has resolved	expansion of gas may compress and damage surrounding tissue

Table 9.2 continued

Condition	Advice	Reason
– ear (e.g. stapedectomy)	do not fly for at least two weeks, preferably not before two months	expansion of gases may cause severe damage
– facial	must be accompanied by someone trained to release the wires holding the jaws together in the event of vomiting	if the jaws are wired, vomiting as a result of motion sickness may asphyxiate
– intracranial	do not fly for at least seven days	expansion of gases may damage brain tissue
– pulmonary	do not fly for at least 21 days	expansion of gases may impair lung function
Terminal illness	at the discretion of the airline, provided that death is not likely to occur on board	death on board presents difficult legal problems and is distressing to other passengers

are maintained so as to be equivalent to those at 2000 metres above sea level. The partial pressure of oxygen at 2000 metres is about 80% of that at sea level, which may have adverse effects on some individuals as a result of hypoxia. This fall in cabin pressure would have little effect on healthy individuals, who would be able to compensate through various physiological homoeostatic mechanisms. Those more sensitive to a reduction in oxygen pressure would include individuals with severe chronic obstructive airways disease or cardiac disease (e.g. heart failure or angina). Sufferers of these conditions should seek medical advice before flying. The air in the cabin is very dry, and all passengers on long flights are at risk of dehydration; regular drinks should be taken, avoiding tea, coffee and alcohol, which cause dehydration. Contact lens wearers should be warned that both hard and soft contact lenses may appear to feel dry.

Prolonged sitting during a flight results in postural oedema, which causes swollen legs and feet; difficulty may be experienced in replacing shoes at the end of a flight. Oedema and venous stasis may produce serious problems for anyone predisposed to, or already suffering from, deep vein thrombosis. It is strongly recommended that air passengers should walk about the cabin as often as is practicable. When sitting down, leg exercises involving isometric contractions of the large muscles (*see* Chapter 8, The physiology of exercise) may help reduce venous pooling.

The reduction in total pressure in the aircraft causes expansion of gases within body cavities, which can also produce adverse effects. Expansion of gases in healthy individuals may be felt as tightness of clothes around the waistline. This is exacerbated by carbonated drinks, alcohol and foods that produce a lot of intestinal gas (e.g. cabbage, beans and turnips), which should be avoided before and during flight. The wearing of loose-fitting clothes may help to minimise the feelings of discomfort.

Air in the sinuses and middle-ear cavities expands during ascent and escapes passively via the Eustachian tubes, producing the familiar feeling of 'popping'. As the aircraft descends, gas in the sinuses and middle-ear cavities contracts, and air must pass in from outside the body via the Eustachian tubes to equalise the pressure. Venting may be assisted by various techniques, including swallowing, yawning, moving the jaw from side to side or opening the mouth wide; some people find that chewing or sucking sweets is helpful. Valsalva's manoeuvre involves holding the nose and venting the oesophagus into the postnasal space. If this does not clear the Eustachian tube, Toynbee's manoeuvre should be tried instead, which involves holding the nose and swallowing with the mouth closed. Sleeping should be avoided during descent so that Eustachian tubes can be vented. If the air passages are blocked (e.g. if they are swollen and inflamed as a result of infection), it is difficult to equalise the pressure and this may cause mild deafness, discomfort, pain and a feeling of fullness. Babies and young children are less likely to be affected by pressure changes because of anatomical differences in the middle ear.

SCUBA divers must be aware that decompression sickness (the 'bends') may occur during high altitude air travel if a flight is taken too soon after a deep dive, because reduction in pressure allows nitrogen to be released too rapidly from body tissues. Divers should check with their diving clubs for the exact rules to be observed when flying after diving. A general rule is that the maximum depth of any dive in the 24 hours before a flight should be nine metres, and diving should cease at least two to three hours immediately before the flight (deep diving should cease much longer before).

Almost all airlines have imposed a ban on carrying pregnant women on long-haul flights if they are more than 34 to 35 weeks into confinement, and after 36 weeks on short-haul flights, because of the risk of early labour and foetal hypoxia; flying is also contra-indicated until seven days after delivery. Neonates under 48 hours of age should not be subjected to the pressure changes within aircraft because of the poor development of the alveoli and the associated risk of hypoxia.

Hypoxia and expansion of gases in body cavities may produce additional problems for those with specific medical conditions. Any weakened tissue (e.g. recent surgical incisions or blood-vessel damage) may be further weakened by distension, particularly in the abdominal region. Flying should be avoided if there is a recent history of gastro-intestinal haemorrhage (e.g. as a result of peptic ulceration) as this may be exacerbated; there is also a danger of hypoxia if haemorrhage has been sufficient to produce anaemia. Air travel should be avoided during the period following introduction of gas into the body for whatever reason (e.g. fractured skull or intracranial surgery, laparoscopy, pneumothorax or surgical emphysema). Air entrapped within a plaster cast may expand and cause compression damage to enclosed tissues, which is exacerbated by the effects of postural oedema (*see above*). Recent dental work may produce pain during a flight as a result of expansion of air trapped beneath fillings.

MEDIF (Medical Information) forms are available from travel agents for patients who are not sure if they are fit to fly. The first part is filled in by patients wishing to travel; the second is completed by their doctor; the final decision is, however, the carrier's. The settings on body scanning security checks used in some countries may induce changes in the electrical components of pacemakers, and patients fitted with a pacemaker should notify the airline at the time of booking. If a patient with a pulmonary disorder is likely to require oxygen during a flight, the airline must be notified in advance, as there is a limit as to how much oxygen may be carried on board; for safety reasons, patients may not take their own cylinders.

First-aid and medical kits

There is an almost never-ending list of preparations and materials that could be recommended to prospective travellers to local and foreign destinations. Indeed, many international companies issue their own special medical packs to travelling employees, although these comprehensive products are not usually necessary for short term travel. A selection of some of the items that may be recommended for inclusion in first-aid kits for travel is listed in Table 9.3. The initial choice will depend on a number of factors, including destination, length of time away and types of activity to be undertaken. Antibiotics may need to be carried by those travelling to remote destinations or where medical facilities are very poor. A general principle should be that, wherever possible, medicines should be obtained before departure. This is because in many developing countries, medical supplies have been shown to be of variable quality. In addition, it may be difficult to obtain certain items, and language could be a barrier in understanding instruction and communicating with health workers.

There may be additional specific requirements for those with pre-existing medical conditions,

Table 9.3 General items that may be considered for inclusion in a traveller's first-aid kit

Analgesics, non-opioid
Antacids
Antibiotics, broad-spectrum (for emergency use in remote regions)
Antidiarrhoeal drugs
Antihistamines, oral
Antifungal preparations
Antiseptic preparations
Calamine lotion
Condoms
Forceps or tweezers (fine-pointed)
Hydrocortisone 1% cream or ointment
Insect repellents
Laxatives
Magnesium sulphate paste
Malaria prophylactics (where appropriate)
Motion sickness prophylactics
Needles and syringes, sterile
Oral rehydration salts
Scissors
Sunscreens
Water purification products
Wound cleansing products
Wound dressings (including bandages and self-adhesive plasters)

Travellers should check the legal status of drugs that they wish to carry in the countries they intend to visit from the embassy, and if necessary obtain a doctor's note or substitute with another product.

and travellers must ensure that they take sufficient supplies. Those planning to travel for longer periods should note that a general practitioner cannot supply more than three months' medication on the NHS. This is because, after this time, the patient may officially become deregistered from the practice list. Also to be considered is a history of medical conditions that could potentially cause problems whilst away (e.g. cystitis or vaginal thrush).

Travellers should be aware of the legal status of any drugs that they wish to carry in the countries they intend to visit. It may be necessary to carry a doctor's note or certificate covering essential drugs, or choose suitable alternatives for non-essential drugs likely to pose problems at customs.

The risk of contracting HIV infection and hepatitis B from injection of contaminated blood products and use of contaminated injection equipment has led to the availability of kits containing sterile needles, syringes, disposable gloves, giving sets, cannulae and plasma substitutes (e.g. modified gelatin preparations). Certain kits contain prescription-only preparations and can only be supplied against a doctor's prescription.

All airliners should carry a medical emergency kit in order that sick passengers may be assisted. Ideally, medical kits should contain diagnostic equipment, first-aid supplies and a range of drugs; some can be given by the crew; others can only be used by a travelling doctor prepared to give assistance.

Prevention and management of conditions associated with travel

Motion sickness

Anyone who has experienced the trauma of sickness while travelling is understandably keen to prevent its recurrence. Motion sickness can occur on land, in the air or at sea. It is thought to be caused by excessive stimulation of the vestibular apparatus by motion, but treatment is merely palliative. The condition can be severe enough to devastate holidays or business trips.

Symptoms of motion sickness follow a characteristic cascade pattern. Stomach discomfort, facial pallor and cold sweating of the hands and face are common early symptoms. Increased salivation, lightheadedness and lethargy may also precede vomiting and, in the event of continued exposure to the motion, the cycle of symptoms may be repeated. Vestibular stimulation can be severe enough to produce symptoms for hours or sometimes days after the journey.

Airsickness commonly occurs when an aircraft cannot rise above turbulent weather or while ascending to, or descending from, cruising altitudes. People's susceptibility to seasickness varies tremendously; some may experience symptoms on the calmest of seas, whereas others are not affected by seas whisked up by force 10 gales. The introduction of stabilisers, especially on cruise liners, has reduced the incidence of symptoms, although roll-on roll-off ferries may not be similarly equipped. Passengers aboard ships should be advised to stay on deck whenever the weather conditions allow this. In aircraft, and in sea conditions that preclude decktop travel, travellers should sit with their eyes closed and their heads fixed in one position. Occupying the mind may assist in the prevention of symptoms.

Drug prevention of motion sickness requires dosage at least half an hour before travel (two hours for cinnarizine). Doses may be repeated according to the regimen of individual drugs. Hyoscine is the most effective drug in preventing motion sickness, but antihistamines (e.g. cinnarizine, cyclizine and dimenhydrinate) are better tolerated; cyclizine and cinnarizine are the least-sedating. Antihistamine preparations are, however, best avoided during pregnancy. Care must be taken in the administration of sedating drugs if driving is to be undertaken immediately after a flight or sea-crossing. Once the symptoms of motion sickness have started, further treatment is ineffective, and the importance of strict adherence to the recommended prophylactic dosage schedule must therefore be stressed; this is particularly important in the event of flight or ferry delays. Children under two years of age do not generally suffer from motion sickness and are, therefore, unlikely to require prophylactic treatment.

Jet lag

Long-distance air travel in an easterly or westerly direction can result in passage across several time zones. Disturbances to physiological systems, and, in particular, to sleeping, waking and mental activity, occur as a result of disruption of normal circadian rhythms, which are governed by the periods of light and dark, temperature and time. The relationship between jet lag and light exposure has led to the use of melatonin to help relieve the condition. Current evidence suggests that it acts as a mild sedative to aid sleep. In the UK, melatonin is classed as a medicinal product, but no marketing authorisation has yet been granted for this indication. Symptoms of jet lag, which are often worse when travelling from west to east, include decreased mental and physical performance, disturbances to appetite and bowel function, disrupted sleep and lightheadedness. Excessive alcohol consumption and dehydration can aggravate symptoms.

Jet lag can be minimised by a combination of the following measures: sleeping for as long or as frequently as is practicable during the flight and on arrival; adopting local sleeping patterns as quickly as possible; and avoiding food at times when sleep should be taken.

Infectious diseases

There are many ways that infectious diseases may be contracted, and it is essential to be familiar with the different modes of transmission in order to give advice to travellers about effective means of prevention. Immunisation has already been discussed (*see* Action to be taken before travelling *above*) but, in some cases, these measures are not completely effective and travellers should be advised of extra precautions. Additional precautions are strongly recommended, and are essential to prevent those infections for which no vaccine is available. A knowledge of infections endemic in the areas to be visited is necessary, and it is important not to assume that all infectious diseases are confined to tropical countries.

All of the infections discussed here require medical attention, and any untoward, chronic or recurrent symptoms should not be ignored. Some of these diseases are life-threatening emergencies; others are generally debilitating and only fatal in vulnerable groups (e.g. infants, immunocompromised patients and the elderly). Some are insidious in onset or have long incubation periods and may not present until some time after the traveller has returned home (*see* Advising travellers on their return *below*). Traveller's diarrhoea (*see below*) may be caused by micro-organisms present in food or water, but it is generally a self-limiting condition and does not necessarily require medical referral.

Food and water-borne infections

A common mode of transmission for many infections is via food or drinking water. Traveller's diarrhoea affects 25 to 50% of those travelling abroad, and sometimes even more to certain destinations. In the majority of cases, the diarrhoea will be self-limiting, lasting no longer than a few days. In this case, the most likely implicated organisms will be certain strains of *Escherichia coli*. Food poisoning from other bacteria (e.g. *Salmonella* spp.) is also possible where food hygiene is inadequate. In other rare cases (about 5%), the diarrhoea may last longer than a week due to dysentery (bacterial or amoebic) or giardiasis. In the case of dysentery, blood may be present in the stools.

Many micro-organisms are excreted in faeces, and in areas where poor sanitation exists or human faeces are used to fertilise crops, pathogenic species may enter the food chain. Faecal contamination of food or water may also deposit the eggs of some species of helminth. Direct contamination of food by foodhandlers may occur if strict standards of hygiene are not observed, and flies may also be responsible for transporting micro-organisms from faeces to food. Other examples of infections contracted via the faecal-oral route include:

- cholera
- hepatitis A
- poliomyelitis
- typhoid fever
- worms (e.g. ascariasis, tapeworm).

Contaminated food may also be derived from an infected animal: unpasteurised milk, or dairy products made from it, may contain the bacteria that cause brucellosis and tuberculosis. Transmission of some helminthic infections (e.g. fish tapeworm) may be effected by consumption of meat or fish containing the larval stages of the parasite.

Dracontiasis (guinea worm) is a helminthic infection contracted via drinking water that has been contaminated by adult worms discharging embryos directly into environmental water through the skin of the host's leg.

The general principles relating to food hygiene and safety have been discussed previously (*see* Chapter 2, Food safety) and these also apply to travellers. However, in view of the low standards of sanitation and hygiene prevalent in some countries, travellers to such destinations may need to take additional action.

Food and water-borne infections may be prevented by ensuring that all food is thoroughly cooked before eating. It should be freshly prepared and not reheated; pre-cooked food should only be eaten if it has been properly refrigerated. The old adage 'cook it, peel it or forget it' should be remembered; generally, any food that is hot and freshly prepared will be the safest. A dish cooked in front of you in a wok may prove to carry less risk than one prepared unseen in the best of hotels. Strict rules of personal hygiene must be observed before handling or eating food, and anyone suffering with diarrhoea should not prepare food for others. Food and drink should be kept covered at all times before consumption to prevent access to flies; this is particularly important when eating in the open air. All unpasteurised milk, and dairy products made from it, should be avoided.

Drinking water is a potential source of pathogenic organisms, but contaminated water may also be ingested from unexpected sources (e.g. ice cubes, when brushing teeth, during a shower or when swimming in polluted water). Water should be boiled or treated with chemicals before drinking, and treated water should be used to wash all food before cooking. Boiling is practicable only for small quantities, and it should be stressed that the water must be maintained at 100°C for at least five minutes. Once boiled, the water can be stored for up to two hours if covered and kept in the vessel in which it was boiled.

Chemical treatment of water by chlorine liberated from chlorine-based disinfectants (e.g. chloramine) is an alternative means of disinfecting water in the absence of facilities for boiling. However, the vessel used for disinfection must be free from organic matter to prevent inactivation of the disinfectant. The water itself should also be free of organic matter and should, where possible, be filtered before disinfection. The manufacturers' recommendations on rate of use and standing time must be followed. Some manufacturers recommend a higher concentration of disinfectant for water used to wash food than for drinking. However, it is necessary to ensure that washed food is subsequently rinsed in water containing a lower concentration of disinfectant. Iodine is an alternative to chlorine for disinfection. Five drops of the 2% tincture are added to one litre of clear water and allowed to stand for 20 to 30 minutes; if the water is cloudy, ten drops are necessary. Tablets that release iodine are also available, although they can be slow to dissolve in cold water.

The efficacy of chemical disinfectants is dependent upon a number of variables, including:

- concentration of chemical
- contact time
- pH
- organic matter
- organisms present (e.g. giardia are more difficult to eradicate than bacteria)
- temperature.

Iodine may have some advantage over chlorine as it is less sensitive to pH and the presence of organic matter. It is also claimed by some to be more effective against protozoa and their cysts. However, it has been shown that continuous consumption of water treated with iodine can result in a reversible enlargement of the thyroid (goitre). A major drawback to both halogens is the taste imparted to the water. This can be removed by adding ascorbic acid to iodine or sodium thiosulphate to chlorine, although this will inactivate the chemical, so should only be used in the final receptacle just before drinking.

The only other chemical in popular use is katedyne silver which, whilst not imparting taste to the water, is not effective against protozoa and viruses. There are also a large range of pumps available, usually supplied through camping and outdoor shops. Some have limitations (e.g. they are slow, need constant cleaning, have a short life and are expensive). Travellers should, therefore, consider the need for such devices carefully.

Traveller's diarrhoea may be treated by the administration of oral rehydration salts, ensuring that only boiled or treated water is used to make up the solution. Antidiarrhoeal drugs may be used if necessary, but it must be emphasised that they are of secondary value, and must not detract from oral rehydration therapy. This is particularly important in infants because of the serious adverse effects of dehydration. Medical assistance should be sought if diarrhoea lasts longer than five days, is recurrent or is associated with the passage of blood or mucus.

Where antibiotics are required, ciprofloxacin is useful for bacterial infection and metronidazole for protozoa.

Infections transmitted by insect vectors

Many pathogenic micro-organisms have a complex life-cycle that involves insects and man. In some cases, there are several possible mammalian hosts, and man becomes an incidental host when entering areas where the infection exists in animals. Examples of insect-borne infections include:

- African trypanosomiasis (tsetse flies)
- American trypanosomiasis (bugs)
- dengue haemorrhagic fever (mosquitoes)
- filariasis (mosquitoes, black-flies, deerflies)
- leishmaniasis (sandflies)

- Lyme disease (ticks from deer and other forest animals)
- malaria (mosquitoes)
- plague, bubonic (fleas from rats)
- typhus fevers (human body louse, fleas from rats and ticks)
- yellow fever (mosquitoes).

In many cases, these diseases are of far greater significance to the local population than the casual traveller. For instance, only around a dozen cases of leishmaniasis are reported per annum in those returning to the UK. The important exception is malaria (*see below*). Dengue is also a growing problem in parts of Asia and the Pacific. Whilst dengue is rarely fatal in otherwise healthy travellers, it can cause a debilitating illness for some weeks.

Mosquitoes that carry malaria are active between dusk and dawn, and the preventive measures to be undertaken need only be applied during these hours; however, this may not be true for all insects, and the general principles outlined may need to be applied at all times. Clothes that cover as much of the body as possible should be worn, choosing fabrics with a close weave and light colour; wet clothing should be replaced immediately as insects may bite through it.

Topical insect repellents interfere with the sensory apparatus of insects. The main active ingredients in commercially available repellents are diethyltoluamide (DEET), extract of lemon eucalyptus, Bayrepel and Merk 3535. Of these, DEET is probably the most reliable, and products containing over 20% (depending on formulation) are to be recommended when visiting malaria endemic areas. DEET has a good safety profile when used according to the manufacturer's directions. Most insect repellents should be reapplied at least every four hours to maintain adequate levels of repellence. Travellers should be warned that DEET insect repellents soften plastics.

Where insect-borne diseases might be a risk, it would also be advisable to treat clothing with permethrin, as the use of a repellent applied to the skin together with clothing treatment gives a higher level of protection than skin treatment alone.

Netting (which may be impregnated with an insect repellent) should be used around beds, and it should be inspected regularly for holes. It should completely cover the bed and be tucked in all around; there should be no point of contact with the skin. A knock-down insecticide should be sprayed in the bedroom before retiring for the night, and the netting examined to make sure that there are no insects inside it.

Infections acquired directly from the environment

Some infections (e.g. hookworm infection and strongyloidiasis) may be acquired directly from the soil as a result of walking barefoot, and footwear should be worn at all times in endemic regions. Soil is also contaminated with tetanus spores, and penetrating wounds pose a risk for non-immunised individuals. All wounds should be cleansed thoroughly and medical attention sought as soon as possible.

Anthrax is still endemic in some parts of the world, and spores present in the environment are a potential risk for travellers. Anthrax is also transmitted from spores present in the products derived from infected animals (e.g. bones, hair, hide, wool and meat), and these should be handled with extreme care in endemic regions.

Schistosomiasis (bilharziasis) is contracted by swimming or washing in fresh water harbouring certain species of snail that are intermediate hosts in the life-cycle of *Schistosoma* spp., and such activities should be avoided in endemic regions (e.g. Africa, Asia and South America). In general, to avoid contracting any water-borne infection, bathing should be confined to chlorinated swimming pools or the sea.

Lassa fever is acquired by contact with urine from infected rats (who represent the reservoir of infection), although the exact mode of transmission is unknown.

Infections acquired directly from animals

The most notable example is rabies, and contact with domestic and wild animals should be avoided in endemic regions. The virus is present in the saliva of an infected animal and is transmitted to man during a bite. Rabies may also be acquired by inhalation of infected secretions in bat caves. Any animal bite should be thoroughly washed with detergent and running water, and any residual debris removed. The application of 40 to 70% alcohol (e.g. in an emergency, whisky or gin is an alternative) or povidone-iodine may help to inactivate the virus, but urgent medical attention is essential. If the animal can be safely captured, it should be handed over to the local authorities for examination. The potential seriousness of animal bites is emphasised by the invariably fatal outcome of rabies once symptoms are seen. Post-exposure vaccination may be successful if the treatment course is started as soon as possible after a bite.

Infections transmitted directly from person to person

Some infections are contracted directly from other people via airborne droplets or by contact with body fluids and secretions (e.g. blood and blood products, seminal fluid, breast milk or nasopharyngeal secretions). This may represent the only form of transmission for some infections, or it may be a secondary mode for those that were primarily acquired from other sources. Examples of infections that may be transmitted directly between people include:

- Ebola fever
- hepatitis B
- HIV infection
- Lassa fever
- leprosy (from untreated persons)
- Marburg disease
- meningococcal infections
- plague, pneumonic
- poliomyelitis
- sexually transmitted diseases
- tuberculosis.

It is absolutely essential to avoid unnecessary surgery, dental treatment, acupuncture, tattooing, ear piercing or any other invasive technique in developing countries. First-aid kits for travel containing sterile syringes and needles (*see* Action to be taken before travelling *above*) are available, and should be carried by travellers to countries where the standards of medical hygiene are questionable. In some countries, screening of blood and blood products is not routinely carried out; however, blood transfusion may be essential in emergencies. Travellers should not indulge in casual sex (especially with prostitutes) or at least use condoms (*see* Chapter 4, Barrier methods and spermicides). The only means of preventing transmission of airborne micro-organisms is by isolation of infected cases. However, there is no guarantee that all cases will be isolated, particularly in remote rural areas; and for many infections, a patient is infectious during the incubation period, which is often asymptomatic. An unsuspecting traveller may therefore unwittingly come into contact with infected individuals. The only means of protection is by immunisation, where possible, and immediately reporting to a doctor any symptoms or general feelings of malaise.

Malaria

Travellers at particular risk from being bitten by mosquitoes infected with *Plasmodium* spp. are those going to Africa, Central and South America and Asia. Infected mosquitoes may also occasionally be transported to non-endemic areas in luggage and aircraft, and pharmacies in the vicinity of airports should be alert to this possibility. Approximately 2000 people return to the UK every year with confirmed malaria, resulting in around a dozen fatalities. In a high proportion of these cases, the affected individuals are returning from a visit to their country of origin without having taken adequate prophylaxis in the mistaken belief that they have resistance to malaria. The main problem is the form of malaria caused by *Plasmodium falciparum*, which can lead to cerebral malaria and death, sometimes just 24 hours after the initial symptoms. Those who live in areas where *P. falciparum* is prevalent can develop resistance to it, but this resistance is lost over a period of time if the individual moves away from the endemic area. Thus, it is particularly dangerous to any non-immune traveller.

For the 'benign' malarias (e.g. that caused by *P. vivax*), the outcome is rarely fatal in otherwise healthy adults. However, resistance cannot be developed and the disease can be difficult to eradicate, returning periodically over many years.

P. falciparum malaria can take up to three months to appear, and longer with other forms of the disease. It is important to be aware of this in returned travellers. It is also important that travellers should be able to recognise the early symptoms of malaria. These can be 'flu-like', sometimes with gastro-intestinal symptoms.

Those travelling to remote destinations, more than 24 hours from medical facilities, may need to carry emergency standby treatment. Such a regimen might include a course of quinine, followed by Fansidar, but specific advice should be sought from a specialist centre before travelling.

The potential role of pharmacists in issuing advice about malaria chemoprophylaxis is complemented by the classification of chloroquine and proguanil in the UK as pharmacy medicines for that indication. However, drug resistance varies considerably between endemic areas and the latest advice in BNF 5.4.1, or from one of the telephone advice lines listed in BNF 5.4, should be given. Chemoprophylaxis should, ideally, be started one week before departure, but not later than the first day of exposure. The course should be taken regularly and continued for four weeks after return without fail, except for mefloquine (*see below*); all tablets should be taken with or after food. Mefloquine is a prescription-only medicine indicated for use in areas where chloroquine-resistant *P. falciparum* malaria is endemic. Weekly doses of mefloquine should be taken three weeks before travel, whilst away and on return for a further four weeks. It is not usually prescribed for journeys shorter than two weeks in duration or for longer than a year. There is some controversy regarding the side-effects of mefloquine, and anxious travellers may ask pharmacists for their opinion. The following points should be borne in mind:

- there is good evidence that mefloquine can provide a better level of protection than chloroquine/proguanil in some parts
- overall the incidence of side-effects is no higher than for chloroquine/proguanil. Occasional dizziness and nightmares appear the most common
- very rarely (about 1 in 10 000), serious debilitating neuropsychiatric or other reactions do occur, and the drug is contra-indicated in anyone with a personal or family psychiatric history
- less serious neuropsychiatric reactions which cause mefloquine to be stopped are seen in around 1 in 200 people taking the drug. However, in 75% of cases, the reaction will be apparent within the first three doses, hence the recommended pre-travel course.

For those who cannot take mefloquine, chloroquine/proguanil might be recommended and stringent bite avoidance measures taken. An alternative prophylactic to mefloquine is doxycycline, but it is not licensed for this indication and there are some drawbacks (e.g. adverse effects and spectrum of activity).

Pharmacists must be aware that no prophylactic is 100% effective. When they are supplied, advice regarding bite avoidance should always also be given.

Pregnant women and immunocompromised patients should be referred for medical advice on malaria chemoprophylaxis. Chloroquine and proguanil may be used during breast-feeding, but mefloquine is contra-indicated. Chemoprophylaxis is necessary in breast-fed infants since the amounts of antimalarial excreted in breast milk is very variable and does not provide therapeutic doses.

Bites and stings

The unwary traveller may be prone to a wide variety of bites and stings that will, in most cases, be no more than a source of minor irritation. However, pharmacists should be particularly aware of the potential hazards in hypersensitive individuals.

Bites

Some infectious diseases are transmitted to man during an animal or insect bite (e.g. rabies, malaria or yellow fever). There is an additional hazard, even if bitten by a non-rabid animal, of contamination of a penetrating wound by micro-organisms present in the animal's saliva. Insect bites may also result in infection if scratched excessively.

Insect bites

Insect bites may be caused by flies, gnats, midges or mosquitoes, which suck up blood from below the skin surface. Simultaneously, insect saliva, which contains substances that are pharmacologically active and capable of provoking allergic reactions of varying degrees, is deposited. Insect bites should be treated by cleansing the area followed by application of a cooling lotion (e.g. calamine lotion). Administration of topical antihistamine preparations is not recommended because of the occasional risk of allergic contact dermatitis in sensitive individuals. Topical hydrocortisone (*see* Box 9.1) or oral antihistamines may be beneficial. For preventive measures to avoid insect bites, *see* Infections transmitted by insect vectors *above*.

Box 9.1 Sale of over-the-counter hydrocortisone preparations in the UK.

Proprietary brands of hydrocortisone cream (0.1 and 1.0%) and ointment (1.0%) may be sold to the public for treatment of:

- allergic contact dermatitis
- irritant dermatitis
- insect bite reactions.

It is unlawful to sell any hydrocortisone preparation if it is to be used

- on the eyes or the face
- on broken or infected skin (including cold sores, acne, athlete's foot)
- on children under 10 years of age
- in pregnancy.

Preparations should be applied sparingly over a small area once or twice daily, for a maximum of one week.

The label must include 'If the condition is not improved, consult your doctor'.

Snake bites

Snake bites occur more commonly in remote regions of travel, although it should not be forgotten that a venomous snake, the adder (*Vipera berus*), inhabits some regions of the UK. Snakes only attack humans as a means of defence, and it is, therefore, prudent to avoid deliberately provoking a snake. Bites as a result of accidental contact with a snake may be avoided by:

- wearing boots, socks and trousers in areas known to be inhabited by snakes
- carrying a torch when walking at night (when snakes are most active)
- inspecting bedding when sleeping on open ground
- not disturbing boulders, brushwood, burrows, or other similar places where snakes may be resting, without first checking the area carefully and protecting the arms, hands and face.

Almost all venomous snakes secrete their poison through fangs located on the upper jaw. Venoms are mixtures of enzymes, peptides and metalloproteins, and produce a wide variety of effects, including haemolysis, haemorrhage, neurotoxic signs, oedema, shock, myonecrosis, pituitary failure and renal failure. However, about 25% of snake bites fail to envenomate. The most common immediate reaction on having been bitten is fear and panic, and there may be breathlessness, dizziness and chest pain. Tenderness and pain may develop at the site of the bite, indicating envenomation, and may be followed by lymphadenopathy and swelling of the distal limb.

The most appropriate action after a snake bite is to calm the patient and immobilise the limb. The age-old remedy of applying a tourniquet is not recommended because, in inexperienced hands, it may lead to gangrene; however, a tight crepe bandage over the whole limb may be of value. Leaching blood by cutting tissue from an area around the wound is also no longer advocated because haemorrhage may occur, the site may become infected and further damage may be caused to surrounding tissues. Aspirin should not be given as it may exacerbate gastro-intestinal haemorrhage. First-aiders should ensure that an adequate airway is maintained, and regularly check that the patient is still breathing. Signs of systemic poisoning, which may appear within 30 minutes or up to 24 hours later, include loss of consciousness, spontaneous bleeding from the gums and muscle paralysis. Because of the wide variety of clinical syndromes produced by the venom of different snake species, the dead snake (held by the tail) should, whenever possible, be transported with the patient to a local hospital to aid identification of the venom; attempts should not be made to capture live snakes. Gloves must be worn at all times when carrying a dead snake because venom can ooze from the body, especially if the head has been severed.

Spider bites
Almost all spiders are venomous, but only a few species are dangerous to man. Spiders possess a small pair of fangs attached directly to venom glands. Spider bites are particularly common in Australia, South America, the USA, Israel, North Africa and Mediterranean areas. Spider venoms may be neurotoxic (e.g. black widow spider) or produce local necrosis and haemolysis (e.g. brown recluse spider). As with snake bites, first-aid measures include immobilisation of the limb and immediate transportation to hospital; neurotoxic symptoms may develop rapidly.

Ticks
Ticks are commonly carried by domestic pets, especially in North America and Australia, and usually bite in hairy crevices or orifices and on the scalp. The tick embeds itself in the skin by a barbed protrusion (the hypostome), which injects saliva containing a neurotoxin.

Stings

Many creatures have developed highly specialised stings. Most social insects (e.g. honeybees, wasps, hornets and ants) will only sting if they perceive a threat to themselves or their colony; accidental disturbance of a nest or of a feeding insect may provoke attack. Insect venom contains a variety of pharmacologically active substances (e.g. dopamine, histamine, acetylcholine, serotonin, formic acid and noradrenaline).

Bee and wasp stings
Having delivered its sting, a honeybee may remain attached to the victim's skin by its barbed sting. Brushing the insect away invariably leaves the sting with its venom and appendages embedded in the skin, and these must be carefully extracted. The location of the pocket of venom at the distal end of the barb demands that only tweezers with fine tips should be used for extraction; theoretically the venom sac should not be squeezed, which will inject more venom into the wound. Scraping away the sting with a blade or fingernail may be a more effective means of removal. A recent study has suggested that it may be more important to remove the sting quickly, rather than worrying about the correct technique. By comparison, wasp stings are smooth and are usually extracted from the skin by the insect itself after attack.

Symptoms include immediate local pain followed by erythema and oedema. In most cases, the swelling lasts for a few hours only, although more severe reactions may result from stings on the face: gross oedema resulting from stings in the mouth may cause respiratory distress and asphyxiation. One in 200 people appear to develop hypersensitivity to bee and wasp stings, and fatal anaphylactic responses may occur in a small minority of cases on subsequent exposure to the allergen. An initial symptom of a hypersensitive reaction after stinging is bronchoconstriction, which may be followed by generalised erythema, nausea and vomiting, oedema, hypotension and shock. Serious systemic reactions generally occur within the first 30 minutes after a sting, and most fatalities occur in the middle-aged or elderly, presumably as a result of associated conditions (e.g. ischaemic heart disease).

If stung within the mouth, ice should be used to reduce the swelling and medical attention sought as soon as possible.

Atopic individuals may be particularly susceptible to developing hypersensitivity reactions and should, where possible, avoid contact with stinging insects. Anyone known to have experienced hypersensitivity to a previous insect sting may benefit from carrying oral antihistamines and an adrenaline inhalation, or pre-filled adrenaline syringe, to relieve bronchoconstriction, which is the primary cause of anaphylactic death. Carrying identification that can alert others to a known history of hypersensitivity (e.g. in the form of a medallion or bracelet) can also be life-saving. Full measures for the treatment of allergic emergencies are described in BNF 3.4.3.

Ant stings
Ant stings contain a high concentration of formic acid, the effects of which can be neutralised by

the application of alkaline solutions containing sodium bicarbonate or 1% ammonia.

Scorpion stings

Travellers to the Americas, the Middle East, India, South Africa and North Africa are liable to scorpion stings. Different species produce different venoms with varying clinical symptoms, and stings from some species may be fatal, especially to young children. A scorpion sting may cause intense local pain, oedema and lymphadenopathy. Symptoms of systemic distribution of the venom may be produced almost immediately, or up to 24 hours later. Overactivity of the autonomic nervous system produces a wide range of symptoms, including dilated pupils, excessive salivation and sweating, diarrhoea and vomiting. Increased release of catecholamines produces cardiovascular hyperactivity, hypertension and arrhythmias. Urgent medical attention is essential, although the onset of systemic effects may be delayed by immobilisation of the affected part.

Stinging fish

Some fish (e.g. scorpion-fish, sting-rays, stone-fish and weeverfish) have bony spines that are covered in venom-secreting tissues. Weeverfish may be found in waters around the UK, although most other species inhabit tropical waters. Swimming should be avoided in infested waters and attempts to handle fish (either dead or alive) should only be made by swimmers who are confident in their identification. The venom causes intense local pain, but may be inactivated by heat. The affected area should first be irrigated with cold salt-water, and then immersed for a few seconds in the hottest water that is bearable (but not so hot as to scald and blister). The process should be repeated until the pain no longer recurs, which usually takes about 30 minutes. If it is not practicable to immerse the wound, hot compresses should be applied. Stone-fish stings may require the administration of an antivenom to prevent potentially life-threatening systemic reactions.

Jellyfish

Jellyfish are equipped with stinging capsules (nematocysts) which release vasoactive substances (e.g. histamine and kinins) that cause erythema, wheals and local pain. Most jellyfish are harmless, but death has occurred following a sting from a Portuguese man-of-war; the most dangerous of all is the box jellyfish (sea wasp) found in seas off north-east Australia. Under-water clothing can act as a barrier to the dermal penetration of nematocysts. Tentacle remains should be removed, although great care must be taken not to discharge more of the venom in doing so. Application of vinegar, dilute acetic acid or calamine lotion may also be beneficial. Intensive supportive therapy may be necessary for serious cases.

Sunburn

The most harmful component of sunlight that reaches the earth's surface is ultraviolet (UV) radiation, which has a wavelength between 200 and 400 nm. UV radiation is made up of three components:

- UVA radiation (wavelength 320 to 400 nm), which represents about 80% of the UV radiation that reaches the earth's surface
- UVB radiation (wavelength 290 to 320 nm), which is partially absorbed by the earth's atmosphere and only constitutes about 20% of the total UV radiation reaching the earth's surface
- UVC (wavelength 100 to 290 nm), which is totally absorbed by the earth's atmosphere, particularly by the ozone layer.

UVB is more energetic than UVA, but is less capable of penetrating human epidermis.

Melanocytes in the basal layer of the epidermis are responsible for the formation of a pigment, melanin, which develops as a protective response to exposure to UV radiation. The number of melanocytes is constant, and the varying rates at which different people tan is a function of the rate of production of melanin, which is genetically-determined. UVA radiation causes oxidation of melanin already present in the skin, producing an immediate but transient tan. UVB radiation stimulates the melanocytes to produce melanin granules, which move to the surface layers of the skin. This process takes 24 to 48 hours and accounts for the delay in tanning after exposure. UVA radiation is less effective than UVB in producing a tan by this mechanism. A further protective mechanism is skin thickening, which is only initiated by UVB radiation. Sunbeds utilise UVA radiation and do not, therefore, offer protection against subsequent exposure to UVB radiation. The tanning and thickening mechanisms are a response to an adverse stimulus, and only occur after the skin has already been damaged (i.e. sunburn). A tan does not completely protect the skin from further damage. Therefore, those who develop tans on a regular basis are more likely to experience an accelerated skin ageing. For this reason, and the potential for malignant skin disease (*see below*), it is recommended that people avoid tanning. Previous advice regarding slowly developing a tan to avoid sunburn does not protect against the problem of skin ageing and some malignancies.

Sunburn is an inflammatory reaction and is not immediately apparent during exposure; the first symptoms may not be felt until two to eight hours later. The most common symptom is erythema, which usually fades within 36 to 72 hours. Severe sunburn may result in bullae, oedema, pain and tenderness, which generally reach a peak on the second day. Peeling starts after about 72 hours and lasts for up to five days. Extensive areas of sunburnt skin may produce constitutional symptoms (e.g. fever, chills, malaise and headache). The symptoms of sunburn can be severe enough to ruin part or all of a holiday or trip. If preventive measures (*see below*) have not been adopted or have been unsuccessful, sunburn may be relieved by cooling the skin with cold-water compresses or by sponging. A cooling lotion (e.g. calamine lotion) may be of value, but administration of topical anti-histamine preparations is not recommended because of the risk of allergic contact dermatitis in sensitive individuals. Non-opioid analgesics may be used for pain relief. Further exposure to UV radiation should be avoided until all symptoms have subsided.

Sunburn is caused by both UVA and UVB radiation, although the dose of UVA radiation required is 1000 times that of UVB; however, more UVA radiation reaches the earth's surface than UVB (*see above*). Prolonged and repeated exposure to UV radiation may, in time, cause premature ageing of the skin and the development of malignant skin diseases. There are three forms of skin cancer believed to be related to UV exposure: basal cell carcinoma, squamous cell carcinoma and malignant melanoma. The exact relationship between these malignancies and exposure to UV is much debated, with a number of factors believed to contribute (e.g. number of episodes of sunburn, skin type and genetic disposition). Of the three, malignant melanoma is potentially the most dangerous. People most susceptible to the harmful effects of UV radiation are fair-skinned, and tend to have red hair, freckles or both. Infants and children are particularly vulnerable to the damaging effects of UV radiation. To prevent the long term consequences of damage by UV radiation, children should be protected from overexposure and should be educated about the dangers. People at risk should examine their skin regularly for any sudden appearances of sinister skin lesions, or changes in existing moles, freckles or birthmarks.

Photosensitivity reactions may occur in those taking some medicines (e.g. griseofulvin, immunosuppressants, nalidixic acid, non-steroidal anti-inflammatory drugs, sulphonamides, tetracyclines or thiazide diuretics) or using topical preparations containing coal tar; contact with some plants or use of perfumes may also have the same effect. Photodermatoses may also occur in individuals suffering from some medical conditions (e.g. systemic lupus erythematosus, porphyrias or chronic actinic dermatitis). These adverse reactions are caused predominantly by UVA radiation and can develop from exposure to even normal amounts of sunlight. All those at risk should be advised to avoid any exposure to UV radiation, or to cover exposed areas; use of sunscreens (*see below*) that absorb both UVA and UVB radiation or total sunblocks may be necessary.

Throughout most of the year, the majority of people living north of the tropic of Cancer and south of the tropic of Capricorn are exposed to only limited quantities of sunlight. Sunlight received at these latitudes is generally of low intensity because of the relatively low angle at which the rays impinge on the earth's surface. Holidays in sunnier regions mean that, for two or three weeks each year, people are exposed to increased amounts of high intensity UV radiation. There is also an increased risk of sunburn at high altitude, even during the winter, because the atmosphere is less capable of filtering UV radiation than at ground level.

The skin-damaging effects of UV radiation may be minimised by observing the following simple rules:

- keep out of the sun as much as possible, and wear a hat and clothes that offer adequate protection
- if tanning, increase exposure times gradually to avoid sun burn (but *see above*)
- always use a sunscreen (*see below*) on exposed parts.

Unless the sun is completely blocked, sunburn can occur on cloudy days, because clouds scatter radiation over a wide area. There is the additional danger that, as clouds absorb infra-red radiation (the heat-producing rays), people may stay out of doors for longer periods, increasing the time of exposure to UV radiation. It is also important to recognise that sitting in the shade may afford little protection because ultraviolet rays may be deflected by sand, snow or concrete; the sun's rays can also penetrate water and thin or wet clothing.

If individuals insist on developing a tan, it is recommended that the maximum time of exposure during periods of high intensity UV radiation (i.e. between 10:00 and 15:00 hours) should not exceed 15 minutes on the first day. This may be increased to 30 minutes on the next day, and to one hour on the third day; thereafter, exposure may be increased by one hour per day.

Sunscreens

Sunscreens protect the skin from receiving high doses of UV radiation by either a physical or a chemical mechanism. In total sunblocks, the active ingredient (e.g. finely divided calamine, talc, titanium dioxide or zinc oxide) completely blocks skin absorption of UV radiation (both UVA and UVB) by scattering and reflecting the rays. These compounds are thick and opaque, and cosmetically too conspicuous for general use. They may, however, be useful in areas that are more prone to sunburn than others.

The most commonly used sunscreen preparations contain agents that act by a chemical mechanism and absorb UVB radiation (e.g. aminobenzoates and salicylates); some also absorb UVA radiation (e.g. benzophenones and cinnamates). Titanium dioxide is particularly effective against UVA and acts by reflecting UV radiation, giving the skin a slight silvery appearance.

The rational selection of sunscreens has been assisted by the development of the Sun Protection Factor (SPF), which is the ratio of the minimal dose of UVB radiation necessary to produce delayed erythema in skin protected by the sunscreen to that in unprotected skin. The higher the SPF value, the greater protection afforded by the sunscreen (i.e. the longer the period of exposure necessary to cause a similar degree of erythema). For example, if delayed erythema occurs in unprotected skin following 15 minutes exposure to UV radiation, then applying a sunscreen with a SPF of 4 would allow 60 minutes exposure to elicit the same reaction (Table 9.5). However, the actual exposure time required to produce delayed erythema is an individual variable and also depends on the intensity of UV radiation. It is also difficult, in practice, to control the amount of sunscreen applied. Previously, tables have been produced to aid in selection of an appropriate sunscreen for a particular skin type and potential UV exposure. It is now recommended that all Caucasians choose a sunscreen with at least an SPF 15, with children and others at higher risk opting for SPF 25.

It should be remembered that SPFs generally refer to protection against UVB, not UVA radiation. A star system is used to indicate comparable efficacy of sunscreens against UVA and UVB: those with four stars have an equal efficacy against both UVA and UVB. A sunscreen that offers good protection against both UVB and UVA radiation should always be chosen. It may be necessary to choose a sunscreen with a high SPF for particularly vulnerable areas of the body (e.g. breasts, buttocks, lips, nose, ears or a bald head); people susceptible to cold sores, which may be triggered by sunlight, should use lipsalves with a high SPF. It should be noted that benzophenones might cause photoallergic contact dermatitis in sensitive individuals. Choosing a product with protection against UVB radiation only effectively increases the exposure time to UVA radiation, which is particularly hazardous to those at risk of hypersensitivity reactions (*see above*).

Sunscreens should be applied evenly and

Table 9.5 Classification of skin types and recommended sun protection factors

Class	Skin type category	Recommended sun protection factor (SPF)
I	Always burns; never tans	10 to 15
II	Always burns; minimal tan	8 to 9
III	Burns moderately easily; gradually tans	6 to 7
IV	Never burns; tans well	4 to 5
V	Asian and Mongoloid skin	2 to 3
VI	Afro-Caribbean skin	none

It may be necessary to use a higher SPF than recommended above at high altitudes and for travel to sunny regions from a winter climate.

thickly to be effective; studies have shown that, in many cases, too little is applied and the actual SPF value may be reduced by up to 50%. For maximum effect, they should be applied at least 30 minutes before exposure to allow time for absorption into the skin; for preparations containing para-aminobenzoic acid (PABA), application should be two hours beforehand. Sunscreens must be reapplied after swimming or during profuse sweating; reapplication does not, however, prolong the protective time (i.e. it does not increase the SPF value). PABA penetrates the skin and binds with keratin, and is therefore less easily removed by water than other sunscreens. However, it only protects against UVB radiation. It must be emphasised that sunscreens are to be used as an adjunct to other sun protection measures. To adequately cover a whole body in sunscreen over a two-week holiday, would involve using far more sunscreen than most people are prepared to purchase.

Sunscreens are generally available throughout the year because of the demand generated by winter holidays, either in the sun or snow. Travellers to sunny regions from a winter climate should initially select products with a higher SPF value than they would for a summer holiday, to allow for the fact that their skin is unlikely to have had any exposure to UV radiation for several months. The reflectant property of snow is strong, and skiers should likewise select a sunscreen with a high SPF value. The choice of sunscreen product for those at higher altitudes and in colder regions should also be determined by the vehicle containing the active ingredient. Many water-based sunscreens will freeze at low temperatures, and this has prompted the manufacture of a range of products specifically for use in colder temperatures.

A limited range of sunscreening preparations (BNF 13.8.1) is prescribable for a range of dermatoses, and for patients at risk of photosensitivity reactions (*see above*). Items cannot be prescribed for any other groups, but the choice for the majority of holidaymakers and business travellers is considerably wider, and pharmacists are often asked to advise on the selection of appropriate products.

The role of the pharmacist

Advising travellers before departure

As will be clear from the information above, there are myriad ways in which pharmacists can become involved in advising travellers prior to their journeys.

Advising travellers on their return

Travellers who have experienced illness while away will, in all likelihood, be prompted to seek medical attention on returning home if symptoms persist or recur. The greatest danger lies with those who felt perfectly fit while away, but develop symptoms on return; the patient may not realise that the symptoms could be related to an infection contracted abroad, and fail to alert the doctor to this possibility, or not seek medical attention at all.

A change in temperature and humidity on returning home may provoke symptoms of the common cold and nasal congestion. However, the presence of a cough or other respiratory symptoms may suggest that a viral or bacterial infection has been contracted, and such patients should be referred to their general practitioner. Feverish, influenza-like symptoms may be early signs of malaria in travellers returning from tropical or subtropical regions. Fever or chills may also be the presenting symptom of many other infectious diseases, and returning travellers reporting such symptoms to pharmacists should always be referred. Some infectious diseases, particularly helminthic infections, may remain silent for years before symptoms present.

Pharmacists should, as a matter of routine, ask all patients with gastro-intestinal symptoms or fever, or any unusual symptoms, if they have recently travelled; if the answer is in the affirmative, referral is strongly recommended, and the patient should be asked to tell the doctor where they have travelled. Some authorities recommend routine tropical screening for travellers returning from high-risk areas if they have been away a long time or if their lifestyle put them at risk of contracting endemic infections.

Further reading

Dawood R (1992). *Travellers' Health*, 3rd edn. Oxford: Oxford University Press.

Department of Health (1998). *Health Advice for Travellers* (T6). London: Central Office of Information.

DuPont S (1997). *Textbook of Travel Medicine and Health*. Ontario: R C Decker.

McIntosh I B (1998). *Travel, Trauma, Risks and Health Promotion*. Dinton, UK: Mark Allen.

Wilson-Howarth J (1995). *Bugs, Bites and Bowels*. London: Cadogan.

World Health Organization (1997). *International Travel and Health*. Geneva: WHO.

Useful addresses

See BNF 5.4.1 for contacts regarding malaria prophylaxis and vaccination. Other useful numbers include:

Diabetes UK
10 Queen Anne Street
London W1G 09LH
Tel: 020 7323 1531

The Royal Association for Disability and Rehabilitation (RADAR)
Unit 12, City Forum
250 City Road
London EC1V 8AF
Tel: 020 7250 3222

10

Contact lens care

Susan Shankie

Contact lenses were first designed more than 100 years ago and consisted of large corneoscleral glass shells that covered both the cornea and the conjunctiva. In the 1940s, hard lenses made of Perspex became available and were followed 20 years later by the introduction of soft hydrogel lenses. Further developments have included gas permeable hard lenses, which allow the movement of oxygen through the lens to the cornea, soft lenses for extended wear and, most recently, disposable lenses.

Approximately 4 to 6% of the UK population are regular contact lens wearers. Primarily, adults wear contact lenses, although a baby can be fitted with lenses if clinically necessary. Lenses are obtained from an optometrist (ophthalmic optician), who will advise on the type of lens that will be suitable after considering the individual's visual requirements, daily environment, leisure activities and personal choice. Some optometrists have an additional qualification in contact lens management.

Contact lenses are often preferred to spectacles for cosmetic reasons, and may also provide better peripheral vision. Visual defects that can be corrected by contact lenses include myopia (short sight), hyperopia (long sight) and corneal astigmatism (irregularly shaped cornea). Contact lenses are not available at NHS expense unless they are indicated for a serious eye disorder as determined by a hospital ophthalmologist. Contact lenses may be used following removal of the lens of the eye in cataract surgery, and can also be fitted to protect the eye in diseases affecting the cornea, including bullous keratopathy (a severe form of corneal oedema), dry eye and recurrent corneal ulceration. Cosmetic contact lenses are sometimes used to disguise eyes that have developed unacceptable appearances, usually following injury or surgery. Contact lenses are also indicated for severe refractive errors where suitable spectacles cannot be made, or are impractical; in these cases, contact lenses provide effective correction of vision and are cosmetically acceptable.

Contact lenses are contra-indicated in certain conditions, particularly active eye diseases. People unable to wear contact lenses include those with a history of allergy, or disease presenting with eye symptoms. Patients with hayfever may not be able to wear contact lenses during the period in which they are affected. People with conditions associated with dry eye or poor tear flow (e.g. hyperthyroidism or Sjogren's syndrome, which often occurs in association with rheumatoid arthritis) have poor lens tolerance. People who are diabetic or immunocompromised are at greater risk of developing eye infections, and should be advised of this if contact lenses are considered. Some skin conditions may also increase the possibility of eye infections. Patients with cold sores should not wear lenses during the course of the infection because of the risk of transferring infection to the eyes. Manual dexterity is important in insertion and removal of contact lenses, and for effective care. Consequently, patients with arthritis, stroke victims, young children and the elderly may not be able to use contact lenses. Tolerance to contact lenses tends to become reduced during pregnancy, but should not necessarily mean that women have to stop wearing their lenses; all that may be required is a reduction in wearing time or allowing an hour or two during the day without lenses.

Contact lenses and care regimens

Contact lenses are broadly classified as either hard lenses, which include gas permeable hard lenses, or soft lenses. Special lenses may be required in certain circumstances (*see below*). Soft lenses are less durable and need to be replaced every six to 18 months; hard lenses and gas permeable hard lenses tend to last for a number of years.

At the time of fitting, contact lens wearers are instructed how to take care of their lenses. This includes the correct techniques for insertion and removal of lenses, and appropriate methods for cleaning and storing them. Meticulous care, allied to strong commitment, is essential in order to obtain the maximum benefit from contact lenses, ensure maximum life of the lenses and prevent eye infection. These objectives are primarily achieved by using an effective care regimen designed for the particular lens type.

Some solutions are suitable for use with all lens types; others are designed for one particular lens type. Solutions labelled for use with one type of contact lens are not usually intended to be used with another lens type, although there are exceptions. Some solutions for hard lenses and gas permeable hard lenses contain preservatives that may be absorbed by soft lenses and slowly released onto the eye; these solutions should not, therefore, be used for soft lenses. While solutions labelled for use with soft lenses can be used for hard/gas permeable lenses, they are not as effective as those formulated specifically for hard/gas permeable lenses. Some people are sensitive to the preservatives used in contact lens solutions, therefore preservative-free solutions are available.

In addition to caring for the contact lenses, lens storage cases need to be rinsed regularly with sterile saline solution, or disinfecting solution, and air dried between use to remove contaminants. Soap and detergents should not be used to clean storage cases. Storage cases should be changed regularly, preferably every month.

When contact lenses are first fitted, there is a period of time during which the eyes adapt to the presence of lenses – the adaptation time. Initially, the lenses are worn for short periods and the wear time gradually increased in increments until lenses can be worn comfortably for the desired duration. The adaptation time is generally shorter for soft lenses than for hard or gas permeable lenses. The adaptation time is often associated with transient symptoms, which include:

- awareness of the lenses in the eyes
- blurred vision (momentary episodes)
- discomfort from exerting extreme eye movements (to the left or the right) and when looking upwards
- discomfort in a smoky or dry atmosphere
- excessive blinking
- excessive lachrymation
- reflections from light (prominent at night)
- temporary blurred spectacle vision after lens removal.

Hard contact lenses and gas permeable hard contact lenses

Hard contact lenses and gas permeable hard contact lenses are both rigid in nature. Hard contact lenses are made of polymethylmethacrylate (PMMA, Perspex). They are inert, hydrophobic and have a very low water content; they are also impermeable to oxygen. Gas exchange with the corneal epithelium is, therefore, dependent on tears flowing behind the lens. The initial tolerance to hard lenses is poor, with a failure rate of about 30%. Hard lenses have now been almost completely replaced by gas permeable hard lenses, although in some cases they may be the most appropriate type of lens for large refractive errors (high prescription lenses).

Gas permeable hard lenses were developed to try and overcome the disadvantages of hard lenses, and to include some of the advantages of soft lenses. The lenses are hard, hydrophobic and have a low water content. They allow the transmission of oxygen through the lens to the cornea, facilitating more normal metabolism. All gas permeable hard lenses are smaller than the diameter of the cornea, and float freely in the tear film. Gas permeable hard lenses may be made from one of the following polymer materials:

- CAB (cellulose acetate butyrate) (low gas permeability)
- siloxane/methylmethacrylate copolymers (medium gas permeability)
- fluorocarbons/siloxane copolymers (high gas permeability).

CAB was the earliest material available, but is rarely used now because of its low gas permeability.

The silicone content of the lenses controls the oxygen permeability. Modern gas permeable lenses scratch less easily than the early types. Compared with soft lenses, they attract fewer deposits and carry the least risk of infection. They provide good correction of vision defects, including astigmatism. However, compared with soft lenses, the fitting is more complex and they are more uncomfortable in the initial stages and require longer adaptation times. The small lens size means that foreign bodies can get behind the lens (causing discomfort), there is risk of loss of the lens from the eye and the lens edge produces reflections.

The following solutions are needed in the care of hard lenses and gas permeable hard lenses:

- daily cleaning solutions
- rinsing and soaking (disinfecting) solutions
- wetting solutions
- rewetting and comfort solutions
- protein removal preparations.

Individual solutions are available for each function, and the properties of these solutions are described below. In order to simplify contact lens care, solutions are also available that perform more than one function (e.g. solutions are available that are used for the combined tasks of rinsing, soaking and wetting) and a multipurpose (or all-purpose) solution is available that cleans, rinses, soaks and wets. These solutions may be less effective overall than individual solutions because some properties may be compromised in their formulation. However, the convenience of their use, and, therefore, greater compliance with the cleaning regimen, make these systems preferable for some people, and they are commonly used.

Essentially, the solutions used for the care of gas permeable hard lenses are the same as those used for hard lenses. However, the converse is not always true: solutions for use with hard lenses may not be compatible with gas permeable hard lenses. For this reason, an optometrist's instructions must be followed, and only those solutions labelled for use with the particular lens type should be used.

Cleaning

Hard lenses and gas permeable hard lenses need to be cleaned daily to remove environment-derived and tear-related deposits from the lens surface and break down the microbial biofilm that collects during wear. The type and amount of deposit varies with the type of lens material. Lipids tend to accumulate on PMMA and CAB lenses, whereas both proteins and lipids are attracted to silicone acrylates. The cleaning solution should be applied to both surfaces of each lens and gentle digital pressure used in a rotating manner in the palm of the hand. Solutions for daily cleaning are isotonic, and usually consist of a nonionic or amphoteric surfactant and a preservative. Some cleaning solutions contain a chelating agent (e.g. disodium edetate), which is present to remove calcium deposits. Disodium edetate also acts as an antimicrobial synergist.

A preservative-free preparation containing isopropyl alcohol 20% is available, and this is suitable for cleaning both rigid and soft lenses.

Rinsing and disinfection

In general, following cleaning, contact lenses are disinfected by placing them overnight in their storage case containing fresh soaking solution. Before soaking, the cleaning solution should be rinsed off each lens (using some of the soaking solution) to reduce contamination of the soaking solution. Soaking solutions are isotonic and consist of wetting agents, disinfectants and a chelating agent. Daily replacement of the soaking solution is essential to prevent micro-organisms from proliferating in the storage case. An alternative method of disinfection is to use hydrogen peroxide 3% (*see* Soft contact lenses *below*).

Heat disinfection (*see below*) is not a suitable method for disinfecting hard or gas permeable hard lenses.

Wetting

Wetting solutions are used for hard lenses and gas permeable hard lenses to reduce the contact angle of tears with the contact lens. They are formulated to be slightly viscous so as to cushion the lens on the eye for greater comfort. Wetting solutions are isotonic and consist of wetting agents, viscosity increasing agents and preservatives. Polyvinyl alcohol or cellulose derivatives, or both, are commonly used in the formulation of wetting solutions. Generally, wetting solutions increase the comfort of contact lens wear and prevent the accumulation of deposits.

Saliva should not be used as a wetting substance on contact lenses because serious eye infections may be caused by micro-organisms present in saliva.

Rewetting and comfort solutions

The purpose of these solutions is to improve comfort when lenses are being worn, reduce lens irritation and augment tear flow. They are administered directly onto the eye with the contact lens in place. These solutions are formulated on similar principles to wetting solutions (*see above*). Hypertonic solutions may be used in some cases to reduce lens irritation caused by slight corneal oedema associated with lens wear.

Protein removal

Periodic cleaning with protein-removing preparations is necessary for all types of contact lenses. Protein removal is carried out as an extra stage after cleaning the lenses (*see above*) and before disinfection. Protein-removing preparations containing proteolytic enzymes (e.g. papain or subtilisin A) are capable of removing stubborn deposits from the lenses. Pancreatin, a preparation containing enzymes having protease, lipase and amylase activity, is included in some cleaning products used periodically. Periodic cleaning preparations are usually presented as tablets for reconstitution. The tablets are generally dissolved in sterile sodium chloride 0.9% solution or in all-in-one solution, and the lenses are soaked for a length of time that varies according to the type of lens and the particular preparation. It is advisable to clean and rinse the lenses again afterwards, before disinfecting them, as the enzymes may only loosen the deposits and a mechanical action may be necessary to complete their removal. The frequency of periodic cleaning varies according to the instructions of the product manufacturer. These preparations are usually suitable for both soft lenses and gas permeable hard lenses. The use of protein removal preparations is not an alternative to daily cleaning; the two processes are complementary.

Soft contact lenses

Soft lenses (also known as hydrogel lenses) are made of materials based on polyhydroxyethylmethacrylate (poly-HEMA), and are the most popular types of contact lens in use. They are larger than hard/gas permeable lenses and cover the cornea and part of the sclera. Soft lenses are hydrophilic and have a water content of 30 to 80%. They can be broadly categorised as low water content (<55%) or high water content (>55%). They allow the transfer of oxygen to the cornea through the lens, with the oxygen dissolving in the liquid in the lens and diffusing through. The higher the water content, the better the oxygen transmission of the lens, although this is usually accompanied by problems of greater fragility and accumulation of dirt in and on the lens.

There are two main types of soft lens:

- daily wear soft lenses, designed to be removed for cleaning each night
- disposable lenses, that are usually removed each night for cleaning, but are discarded and replaced at regular intervals (for example monthly, fortnightly or weekly), thus reducing complications associated with the accumulation of deposits.

There are some disposable lenses available for a single day's use and then discarded, thus removing the need for any cleaning/disinfecting procedures. Disposable lenses are becoming increasingly popular. They were originally developed for continuous wear (known as extended-wear lenses) for a minimum of 24 hours and usually several weeks. However, because the risks associated with overnight wear are now more clearly understood, this practice is not generally recommended.

Compared with gas permeable hard lenses, soft lenses are well tolerated and more comfortable; as the adaptation time is short, they are suitable for occasional use. Soft lenses are larger than gas permeable lenses and cover the cornea and part of the sclera. This property makes them less prone to problems with dust/foreign bodies trapped behind them or to dislodgement; it also removes edge reflections. Soft lenses are suitable for use during sport and exercise. However, soft lenses are less resilient to damage and more readily accumulate deposits. They may cause more problems with lens dehydration and dry eyes. In addition, they are not able to provide the same degree of visual acuity.

The care of soft lenses involves cleaning, rinsing and disinfection. Non-disposable lenses also require regular protein removal. Contaminated soft lenses are considered to be primarily responsible for the complications associated with the use of soft lenses.

In common with the care regimens for gas/hard lenses described *above*, solutions are available which perform single functions (these are described *below*) or there are multi-purpose solutions that perform more than one function. The antimicrobial efficiency of these multipurpose solutions is debated, although their ease of use overcomes many of the compliance problems associated with the more complicated cleaning regimens. Most of the multi-purpose solutions incorporate polyhexanide (polyhexamethylene biguanide) as the disinfectant agent. They are not consistently effective against *Acanthamoeba*. Usually, a chelating agent and a poloxamer/poloxamine surfactant are also included.

Cleaning

The routine for cleaning soft contact lenses is similar to that described for hard lenses (*see above*). Cleaning is one of the most important aspects in the effective care of soft lenses; it is also one of the most neglected. Daily cleaning is necessary to remove fresh deposits of lipids, proteins and other contaminants. Daily-use cleaning solutions are isotonic, and usually contain surfactants, preservatives and a chelating agent. A preservative-free preparation containing isopropyl alcohol 20% is available for cleaning both rigid and soft lenses.

Rinsing and disinfection

Soft lenses must be disinfected daily to eliminate potentially pathogenic microbes. There are two methods that may be used: chemical disinfection or heat disinfection. Chemical disinfection is almost always the method used. Chemical disinfection solutions (soaking solutions) contain disinfectants and a chelating agent. Soaking solutions for soft lenses usually contain the same preservatives that are used in solutions for hard lenses, with the exception of benzalkonium chloride. Following cleaning, the lenses are rinsed and placed in fresh soaking solution, ideally for overnight storage. Soaking solutions are commonly used for rinsing soft lenses after cleaning. Sterile sodium chloride 0.9% solution may also be used. Sodium chloride 0.9% solutions may contain preservatives, but unpreserved solutions are available in unit-dose packs and aerosol formulations. The use of home-made saline solutions is strongly discouraged because of the likelihood of contamination, which may cause serious eye disorders (*see* Complications related to contact lens wear *below*).

Soft contact lenses should never be rinsed or soaked in water, as changes to the structure of the lens may occur. After overnight soaking, the lenses can be inserted into the eyes without further rinsing, although it is commonly recommended that the lenses be rinsed before insertion. Disinfecting solutions often contain a preservative. A preservative-free disinfection method is provided by the use of hydrogen peroxide 3%, and is considered to be the most effective method of lens disinfection. It is necessary to clean the lenses before disinfection, although this may be contrary to some manufacturers' instructions. In addition, although a ten-minute disinfection cycle may be specified in the instructions, a soaking time of at least two hours has been reported to be necessary to eliminate *Acanthamoeba* trophozoites and cysts, and overnight soaking is therefore recommended. Only hydrogen peroxide solutions that are specifically formulated for contact lenses should be used. Contact lenses must be neutralised after soaking in the hydrogen peroxide solution. This neutralisation process is usually achieved by adding sodium pyruvate, sodium thiosulphate, or the enzyme catalase or by using a platinum disc. The neutraliser may be added as a separate step after the overnight soak; alternatively, one-step systems are available in which the neutraliser is added in a delayed-release tablet form at the same time as the hydrogen peroxide solution is added to the storage case. Hydrogen peroxide disinfection is suitable for gas permeable and hard lenses as well.

Heat disinfection requires the use of units designed specifically for the purpose. It is a technique suitable for use with low water content soft lenses. Preserved sodium chloride 0.9% or non-preserved sterile sodium chloride 0.9% solutions may be used to store the lenses during the heating process. It is essential to follow the method of disinfection outlined by the manufacturer of the disinfection unit. Heat disinfection is more detrimental to the lenses than chemical disinfection, and can reduce the lens-life considerably. Soft contact lenses that are subjected to heat disinfection may last as little as six months. The need for special equipment and the reduction in the life of the lenses has made heat disinfection a little-used method. It may be useful for people sensitive to preservatives.

Heat disinfection is not a suitable method for disinfecting hard or gas permeable hard lenses.

Comfort solutions

These solutions are formulated for instillation directly into the eye with the lens in place. They provide fluid to maintain adequate lens hydration and improve the comfort of soft lenses. They are formulated on similar principles to comfort solutions used for rigid lenses. The regular use of these solutions is important with extended-wear and disposable soft lenses.

Protein removal

Periodic cleaning (usually once a week) with the use of enzymatic protein removal preparations is required (*see under* Hard contact lenses and gas permeable hard contact lenses *above*) to remove tear proteins that are chemically more tightly bound to the lens surface. Protein removal preparations are usually suitable for both soft lenses and gas permeable hard lenses, and should be used according to the manufacturer's instructions.

Special contact lenses

Special contact lenses are used to correct particular problems affecting the eye. Scleral lenses cover the cornea and the sclera, and are used to mask damaged eyes. They can also be used in certain sports (e.g. water skiing) because they are less easily dislodged.

Toric lenses can be made with most materials and are used to correct astigmatism. They have an uneven surface curvature and correct irregular astigmatism and keratoconus (protrusion of the cornea) more effectively than spectacles.

Bifocal lenses in hard or soft lenses can also be fitted for age-related changes to the eye. However, they are difficult to fit and frequently represent a compromise to vision and their success rate is low.

Tinted contact lenses can be used to alter cosmetically the colour of the eyes, or they can be used instead of sunglasses. However, the degree of protection from ultraviolet light is lower since the lens does not cover the entire eye. Contact lenses may be tinted to make them easier to see when out of the eye, but this tinting does not affect eye colour when worn.

Some gas permeable lenses are available with a hydrophilic coating that makes them suitable for people with dry eyes. A combination lens consisting of a gas permeable central lens surrounded by soft lens material is used in certain people with irregular eye shape.

Complications related to contact lens wear

Most complications associated with the wearing of contact lenses are self-limiting if the lens is removed at the first sign of trouble. The problems encountered are usually caused by the reaction of the eye to deposits on the lens or to chemicals absorbed by the lens. In addition, complications may be a result of poor lens care, inadequate hygiene, corneal hypoxia, overwear, poor fitting or allergy to the cleaning solutions.

Daily contact lens wear is associated with accumulation of deposits on the lens surface, which are responsible for many of the complications. Deposits on contact lenses may consist of:

- abraded corneal materials
- cosmetics
- divalent and trivalent cations
- dust
- lysozyme
- mucoproteins
- oils and lipids
- pollutants
- tear proteins.

The type and extent of lens deposits are influenced by tear consistency, flow rate and volume. Increased lens deposits are seen in hot, dry environments as a result of evaporation of tears and increased concentration of constituents. The extent of deposit formation appears to be proportional to the water content of the lens. Accumulated lens deposits are relatively easy to remove from hard lenses by routine cleaning; they are less easily removed from gas permeable hard lenses, and may become chemically bound to soft lenses. The consequences of contact lens deposits include:

- allergy caused by denatured protein accumulation
- irritation as a result of poor wetting
- lens discoloration
- ocular irritation caused by binding of cationic preservatives to lens deposits
- pitting in surface of lens upon removal of calcium deposits
- reduced visual acuity
- reduction of antimicrobial activity of contact lens solutions caused by binding of preservatives to deposits on lens.

Daily wear gas permeable lenses are associated with the lowest incidence of complications and extended-wear soft lenses appear to cause most problems. Soft contact lenses are slightly larger than hard lenses and the long circumference tends to irritate the conjunctival membrane of the eyelid; the high surface area of the contact lens maximises the deposition of potentially antigenic deposits. The most common, and potentially serious, complication associated with daily wear soft contact lenses is corneal ulceration. Extended-wear soft lenses have been associated with a high incidence of suppurative keratitis, the risk of which appears to be related to the number of nights that the lenses are worn.

Contact lenses may cause chronic conjunctival problems. Purulent conjunctivitis is probably more common in contact lens wearers than in the general population. Contact lens-associated papillary conjunctivitis may be caused by antigenic deposits on contact lenses. It occurs in approximately 3% of hard lens wearers and 8% of soft lens wearers. Symptoms include red eye, itching, and mucous discharge, which causes smeared lenses and blurred vision. The condition is similar to allergic conjunctivitis and is thought to be an immune system-mediated reaction to the lens deposits. In the late stages, the condition may be associated with the appearance of giant papillae on the underside of the eyelid.

High water content soft lenses may become tight during wear, particularly if worn overnight. Immediate lens removal is essential to prevent corneal ulceration. A small degree of corneal oedema is inevitable with contact lens wear, but more extensive oedema may increase the risk of other complications. Contact lens removal and refitting with new lenses may resolve the problem, but some people have to stop using contact lenses. Prolonged wear of soft lenses may cause corneal opacities, which occur only infrequently with hard lenses and almost never with gas permeable hard lenses.

Toric lenses may have a thick inferior edge to prevent excessive rotation. The lower portion of the cornea may then become oxygen starved, which can lead to the formation of new blood vessels (neovascularisation).

Ulcerative keratitis is a rare, but serious, complication of contact lens wear; it is more common with soft lenses due to increased microbial adherence to the lens and lens deposits. Other predisposing factors include overnight wear of daily wear lenses and long intervals between cleaning. The risk of keratitis is further increased with extended-wear soft lenses and disposable lenses. Infecting organisms are commonly bacterial (e.g. *Pseudomonas aeruginosa*, *Serratia marcescens*, *Staphylococcus aureus*, *Staph. epidermidis* and *Streptococcus pneumoniae*), although fungal keratitis is occasionally encountered.

Acanthamoeba keratitis is a protozoal infection that is being increasingly encountered, particularly in soft lens wearers. It is a serious, sight-threatening condition, which is also difficult to diagnose since it mimics the symptoms of herpes virus infection. Symptoms include red eye, a purulent discharge, visual impairment and pain. *Acanthamoeba* spp. can cause corneal scarring with partial or complete loss of sight. Home-made saline solutions have been implicated as a source of *Acanthamoeba* infection.

Red eye is a symptom of many complications associated with the use of contact lenses. It can also be caused by accumulated deposits and scratches on the lenses. Treatment involves stopping lens wear until the red eye has subsided and refitting with new lenses. Wearing lenses for longer than the recommended period of time may result in corneal oedema, which causes blurred vision and epithelial necrosis. Symptoms resolve within a few hours of lens removal, although some people may require active treatment.

Allergic reactions to the preservatives and disinfectants included in contact lens solutions may occur. Chemicals used for cleaning and disinfection may be taken up by the lenses and released onto the eye. Symptoms may include itching, stinging and, in more serious cases, severe discomfort and visual impairment. Patients may be advised to use alternative formulations to avoid a particular allergen.

The role of the pharmacist

Contact lens wear demands motivation, commitment and meticulous care to prevent problems. Wearers must realise that it is essential to conform to the recommended regimens of maintenance and use for their particular type of lens. The regimen that is necessary will have been explained to wearers by the optometrist; however, it has been demonstrated that compliance is commonly poor. Pharmacists should emphasise to contact lens wearers that they should visit the optometrist regularly for contact lens after-care. New contact lens wearers will usually be required to visit the optometrist at frequent intervals in the period immediately after fitting. Thereafter, regular visits at six-monthly intervals for soft lens wearers and yearly intervals for those with rigid lenses are recommended. Symptom-free wear does not necessarily mean that the contact lenses are not causing undesirable effects. These visits are important to keep the contact lens prescription updated and identify insidious complications at an early stage. All contact lens wearers should also have their spectacle prescription kept updated, and have a pair of spectacles to use in place of their contact lenses, either in an emergency or on an occasional basis to rest the eyes.

Advice on the prevention of complications associated with the use of contact lenses is essential because inadequate lens care is one of the many causes of eye infections. Lenses should only be worn for the recommended length of time, and should not be worn during sleep, unless they are extended-wear or disposable lenses designed for the purpose. It is important to refer wearers immediately if any of the following are apparent:

- discomfort
- excessive lachrymation
- frequent eye infections
- itching
- pain
- photophobia
- recurrent red eye problems
- visual impairment.

Pharmacists are ideally placed to advise contact lens wearers on contact lens products and effective care regimens. The type or brand of contact lens solutions should not be changed by wearers without first obtaining guidance from optometrists or pharmacists. Lens care products are intended to be used in clean surroundings, and hands should be washed (avoiding perfumed and medicated soaps) and dried before attempting to remove or insert lenses. If working over a sink, it is essential to put in the drainage plug to stop the accidental loss of a lens.

Awareness of circumstances and situations that can adversely affect contact lens wearers will assist pharmacists in advising ways to achieve comfortable and problem-free wear. Adverse environmental conditions (e.g. dry heat, air-conditioning and windy days) may cause burning, stinging and blurred vision; comfort solutions can be used to alleviate discomfort if the stimulus cannot be avoided. The use of cosmetics with contact lenses is acceptable, provided simple guidelines are followed. Generally, contact lenses should be inserted before applying cosmetics; however, hairspray and other aerosol applications should be used before contact lenses are inserted. It is preferable to use water-based, fragrance-free cosmetics, because oily cosmetics tend to stain lenses or bind with lens material. Cosmetics should not be applied to the edge of the eyelids, and mascara should be water-resistant and applied only to the tips of the eyelashes. Contact lenses are fragile, and sharp objects (e.g. fingernails) can scratch hard lenses and gas permeable hard lenses and tear soft lenses.

Contact lens wearers should be advised that lenses cannot disappear behind the eye. They may need to be recentred if they slip out of position, and the techniques, which vary with different lenses, will have been explained to wearers by the optometrist. Lenses can be worn when swimming if certain precautions are taken, although it is advisable to consult the optometrist first; serious eye infections have been associated with contamination from swimming pool water. Swimming in sea water is best avoided, as sea water is often a potential source of infection, and the high salinity can cause difficulties. Goggles should be worn with gas permeable lenses in case they fall out and soft lenses should be cleaned thoroughly after swimming. During illness, the duration of contact lens wear should be shortened and built up after recovery.

Pharmacists should be aware of the effects of systemic and topical eye medication in contact lens wearers (Table 10.1).

Effects of systemic medication

Systemic medication can have adverse effects on the wearing of contact lenses, or on the lens material itself. If the medicinal product must be taken, the use of comfort drops and/or saline may help reduce discomfort. In some cases, though, the lenses may need to be left out. Reduced tolerance to contact lenses has been reported with the use of oral contraceptives and hormone replacement therapy, particularly when higher doses of oestrogen are involved. Reported effects include corneal and eyelid oedema, reduced visual acuity, photophobia, allergic conjunctivitis and altered tear composition. Corneal oedema appears to be less of a problem with low-dose oral contraceptives and modern lenses. Pregnancy can produce the same effects on contact lens wear.

Anxiolytics, hypnotics, antihistamines and muscle relaxants can reduce the blink rate. Adequate blinking is necessary to maintain proper hydration of lenses, particularly with soft lenses. Blinking also removes stale tears and provides a fresh supply.

Antimuscarinic drugs, drugs with antimuscarinic effects (e.g. sedating antihistamines, chlorpromazine and tricyclic antidepressants), some beta blockers and diuretics can decrease tear volume, which may lead to corneal drying and irritation. Reserpine, ephedrine or hydralazine may cause an increase in lachrymation and can adversely affect contact lens wear by impairing the fit.

Conjunctivitis can occur with isotretinoin and it is wise to avoid wearing contact lenses during treatment. Primidone and chlorthalidone may produce ocular or eyelid oedema, causing interference with lens wear. After oral administration of aspirin, salicylic acid appears in tears and may be absorbed by soft lenses, causing ocular irritation and redness. Rifampicin, nitrofurantoin, phenolphthalein, tetracycline, labetalol and sulphasalazine can cause discoloration of soft contact lenses. Discoloration is only likely on prolonged use of the drug. Certain drugs applied topically can also cause discoloration (*see below*).

Table 10.1 Reported drug interactions with contact lenses

Drug	Lens type: Hard	Lens type: Soft	Interaction mechanism
Adrenaline, topical		•	Discoloration
Anxiolytics	•	•	Decreased blink rate
Aspirin		•	Absorption by lens causing irritation and redness
Antihistamines	•	•	Decreased tear volume and blink rate
Antimuscarinics	•	•	Decreased tear volume
Benzoyl peroxide, topical		•	Fading of lens tint
Diuretics	•	•	Decreased tear volume; ocular and eyelid oedema with chlorthalidone
Fluorescein, topical		•	Concentration by lens and subsequent discoloration
Hypnotics	•	•	Decreased blink rate
Labetalol		•	Calculi formation (white dots) on the lens
Muscle relaxants	•	•	Decreased blink rate
Nitrofurantoin		•	Yellow/brown discoloration of the lens
Oral contraceptives	•	•	Ocular and eyelid oedema; altered tear composition
Phenolphthalein		•	Pink discoloration of the lens
Phenylephrine, topical		•	Discoloration
Primidone	•	•	Ocular and eyelid oedema
Reserpine	•	•	Increased lachrymation
Rifampicin		•	Orange discoloration of the lens
Rose bengal, topical		•	Concentration by lens and subsequent discoloration
Sedatives	•	•	Decreased blink rate
Sodium sulphacetamide 10%, topical		•	Lens dehydration due to hypertonicity of solution
Sulphasalazine		•	Yellow discoloration of the lens
Tetracycline		•	Yellow/brown discoloration of the lens
Tricyclic antidepressants	•	•	Decreased tear volume

Effects of topical medication

Generally, topical eye medication should not be used while lenses are being worn. Topical treatment of an eye infection necessitates the removal of contact lenses for the duration of treatment, as the lenses may harbour the micro-organisms. The lenses may need professional cleaning and sterilisation, and this can be done by optometrists. If, for medical reasons, continued wearing of lenses is necessary, eye drops should be administered 30 minutes before the insertion of lenses. Soft lenses require care, since many eye drops are preserved with benzalkonium chloride, which binds to soft lenses and causes irritation; a preservative-free formulation should be used. Ointment preparations should never be used with contact lens wear.

The effect of topically applied drugs on soft contact lenses may be exaggerated due to the following effects:

- absorption and consequent concentration of drug can occur, with gradual release over time
- increased drug absorption due to compromised cornea in contact lens wearers
- lenses can increase contact time of drug medication.

Dark discoloration of soft lenses with repeated use of phenylephrine and adrenaline has been observed. At after-care visits to optometrists, diagnostic stains (e.g. fluorescein sodium) may be used to detect corneal abrasions. Fluorescein is capable of staining contact lenses, and spectacles should be worn following its use in an examination, for a period specified by the optometrist. Acne medications containing benzoyl peroxide can fade tinted soft lenses.

Smokers have a higher incidence of stained soft lenses than non-smokers. This may be due to stimulation of melanin products in tears by nicotine and other aromatic compounds in cigarette smoke. Patients should be counselled about the potential for lens spoilage and the importance of disinfection. Nicotine transferred to lenses by smoke or fingers can reduce their clarity.

Further reading

Bennett I (1994). *Contact Lens Problem Solving*. London: Mosby.

Larke J (1999). *Eye in Contact Lens Wear*, 2nd edn. Oxford: Butterworth-Heinemann.

Lyndon J, Jones D (2000). *Common Contact Lens Complications: Diagnosis and Management*. Oxford: Butterworth-Heinemann.

11

Companion animals and human health

Steven Kayne

In the search for the cause of many human diseases, suggestions implicating animals or animal agents have been made. Infection may result from intended or unintended contact as follows:

- contact through petting a companion animal
- contact through involvement with an animal casualty
- unintended contact with 'friendly' neighbours' animals
- physical damage (mainly bites) resulting from attack.

More than 200 diseases may be transmitted from animals to humans, but comparatively few involve pets. In this chapter, some of the conditions that may be associated with pets are described and the problems most likely to be seen in the pharmacy are highlighted. Some of the physical and psychological benefits to be gained from keeping pets are also considered.

What is a pet and why is it kept?

A pet is a domestic or tamed animal, usually kept in the owner's house for pleasure or companionship and treated with affection. This definition does not cover some of the more exotic pets (e.g. snakes and spiders), which many would find less attractive. Also, it does not recognise that some animals (mainly dogs and sometimes horses) start out as working animals and subsequently become a family pet.

The centuries-old bond between people and animals has satisfied a variety of human needs. Animals first provided basic resources for living: food, clothing, transport and even shelter. Later, the relationship developed to meet psychological needs of humans for companionship and security. Both of these functions still exist.

It is more readily apparent why farmers keep large animals. Farmers run a business and use animals to provide saleable commodities, although the prices being attained for animals has fallen dramatically in recent years. Farmers keep working dogs, horses, beef and dairy cattle, sheep, pigs, chickens and, sometimes, goats. With the possible exception of the sheepdog, decisions on whether to treat or slaughter animals are usually taken on economic grounds. Occasionally, a favourite cow or horse becomes a family pet, and, therefore, return on investment is not the sole factor in its welfare.

The situation with small pets is different. There is evidence that humans have enjoyed the companionship of animals since prehistoric times. The dog is generally thought to be the oldest domestic animal species. The earliest remains found in Iraq and Israel may date from 10 000 BC. Later finds include those in the USA, dated at around 8000 BC, and the UK, dated around 7000 BC. Origins of the domestic cat are less easy to trace, with estimates of the start of its domestication varying from 7000 BC to 4000 BC. There may be a connection between keeping cats and pest control.

Keeping a pet may help to fulfil some of the owner's basic psychological needs. Most owners consider pets to be part of the family, responding to their behavioural profile at any given time. Dogs seem to sense when their owners are unwell or unhappy, and often offer comfort. Pets are taken on holiday or away for the weekend, for which some hotels cater. From early in the year 2000, pets from specified countries (including the

UK) are able to travel to and from other specified countries without having to undergo substantial quarantine requirements.

The companionship that a pet can provide is often seen as something that has special value for the elderly. Ideally, animals should be banned from pharmacies. However, such action may be difficult to enforce with elderly owners who cannot bear to be parted from their pet for even short periods. As with all aspects of pharmacy practice, some degree of flexibility is appropriate. The fixing of hooks on outside walls to which dog leads can be attached has proven effective in some pharmacies.

Reasons other than companionship for which pets are acquired include:

- to perform certain tasks (guide dogs or hearing dogs)
- for protection
- for education of children
- received as a present
- to conform to popular local trends.

The latter two have public health implications that may involve pharmacists. When a decision to buy a pet is made, potential owners usually spend time finding out the scope of their new responsibilities (e.g. the amount of exercise required, special health requirements, the costs of feeding and the costs of healthcare). If a pet arrives unexpectedly, pharmacists may have to suggest the need for worming or flea treatments. General hygiene advice (e.g. washing hands after contact with animal faeces or cleaning fish tanks) can be extremely important. The majority of zoonotic diseases result from contact with animal excreta, but risks can be minimised by good hygiene procedures.

The benefits of keeping pets

There may be significant therapeutic benefits derived from companion animals. In a ten-month prospective study to examine the behaviour and health status in 71 adults following the acquisition of a dog or cat, there was a significant reduction in minor health problems during the first month compared with a non-pet-owning group. This effect was sustained in dog owners to the end of the study. Walking a dog is a compelling stimulus to patients requiring exercise, particularly in cardiac rehabilitation or diabetes.

Pets, and especially dogs, can enhance human emotional, social and relaxation effects, although tendencies towards humanisation are inappropriate. Even at a pre-school age, children derive psychological benefits from rodents, fish and birds.

Pets can influence human development, but whether the effect is due to the presence of a pet or to the person's relationship with the pet is uncertain. Female dog-owners may exhibit less physiological reactivity during stressful tasks than control women who do not own pets. Similarly, fish tanks in dental surgeries are common, supposedly to soothe the nerves of waiting patients.

People publicly identified with a companion animal are making a symbolic statement of their personality and self-image. Similarly, the presence of a pet and the way it is treated can influence the image others form about individuals. The kind of pet that one chooses is a way of expressing one's personality. Thus, the Great Dane dog may be a symbol of masculinity, power, strength and virility; conversely, a Chihuahua dog serves as a symbol of femininity (Hartley and Shames, 1959). Pets can also reflect status, as some pets are expensive or 'fashionable' (e.g. the Vietnamese Pot Belly pig).

A pet may enhance social contact with other people, stimulating conversation. Owners, as 'animal lovers', are often perceived as 'nice' people. There are also social benefits for people confined to wheelchairs, particularly as eye contact, meaningful conversation and social interaction may be enhanced in the presence of a companion dog. Acknowledgements from passers-by when people in wheelchairs have a dog may help reduce feelings of social ostracism. There is considerable evidence that a residential or nursing home pet increases social interaction and alertness among patients and staff.

Physiological benefits that have been demonstrated include reduced blood pressure in a person patting and talking to a dog compared with that experienced as a result of human conversation. The patient and animal must be carefully matched: with the chronically mentally ill, pet therapy is based on the personality and animal experiences of the patient concerned. The inclusion of animals as a positive therapeutic approach for the development, treatment and rehabilitation of people is still a relatively new innovation; however, orthopaedic benefits of horse riding are well known.

As a group, pet owners may have lower blood pressure and lower cholesterol levels than those without pets. One study has shown that people who suffer heart attacks are likely to make a swifter recovery if they have a pet. As a result, a variety of pet therapy schemes have been introduced in the USA (e.g. Pet-a-Pet and Caring Canines in children's hospitals and nursing homes); some are also being introduced in the UK. The Children in Hospital and Animal Therapy Association (CHATA) was founded in 1994 and works principally with terminally ill children in London hospitals. Volunteers must have qualifications associated with medicine or be qualified to work with children in some capacity. Some patients have also claimed that contact with animals has reduced pain.

The enormous assistance given to the blind by guide dogs is widely recognised. Fund-raising to cover the cost of training guide dogs is well organised, and many pharmacies act as collecting depots (e.g. for stamps and newspapers) and have collecting boxes on the premises. Such 'seeing-eye' dogs are exempt from many public health regulations that govern dogs in general. Such animals are allowed into restaurants and public buildings, as well as establishments operated by and for blind people. These exemptions recognise not only that these dogs are vital to their owners' mobility, but also that they are usually in excellent health, highly trained and stay close to their owners. Blind people have a very close relationship with their guide dogs. As well as providing a valuable working function for its owner, a dog can help to decrease anxiety and boost confidence. The support is psychological as well as practical, and enhances a blind person's mobility. Separating the dog from its owner is often confusing and disorienting for both, and should be avoided whenever possible. To promote their special status, organisations for the blind emphasise that guide dogs are safe, hard-working, healthy animals, not merely pets. Owners are encouraged to ensure that the dog is kept in good condition. However, it is recommended that visiting with a guide dog in hospital should be restricted when visiting patients in the following circumstances (Hardy, 1981):

- those in isolation for an infectious disease or who are immunocompromised
- those in intensive care, coronary care, renal dialysis or other restricted areas
- those who suffer from a dog allergy or phobia
- patients in a severe psychotic state.

'Dogs for the Deaf' is a related scheme that provides specially trained dogs for people who are hard of hearing. The animals can warn of a phone, doorbell or a baby crying by touching the owner gently with its paw and then leading them to the source of the sound.

Similarly, dogs and a cat have been reported to be able to warn epilepsy sufferers and their families of an impending seizure. They are thought to be able to detect electrical disturbances or minor body odour and behavioural changes.

The following guidelines to ensure the quality of life of the animals involved in providing practical assistance or therapy were adopted by the International Association of Human–Animal Interaction Organizations at a meeting in Prague in 1998:

- only animals that have been trained using techniques of positive reinforcement and that have been, and will continue to be, properly housed and cared for may be involved
- safeguards must be present to prevent adverse effects on the animals involved
- the involvement of assistance and/or therapy animals must be potentially beneficial in each case.

Basic standards ensure safety, risk management, physical and emotional security, health, basic trust and freedom of choice, personal space, appropriate allocation of programme resources, appropriate workload, clearly defined roles, confidentiality, communication systems and training provision for all persons involved.

The process of incorporating animals as a therapeutic approach for the development, treatment and rehabilitation of people is still in its infancy. Subject to precautions on hygiene, there may be significant health advantages from owning pets. Pharmacists are likely to be an even more important source of pet-care information and advice in the future, given this apparently important link with healthcare.

Disadvantages of keeping pets

Pets can create special health problems for humans. Dogs and cats live in close proximity to their owners and can transmit diseases (e.g. echinococcosis and toxoplasmosis). Even greater danger is associated with exotic pets (e.g. parrots and monkeys) that may harbour potentially fatal infections (e.g. ornithosis and herpes infections). New lifestyles sometimes create special hazards. Both agricultural and urban developments may encroach into previously fallow ground, where new contacts may be made with wildlife that can be a reservoir of infection: plague and various types of viral encephalitis are examples.

Simple advice on hygiene (e.g. recommending pet owners to wash their hands after touching animals and explaining how they can guard against risks from ecto- or endoparasites) may be appropriate. Pet-associated diseases are also contracted through bites, scratches and, with birds, as a result of inhaling feathers. Ensuring that animals do not sleep on or near people's beds can reduce allergic reactions from cat and dog hair. There are similar potential dangers associated with farm animals. The risks from keeping pets are summarised in Box 11.1.

Box 11.1 Risks associated with keeping pets.

Non-infectious disease may be caused by:

- contact with animal secretions
- direct contact with the animal
- exposure to ectoparasites.

Infectious zooonotic disease may be transmitted directly by:

- animal bites
- anthropod vectors (especially fleas, mosquitoes and ticks)
- physical contact with animals.

Infections can also be contracted indirectly by:

- contact with contaminated hides, wool, fur or feathers
- environmental contamination
- ingestion of contaminated food.

People may be injured by:

- behavioural and psychological influences
- direct contact with toxic secretions and venoms
- falling off horses
- involuntary contact or bites
- tripping over small pets.

Conditions associated with ectoparasites

Control of fleas and other related ectoparasites is important. Apart from a direct effect on human health, they can act as vectors in transmitting disease, thus also posing a zoonotic risk (e.g. cat, dog and human fleas, and lice can all act as intermediate hosts for the tapeworm; ticks are implicated in the spread of Lyme disease). The European rabbit flea can cause myxomatosis; in Asia, the Oriental rat flea causes bubonic plague.

Fleas

There are about 2000 species of flea in existence worldwide. They are wingless, with laterally compressed bodies from 1.5 to 4 mm in length. The thick and chitinous covering is dark brown; some species have large or simple eyes. The long legs are strong and adapted to leaping: the flea can jump more than 100 times its own body length. Cat and dog fleas (*Ctenocephalides felis* and *C. canis*) are even more impressive, being able to execute a leap from standing of up to 33 cm.

More than one species of flea may be present on an animal. These variants are not identical in habit, action or antigen. At any one time, *C. felis*, *C. canis* or *Pulex irritans* (the human flea) may be dominant on a dog. Studies have shown that *C. felis* is most common on dogs in London and Denmark; *C. canis* is more prevalent in Dublin. A study of dogs in the London area in 1995 (Kayne, 1995) found that almost half were infested mostly with the cat flea, double the number found in a similar survey in 1981. Cat fleas on cats had increased from 56 to 63% over the same period. Cat fleas are much less specific than dog fleas, but tend to be the only species found on cats. Both cats and dogs pick up fleas from rabbits, hedgehogs and squirrels, but these are host-specific and do not remain on the animal for long.

Adult fleas must obtain a blood meal to become sexually mature and reproduce. At the anterior end of their body, fleas have two pairs of palps to feel the skin surface and two lance-like blades bearing rows of 'teeth' with which they can puncture the skin. Once punctured, saliva is injected to prevent blood clotting, and it is this saliva that causes hypersensitivity in animals.

The female flea lays up to 20 eggs at one time and 400–500 eggs over a lifetime. The oval glistening ova are about 0.5 mm in length and pearly white in colour; they are dropped in dust or dirt, or deposited directly on the host. As the eggs are not sticky, they soon drop off the host.

The rate of development varies greatly, and depends on an ambient humidity and temperature. The creamy-yellow coloured larvae may hatch in two to 16 days. The main source of dried blood that is necessary for larval development are the adult parasites' faeces, often present on pets' bedding. In fact, over 99% of fleas live in the bedding and other soft furnishings around the house. Comfortable furnishings, increased living temperatures and draught-free conditions in modern houses offer suitable conditions for the development of virulent strains. There is evidence that some fleas are developing increasing resistance to the common organophosphate anti-flea preparations. Even non-pet owning households can become infected as a result of people unwittingly transferring the insect's eggs after patting a neighbour's pet. Fleas may also be obtained from hedgehogs, except in New Zealand, where the species there is parasite-free.

Fleas can cause a range of allergies and skin conditions (including eczema) in humans. When infestation gets out of control, hungry fleas may even bite pet owners. Further, fleas can often act as intermediaries in endoparasitic life-cycles, facilitating the transfer of worm infestation between animals. The most usual clinical signs for the presence of fleas include:

- alopecia
- bloody inflammation and other skin conditions brought on by hypersensitivity to the flea saliva during warm weather and the animal's response
- excessive grooming
- pruritis
- scratching
- visual evidence (e.g. fleas and flea faeces in the fur).

Pet owners who seek advice from pharmacists about flea infestation should be advised that cats act as a greater source of infection than dogs. In some cases, a cat living in the same household as a dog may provide a reservoir of fleas for the latter, but is apparently unaffected itself.

Animals should be treated according to the instructions on the product chosen. To obtain effective flea control, an animal and its surroundings must be treated. Careful attention should be given to an animal's bedding, which may need to be destroyed to prevent reinfestation.

Initially, the animal should be washed with an insecticidal shampoo to kill fleas and clean up the animal's hair coat. A topical agent should then be applied. Sprays are the most popular form, probably due to the ease of use; powders are the second preference of animal owners. Flea collars are useful, but, whilst providing insecticidal protection, they can invoke an allergic reaction due to continual contact with the skin. The ingredients are mainly based on pyrethrum and permethrin, although there are also some 'natural' products (e.g. oil of citronella and oil of lime). Care must be taken to avoid toxicity with nursing bitches. Most owners recognise the importance of minimising the risk of transfer of diseases between animals. As a result, insecticidal products have become very popular, and a wide range of different formulations are available, including some herbal varieties.

Some of the more common topical anti-flea products, which are widely available from UK pharmaceutical wholesalers, are listed in Table

Table 11.1 Selection of cat and dog flea products available generally from pharmaceutical wholesalers

Product	Animal	Brand
Flea powders and sprays		
Flea powder	Cats and dogs	Bob Martin
Flea killing powder – natural	Cats and dogs	Bob Martin
Flea powder	Dogs	Johnson's Veterinary
Flea and tick powder – permethrin	Dogs	Johnson's Veterinary
Permethrin flea powder	Cats and dogs	Sherley's
Flea spray	Dogs	Bob Martin
Flea control kit	Cats and dogs[a]	Secto
Vetzyme and Kitzyme flea sprays and powders	Cats and dogs	Seven Seas Vet
Big Red Flea Spray	Cats and dogs	Sherley's
Flea collars		
Flea collars	Cats and dogs[a]	Bob Martin
Natural flea collars	Cats and dogs	Bob Martin
Flea collar	Cats	Johnson's Veterinary
Flea and tick collar	Dogs	Johnson's Veterinary
Herbal flea collars	Cats and dogs[a]	Johnson's Veterinary
Herbal flea collar	Cats and puppies[a]	Secto
Reflective flea collar	Cats	Vetzyme
Vetzyme and Kitzyme flea collars	Cats and dogs	Seven Seas Vet
Flea collar	Cats and dogs[a]	Sherley's
Pour on and solutions		
Flea and tick spot on	Large and small dogs[a]	Bob Martin
Flea spot on	Cats	Bob Martin
Flea and tick solution	Cats and dogs	Bob Martin
Herbal flea drops	Cats and dogs	Johnson's Veterinary
Flea repellents		
Flea repellent – natural	Small cats and dogs	Bob Martin
Flea repellent spray (citrus)	Cats and dogs	Johnson's Veterinary
Flea repellent shampoo	Cats and dogs[a]	Johnson's Veterinary

[a] Separate versions available

11.1. Other products are available from specialist suppliers.

Cyflea tablets are a systemic treatment for cats and dogs over three months of age. The treatment is restricted to veterinary prescription, and works when the flea bites the animal and ingests the medication whilst sucking for blood. It is a useful treatment where resistant strains of fleas do not respond to topical treatments.

Household furnishings should be treated as if they are suspected of being infested. The following can act as a framework:

- thoroughly vacuum the house with a new dust bag in place, ensuring complete disposal afterwards. Concentrate on those areas where fleas and photophobic larvae are known to hide (e.g. dusty corners, under furniture and between sofa cushions)
- if necessary, wash carpets. This will raise the carpet's pile, facilitating more complete penetration of the insecticidal product
- apply a suitable anti-flea spray to all floors, carpets, and indoor rugs
- do not vacuum the house for at least seven to

ten days after application of the insecticidal product
- repeat the procedure twice, at two-weekly intervals; subsequent once-monthly application should be continued for as long as necessary
- repeat the procedure more frequently in warm weather, and alternate products to prevent resistance developing
- if severe infestation is present, it may be necessary to obtain help from local Environmental Health Safety Officers.

A sample of suitable environmental products is given in Table 11.2.

Table 11.2 Selection of environmental flea products available from most main line pharmaceutical wholesalers

Product	Brand
Household flea powder and sprays	Bob Martin
Household flea spray	Johnson's Veterinary
Home fleaguard and spray	Johnson's Veterinary
Defest flea spray	Sherley's
Flego household flea spray	Sherley's

Lice

These small wingless insects lay eggs on the host body and these become glued to a hair or feather. The emergent louse is a miniature form of the adult. They are generally host specific, so cannot live for longer than a few days if transferred to humans. Nevertheless, their appearance can cause considerable anxiety and requests for help from pharmacy staff in whispered tones.

Two distinct families of louse exist on domestic animals. The *Siphunculata* have compressed heads and strong claws with pointed sucking mouth parts. The *Mallophaga* have mouth parts that comprise a set of mandibles to facilitate biting. Symptoms include skin conditions and allergic responses. Important species in the cat and dog include a sucking louse (*Linognathus setosus*) and a biting louse (*Trichodectes canis*). The latter acts as an intermediary in the life-cycle of *Dipylidium caninum*, the canine tapeworm. Treatment is by application of a suitable insecticide and associated procedures.

Mites

The canine strain of the mite *Sarcoptes scabei* causes the highly contagious sarcoptic mange, characterised by scaling, crust formation and hair loss. It is extremely uncomfortable and stressful for the infested animal. The mite may be transferred to humans, causing scabies. *Notoedres cati* from the cat and *S. equi* from the horse can occasionally affect humans too. The latter case has been termed 'Cavalryman's itch'.

In humans, the disease usually appears on the skin between the fingers, in the groin or below the breasts, but it may spread to other sites (Chakrabarti, 1985). Eggs deposited in the epidermis hatch after three to four days and the resultant larvae provoke an intense irritation.

Treatment is with topical benzyl benzoate, benzyl hexachloride or monosulfiram. Animals are first treated with organophosphate lotions, sprays or dips, and benzyl benzoate applied. It is advisable to treat the animal's living environment.

Ticks

Ticks may be seen on dogs that have visited commercial kennels or have been exercised in rural settings. They are subject to infestation with dog ticks (*Ixodes canisuga*) and hedgehog ticks (*I. hexagonus*). Treatment usually involves physical removal and application of an organophosphate ascaricide.

The reaction to tick bites is similar to other ectoparasites. For ticks' involvement in Lyme disease, *see below*.

Non-infective conditions

Allergies

Allergic symptoms resulting from contact with cat and dog dander or bird feathers can range from acute rhinitis and lachrymation to urticarial skin eruptions. Domestic cats in particular are implicated in childhood allergies. A contact dermatitis may erupt in some owners after contact with commercially available flea collars, especially if the collars are wet. Allergic symptoms may prove difficult to treat because of the continuing presence of the stimulus. It is not unusual for owners to self-medicate with antihistamines and then allow the family pet to sleep on their bed at night! Getting people to change this habit can be extremely difficult.

In a study on the consequences of lifestyle on health, 341 adults who had been diagnosed as being allergic to dogs or cats (mean age 38.4 years) were recruited (Coren, 1997). Each recruit had been specifically advised by their doctor to stop sharing their living quarters with their pets, but only 21% had complied. Such low compliance might be expected because of the large human emotional investment in a pet. It was even more interesting that, for a subset of 122 of these people, the allergy had been diagnosed sufficiently long ago that the animal they were living with at the time had died. In this group, 70% had replaced the deceased animal with a new dog or cat, despite the presence of allergies. Thus, some people consider pet ownership to be sufficiently important to warrant ignoring chronic allergy symptoms and medical advice.

Treatment is normally with oral and/or topical antihistamine preparations. Isopathy, in which a sample of the animal's hair is made into a homoeopathic dilution, has also been used orally with some success. Extrinsic allergic alveolitis (bird breeder's lung or pigeon fancier's lung) is a disease caused by the inhalation of antigens found in avian droppings. It is characterised by systemic and pulmonary symptoms of cough, dyspnoea and restrictive lung disease. A similar condition (farmer's lung) has also been described, whose the symptoms usually appear four to six hours after exposure. Diagnosis is with the aid of immunological tests.

Tarantulas are becoming increasingly popular as pets, and ocular injury resulting from them has been reported. Tarantulas are widely available, easily maintained and considered harmless, as many are non-venomous. Unfortunately, the popular American varieties have evolved highly urticarious hairs to leave on their webs and flick at predators. There is evidence to support the theory that the transfer from spider to human hands and then eyes may result in serious ocular inflammation. People who handle Chilean rose tarantulas regularly should wear gloves, avoid rubbing the eyes during handling and thoroughly wash their hands to minimise the transfer of hairs.

Behavioural influences

Some people may inadvertently acquire pets that cannot be easily accommodated at home. To form a bond with a puppy and then have to find it a new home can be extremely traumatic, affecting an owner's health and quality of life.

The death (or loss) of a companion animal can also greatly affect the owner, causing a profound sense of bereavement. Requests for assistance in the pharmacy could include advice on obtaining a new pet or (in severe cases) medical referral. Communicating with an owner whose animal has a chronic illness may be even more difficult.

Cancer

There have been suggestions that keeping pet birds increases the risk of lung cancer. A number of studies in the Netherlands, Germany, Sweden and Scotland have attempted to demonstrate a correlation between lung cancer and keeping pet birds, but more work is required to confirm the findings. There is some circumstantial evidence that pigeons may be implicated, but the keeping of budgerigars, canaries and parrots does not seem to constitute an appreciable risk (Britton and Lewis, 1997).

Physical injuries

In a Swedish study, almost half of human injuries that required hospital treatment and were caused by animals were due to dogs. Horses accounted for about a third of injuries and the highest number of fractures. Cats are also implicated in causing injury in the UK. When either humans or pets are injured, it is important that prompt first aid is administered. A recent case established that owners are legally responsible for their pets' actions with respect to other pets. Proper control must therefore be maintained at all times, particularly with large, powerful dogs. Appropriate immunisation should be considered if the skin is broken.

For the consequences of bites and scratches, *see* Bacterial infections *below*.

Toxins and venoms

People who purchase reptiles, spiders and other exotic pets may be at risk from toxic secretions or venoms. In such cases, owners should ascertain where treatment would be available should an accident occur. In practice, most venomous attacks are no worse than a bee sting, and a pair of sturdy gloves would offer adequate protection.

Infective conditions: zoonoses

Zoonoses are infectious animal-associated diseases that may be transmitted to humans from vertebrate animals by bites, scratches, injection of saliva from ectoparasites and inhalation of airborne agents and direct contact. The definition includes human diseases acquired from animals and those produced by non-infective agents (e.g. toxins and poisons). Strictly speaking, the definition excludes ecto-parasites, which act as intermediate hosts and can both transmit zoonotic diseases and cause them from allergic reactions or bites.

The interaction of agent, host and the external environment determines the degree of susceptibility of the host to infection and subsequent development of the disease. Carrier hosts and asymptomatic infected individuals are important in the persistence of many zoonotic agents. The infecting agent persists in nature (zoonotic reservoirs) in vertebrate animals.

Classification

By life-cycle complexity

The agents may be transmitted either directly (a simple life-cycle) or indirectly by intermediate vectors or environmental contamination (a complex life-cycle). The surrounding environment may be the reservoir of some diseases that may be shared by several animals and humans (e.g. soil is the reservoir for mycoses and mycobacterioses; water supports free-living pathogenic amoebae).

By type of life-cycle

Within this simple/complex life-cycle description, there is a classification based on the type of life-cycle of the infecting organism. It divides the zoonose into four categories, each with important shared epidemiological features of clinical importance:

- direct zoonoses, which are transmitted from an infected to a susceptible vertebrate host by direct contact, and undergo little or no propagative changes
- cyclozoonoses require more than one vertebrate host species in order to complete the development cycle of the infective agent
- metazoonoses are transmitted biologically by invertebrate vectors in which they develop or multiply
- saprozoonoses have both vertebrate hosts and a non-animal development site or reservoir (including soil and water).

By type of causative organism

Another system of classification refers to the causative organism (e.g. bacterium, fungus, protozoa and virus). This classification is used in this chapter.

Factors affecting the emergence of zoonoses

Many elements can contribute to the emergence of a new zoonotic disease (Hugh-Jones *et al.*, 1995):

- microbial/viral determinants (e.g. mutation, natural selection and evolutionary progression)
- individual host determinants (e.g. acquired immunity and physiological factors)
- host population determinants (e.g. host behavioural characteristics and societal, transport, commercial and iatrogenic factors)
- environmental determinants (e.g. ecological and climatic influences).

Emergence of new zoonotic pathogens seems to be accelerating for several reasons, including the following:

- global populations of humans and animals have continued to grow, bringing increasingly larger numbers of people and animals into close contact
- transportation has advanced, making it possible to circumnavigate the globe in less than the incubation period of most infectious agents
- ecological and environmental changes brought about by human activity are massive.

Mode of transmission of zoonoses

Direct transmission involves spread of the infective agent by direct contact with the infected animal. This may occur by:

- a bite or scratch
- a spray of infected urine
- inhalation of discharged respiratory droplets from coughing or sneezing
- contact with infectious reproductive discharges.

Indirect transmission involves an intermediate vector:

- transmission by a flea, mite, mosquito, sand fly or tick
- transmission through environmental contamination
- airborne spread (e.g. droplets or dust)
- food-borne disease (especially foods of animal origin).

Transmission of infective agents directly or indirectly to another susceptible individual of the same generation is said to be horizontal transmission. When transmission occurs from one generation to the next, either prenatally in utero or neonatally via collostrum, it is called vertical transmission. Prenatal toxoplasmosis is a serious disease of human infants.

Exposure to zoonoses

Various methods exist to classify how people may be at risk of exposure to zoonotic agents. One method is illustrated in Table 11.3.

Another method relates to epidemiological factors. In examining the causal factors of potential zoonotic disease, the following risk factors have been identified:

- residence in a pet-owning household theoretically represents the most intimate and prolonged contact many people have with animals. However, some zoonoses can be transmitted without prolonged contact (e.g. rabies) or even without direct contact with the animal (e.g. toxicariasis). People may also interact with pets belonging to relatives or neighbours, and with strays, thus demonstrating that residence in a pet-owning household is not the only factor. Furthermore, residence in a pet-owning household does not necessarily imply intimate or prolonged contact for every family member
- exposure to diseased animals (some investigators have identified a link between human illness and sick animals)
- exposure to a specific animal pathogen
- exposure resulting from a bite wound
- exposure as the result of membership of a high-risk group (e.g. veterinarians, farmers and farm workers)
- residence in a country with large numbers of animals. In some ecological studies, rates of human disease have been correlated with the population densities of particular species in each country.

Table 11.3 Classification of people at risk of zoonotic infection

Grouping	People involved
Group 1 – Agriculture	Farmers, farm workers
Group 2 – Animal product processing	Personnel from abattoirs and food processing facilities
Group 3 – Forestry	Persons visiting wilderness areas
Group 4 – Recreation	Persons in contact with pets or wild animals in an urban environment
Group 5 – Clinics and laboratories	Health care and laboratory personnel working with infected material
Group 6 – Epidemiology	Public health professionals and field researchers
Group 7 – Emergency	People involved in disasters, refugees and people living in crowded, stressful situations

Principles of prevention and control of zoonoses

Prevention and control are sometimes referred to as 'primary prevention' (preventing the occurrence of disease) and 'secondary prevention' (damage limitation after a disease has already occurred). Rehabilitation after the failure of primary and secondary prevention has been called 'tertiary prevention'. The methods for prevention and control of zoonoses include the following:

- neutralising the reservoir of infection, by isolating infected individuals from the healthy population, treating infected individuals to reduce the risk of transmission (this could involve slaughter of animals if treatment is ineffective, impracticable or too costly) or 'cleaning up' the environment in which the animal lives
- reducing the potential for contact with the reservoir (e.g. by isolation) through strict quarantine regulations (e.g. for rabies) or by more drastic population control methods (e.g. reducing the number of stray dogs and cats on the streets)
- increasing host resistance. In veterinary medicine, genetic selection favouring resistance, and reducing stress by improved nutrition or better shelter are routine procedures that ensure increased resistance to disease. Chemoprophylaxis and immunisation are other important measures
- public health protection. Two major weapons against zoonotic disease are prophylactic immunisation (when available) and education. Simple measures (e.g. maintaining personal hygiene, washing hands or wearing protective clothing) can reduce the possibility of disease transmission
- health reporting procedures. These involve passive reporting of disease clusters and active surveillance to identify areas of potential danger.

Examples of the most frequently encountered pet zoonoses

Bacterial infections

The risk of bacterial infection following a bite is high. Infected cat and dog bites have a complex microbiological mix (Talan, 1999). The normal oral flora of dogs includes *Pasteurella multocida*, which is found in almost half the wounds from dog bites, and *Eikenella corrodens*, found in gingival plaque. Two other bacteria, *Capnocytophage canimorsus* and *C. cynoodegmi*, are also found in canine oral flora. In immunosuppressed people, these bacteria can cause severe disease. Other bacteria commonly isolated in dog bite wounds include various species of *Pseudomonas*, *Actinobacillus*, *Streptococci*, *Staphylococci* and *Corynebacterium*.

A bite wound that becomes infected with *Clostridium tetani* may lead to tetanus, but this is relatively unusual. Cats also have a number of organisms potentially harmful to humans.

Because of the rich array of flora in animals' mouths, bites should be treated promptly, cleaned and stitched if necessary. Anti-tetanus and antibiotic treatment should be considered.

Campylobacter jejuni has been known to cause severe disease in animals for more than 70 years, but it is only comparatively recently that modern culture methods have facilitated more intense study. Its main reservoir is probably wild birds, in which it forms part of the normal faecal flora. Domestic animals and poultry may carry the organism for long periods without any symptoms. Surveys carried out in the 1980s showed that around 50% of dogs and cats carry the bacterium. Highest isolation rates are found in animals with diarrhoea. Infection acquired by humans in the home is confined mainly to close contact with a sick puppy and, occasionally, a kitten or caged bird. Most infections are self-limiting and cause abdominal pain and diarrhoea for two to three days. Treatment for humans is fluid replacement, to prevent dehydration and possibly erythromycin.

Prevention of infection is effected by prompt disposal of excreta from sick persons and disinfection of contaminated areas. Keeping pets out of the kitchen and dining areas and frequent handwashing are also important measures, as *C. jejuni* is also acquired by ingesting contaminated raw milk, undercooked chicken or other food contaminated in the kitchen. Recent indications show that the incidence of *Campylobacter* infection is rising, taking over from *Salmonella* as the new food-poisoning villain.

Leptospirosis, or Weil's disease, is a sporadic bacterial disease transmitted by contact with infected urine. The causative agents are *Leptospira* spp., of which there are over 170. Dogs are the main reservoir for *L. interogans canicola*. Some canine infections are sub-clinical; in others, fever, anorexia, vomiting and haemoglobinuria occur. The organism is excreted in the urine and this may continue for many months. Transmission to humans occurs by contact with infected urine or blood, or by exposure to a contaminated environment. After an incubation period of approximately ten days, headache, malaise, myalgia and fever occur. Treatment with high doses of antibiotic (usually penicillin) is effective if given early. Clinical infection in dogs is minimised by the administration of leptospira vaccine, but sub-clinical infection with excretion of leptospires may still occur. Humans should avoid contact with dog urine.

Other zoonotic variants of the bacterium include *L. hardjo* (occurring in cattle) and *L. icterohaemorrhagiae* (in rats). Human leptospirosis is most often seen as an occupational hazard of farmers due to their contact with both these species.

Salmonella infections are chiefly acquired through food-borne sources, but can also be transmitted directly by animals. Many birds, mammals and reptiles harbour *Salmonella* spp. in the gastro-intestinal tract, either as pathogens or as part of the normal flora. Common pets that can serve as reservoirs for the micro-organism include tortoises, turtles, chickens, cats and dogs. The infection is usually characterised by a self-limiting gastro-enteritis, with watery stools that may contain mucus and blood. The acute illness subsides within 24 hours and treatment involves electrolytes and possibly antibiotics.

An unusual pet, the African pygmy hedgehog, has recently made an appearance in Canada. Not only is stroking the animal's spikes unlikely to calm the owner's frazzled nerves, but the hedgehog may also be a source of *Salmonella*. Confirmed laboratory reports have indicated a link between the animal and infection with the bacterium. Salmonellal infection associated with keeping terrapins and tortoises has been reported. Observing strict hygiene would probably prevent such transmission.

Yersinia species are found in wild rodents, birds and pigs. Healthy dogs and cats have also been found to be carriers, and are probably the main source of transmission of human infection. Food-borne infection from unpasteurised milk, cheese, raw pork and water have been reported, and person-to-person spread seems possible. Symptoms include fever, abdominal pain and diarrhoea for one to three weeks; pharyngitis is another common symptom. The overall clinical picture may resemble appendicitis with abdominal pain. The condition is usually self-limiting, but antibiotics may be indicated.

Endoparasitic infection

Endoparasitic infection in farm animals (cattle, sheep and pigs) has important welfare implications and can lead to economic loss. In the companion animal, public health issues are also involved. Worm species are usually specific to an animal species, and many different species can infest one animal at the same time. There are three main groups:

- roundworms or nematodes
- tapeworms or cestodes
- flukes or trematodes.

Roundworms and tapeworms are the most important in dogs and cats, and pose a zoonotic risk to man. Roundworms occur most commonly in pups or kittens, through pre- and post-natal infections. Tapeworms are usually acquired in later life.

Roundworms

Roundworms have a direct life-cycle, with a free-living development phase in the animal environment, a parasitic development phase and an adult phase in the host. Infection of the host group generally occurs by ingestion of the larval stage of the parasite. A typical round worm life-cycle is illustrated in Figure 11.1.

Strongyloidiasis

This is a chronic roundworm infection transmitted by direct contact with faeces. The causative agents are *Strongyloides stercoralis cata* (affecting dogs) and *S. fuellebotni* (affecting non-human primates). The helminth is usually sited in the duodenum, from where eggs are shed in the faeces and develop into larvae.

Young dogs have thin skins that allow large quantities of larvae to penetrate. Humans are also infected by penetration of larvae. On entering the body, they migrate to the lungs and gastro-intestinal tract. Symptoms include skin inflammation and pruritis at the site of entry, followed by bronchial symptoms, fever, diarrhoea and abdominal pain. In animals, severe dermatitis, accompanied by coughing and vomiting, is often present. Both humans and animals may be treated with thiabendazole or its more recent derivatives.

Toxocariasis

There are several Orders of roundworm, but the one that concerns the domestic animal most is from the Order Ascaridida. Ascarids are amongst the largest and most common of nematodes, and the adults are host-specific: *Toxocara canis* infects dogs, *Toxocara cati* infects cats and *Parascaris equorum* affects horses. *Ascaris suum*, specific to pigs, is considered only occasionally to be a zoonose. Dogs and cats also share a second ascarid, *Toxoscaris leonia*. *Toxocara cati* has a similar life-cycle to *T. canis*, but is rarely involved in human disease.

Over 80% of puppies under one year old are thought to be infected with *T. canis*. Most infection is acquired pre-natally from the mother; some are infected through maternal milk. About 2% of the UK's total human population and 15% of dog breeders are thought to be seropositive.

Effective control of *T. canis* depends upon a proper understanding of its highly complex life-cycle. Eggs excreted in faeces (up to 15 000 eggs/g puppy faeces) enter the animal following a period of maturation in the soil. Survival of the eggs depends upon weather conditions. Dry conditions cause dessication; in moist humid climates, however, the eggs can remain viable for several years. After becoming infective (usually within about two to six weeks) and their ingestion, the eggs hatch in the small intestine. In puppies less than five weeks old, second stage larvae penetrate the intestine wall to enter the blood vessels, migrating through the liver, lungs,

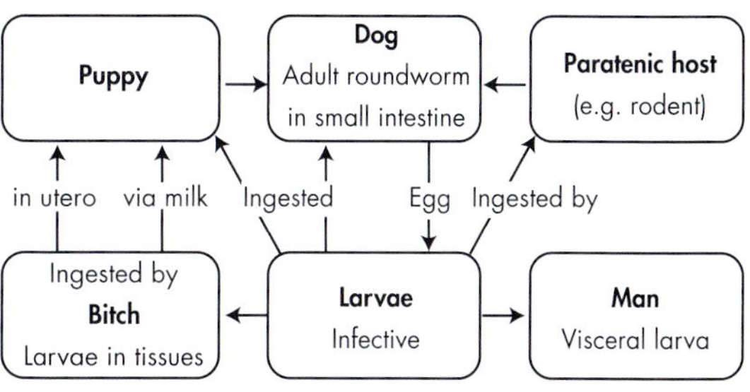

Figure 11.1 Roundworm life-cycle in the dog.

and kidneys to the trachea, where a third larval stage develops. These can be coughed up and swallowed, returning to the small intestine and stomach. The adult parasite then develops in the intestine three to six weeks after ingestion of the eggs. Any larvae excreted by the puppies may mature in the bitch once ingested. Figure 11.1 shows a representation of the Toxocara life-cycle in dogs.

In older dogs, the development ceases at the second stage larvae and these larvae undergo somatic migration into the tissues, where they persist for long periods. The dormant larvae reactivate during pregnancy, possibly due to hormonal changes, and migrate to the placenta to mature in the unborn puppies. Perinatal transmission appears to be highly efficient, as almost all puppies are infected by the time of whelping.

Although puppies and nursing bitches are an important source of human infection, a more significant public health risk comes from embryonated Toxocara eggs in the soil. Freshly voided faeces are not a problem because the eggs need 14 to 21 days under optimal conditions to become infective. The animals may develop substantial worm burdens and pass large numbers of eggs in their faeces, leading to heavy contamination, especially in densely populated urban areas where dog owners walk their pets in public areas. In the UK, a quarter of soil samples have been shown to contain eggs of *T. canis*. In central USA, 16% of samples were positive. Humans are infected when eggs from contaminated soil and grass are ingested.

Toxocara cati is the most common roundworm of cats. It has a wide geographical distribution, and adult forms have been recorded in man. The life-cycle of *T. cati* is similar to that of *T. canis*, except there is no placental transfer of larvae. Although there is less chance of human infection from cat worms compared with those from dogs, the habit of cats burying their faeces can cause children to acquire infections from contaminated soil; sandpits may also be a source of infection. Figure 11.2 depicts the Toxocara life-cycle in cats.

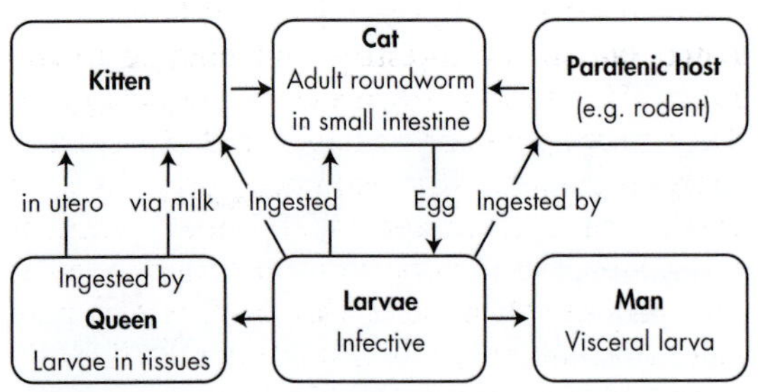

Figure 11.2 Roundworm life-cycle in the cat.

Infection is frequently sub-clinical. The disease has two forms: visceral larva migrans (VLM) affects children of one to four years of age, who develop fever, asthmatic attacks, acute bronchiolitis, nausea and vomiting, and enlarged liver and spleen; sometimes the heart and CNS become involved. Second stage larvae migrate through the tissues and typically present in a young child with a history of pica. The second form, ocular larva migrans (OLM), affects older children and, occasionally, adults. Granulomatous nodules develop in the eye, causing severe ocular inflammation and loss of vision.

Confirmation of the infection is with an enzyme-linked immunosorbent assay (ELISA).

The UK Pet Council have stressed that there are only about two new cases of illness annually due to Toxocara per million of population. There is evidence that people can take active steps to minimise the risk of contracting toxocariasis by regular worming of their pets and 'pooper scooping'. The most recent studies on soil in parks show lower levels of Toxocara eggs than previously recorded; and a study conducted through the University of Glasgow's Department of Parasitology, in co-operation with Canine Control Scotland, found considerably reduced incidence of *T. canis* than in previous studies.

Most infections are self-limiting due to the host inflammatory response, which kills many larvae. Products containing diethylcarbamazine and thiabendazole are effective as treatment. Corticosteroids may be used to control allergic symptoms, especially in the eye. Guidelines for the control and prevention of the disease are:

- routine worming of both young and adult animals (*see below*)
- remove and destroy all voided faeces ('pooper-scooping')
- train dogs to defecate in gutters or on ground not used by children

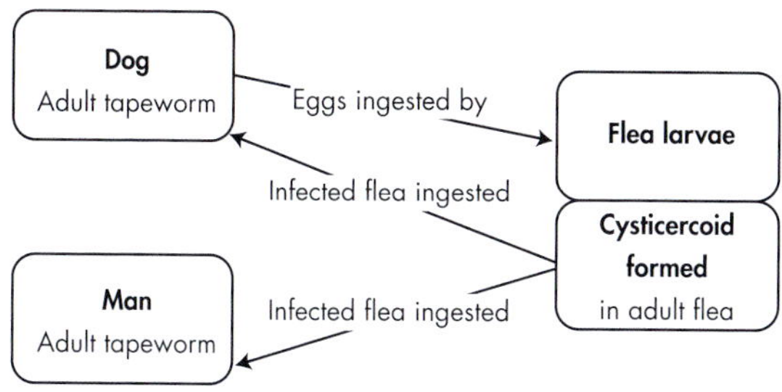

Figure 11.3 Tapeworm life-cycle in the dog.

- wash hands after handling animals and before eating food
- do not allow nursing bitches to lick children's faces and hands.

Tapeworms

Tapeworms are most numerous in the adult species of dogs and cats, with about 10% of animals being infected. Tapeworms require a two-host system: the developmental stages occur in the intermediate host; final development and adult stages occur in the definitive host. Infection is by ingestion, and transmission relates to the carnivorous eating habits of dogs and cats; rabbits, mice, birds and large herbivores (cattle and sheep) provide for completion of the life-cycle. The main vector is the flea, especially in the urban family pet. The main tapeworms in the UK are *Dipylidium caninum* and *Echinococcus granulosus*. A typical tapeworm life-cycle is illustrated in Figure 11.3.

Dipylidiasis

Cats and dogs are the definitive hosts for the infective organism of this disease. The intermediate hosts are the fleas, *Ctenocephalides canis* and *C. felis*. Gravid proglottids, the first stage of a complex life-cycle, are passed in the pet faeces. This permits release of the eggs into the environment, which are ingested by fleas and lice. Infection of cats and dogs is caused by ingestion of the ectoparasites in which cysticercoids have developed; these further develop into adult worms in the cat or dog gut. Accidental human ingestion of fleas infected with *Dipylidium caninum* results in the appearance of diarrhoea and abdominal pain; there may also be anal itching, and there is the characteristic appearance of melon-shaped proglottids in faeces. Children are most frequently affected.

Prevention is by control of fleas on the animal and regular worming. Treatment of humans is with niclosamide and praziquantel.

Echinococcosis (hydatid disease)

Infection is usually caused by the cystic larval form of *Echinococcus granulosus*, the canine tapeworm. Depending on the intermediate host, the bacterium is further differentiated into *E. granulosus granulosus* (sheep and cattle) and *E. granulosus equines* (horses). Other echinococcal species (e.g. *E. multilocularis*, *E. oligarthus* and *E. vogeli*) are restricted to certain geographical regions.

E. granulosus is present throughout most of the world in communities where man, grazing animals and carnivores live in close association; two exceptions are Iceland and Ireland. It is endemic in mid- and south Wales, where the proportion of infected sheep is 37% and 15% respectively and sheep dogs 26% and 12% respectively. In the Western Isles of Scotland, studies have shown that 20% of sheep and 12% dogs are affected.

E. granulosus is a cestode of 3–9 mm in length with three or four proglottides. The terminal segment becomes gravid, and is the broadest and longest. Adult worms may be found in the intestines of dogs, foxes, dingo and wolf as a result of eating raw offal.

Adult tapeworms shed eggs that pass in the faeces of the primary host, often a sheepdog, about six weeks after infection. Ungulates and humans are infected from these faeces by ingestion of eggs that contaminate the environment, dog hairs or growing vegetables. The larval forms hatch out in the intestine and migrate to the lungs, liver or other organs via the bloodstream. The embryo grows into a large vesicle 5–10 cm or more in diameter (the echinococcus or hydatid cyst). The cyst comprises an inner germinal layer, which may burst to form daughter cysts, and an outer laminated cyst wall, which may calcify. Eventually, this will interfere with body function. If it ruptures suddenly, instantaneous death can occur or further cysts may develop.

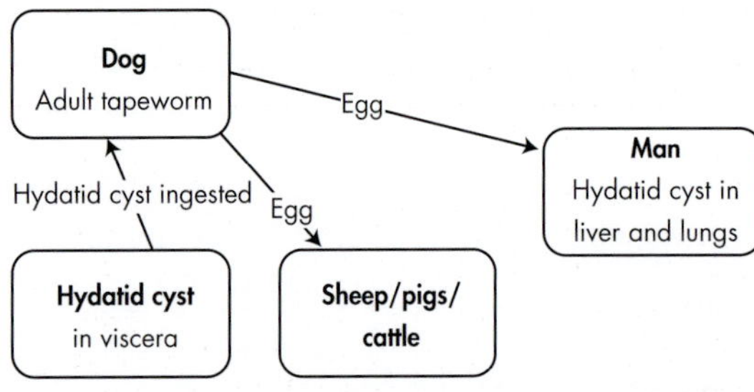

Figure 11.4 Hydatid life-cycle.

The majority of infected humans are more than 25 years of age.

E. granulosus equines infection is common in hunt kennels throughout the UK, but seems to be of low human pathogenicity for hydatid disease.

Apart from the risk to humans, hydatidosis causes condemnation of offal, especially liver and lungs, resulting in financial loss to the meat industry.

The life-cycle of the Hydatid cyst is illustrated in Figure 11.4.

Symptoms in humans depend on the site of the cyst and its pressure on surrounding tissues. Commonly, liver cysts cause abdominal pain and sometimes jaundice. Lung cysts cause chest pain, cough and secondary infection.

The cysts are surgically removed in humans, although mebendazole and albendazole may be useful. Control begins with education of farmers, and their families and workers, on the maintenance of strict hygiene. Several other measures are possible:

- routine worming every three months to prevent infection of pastures by tapeworm eggs
- denial of access by dogs to infected offal
- burning or burying of carcasses, although this may not be possible for hill farmers in winter months.

Worming procedures for cats and dogs

Anthelmintics can be used to eliminate adult parasites from the intestine or to kill larvae in the tissues and break the life-cycle. As with flea products, the list of anthelmintics includes those brands most usually available from pharmaceutical wholesalers (Table 11.4).

In roundworm infection, piperazine is usually the drug of choice: it is well tolerated by dogs and cats and can be given to young animals, either over a period of five days or as a single dose. Adult worms in lactating bitches and puppies are central to the parasite's life-cycle. Therefore, an effective control measure is to treat lactating bitches, and then the puppies until three months of age, to eliminate the successive waves of prenatal transmission, transmammary transfer of larvae and the ingestion of infective puppy faeces. The bitch is wormed from day 45 to 50 of pregnancy through to day 21 after whelping with high daily doses of a broad-spectrum preparation (e.g. fenbenazole, 50 mg/kg or mebendazole). This kills migrating larvae in the bitch and minimises transmission of infection to the puppies. To control infection adequately, puppies should be treated at two, four, eight and twelve weeks of age; adult dogs should be wormed every six months.

Tapeworm infection is often treated with diclorophen, but new drugs are being developed to offer a broader spectrum of activity. Regular dosing at three-monthly intervals is recommended for the treatment of worms in older animals.

Various factors should be considered when recommending appropriate anthelmintics to pet owners (e.g. resistance, spectrum of effectiveness, safety in young animals, dosage form – tablets, granules, powders, pastes or liquids – and cost). For maximal effectiveness in eliminating intestinal worms and preventing excretion of eggs, the correct therapeutic dose of the selected drug should be given at strategic intervals. If uncertainty exists as to which type of helminth exists, or if both are likely to be present, dual-purpose wormers should be used (*see* Table 11.4). When calculating the dose, it is important that the manufacturer's instructions are followed carefully. Doses are usually based on the animal's weight, and pet owners may require help in estimating the size of their animal.

Table 11.4 Selection of cat and dog anthelmintics generally available from pharmaceutical wholesalers

Product	Animal	Brand
Roundworm anthelmintics		
Roundworm tablets	Dogs and puppies (6+ weeks)	Bob Martin
Cats' roundworm tablets	Cats and kittens (6+ weeks)	Bob Martin
Easy wormer – roundworms	Cats and dogs (2+ months)[a]	Johnson's Veterinary
Easy worm syrup	Kittens and puppies	Johnson's Veterinary
Palatable roundworm tablets	Cats and dogs	Johnson's Veterinary
Worming cream and syrup	All	Sherley's
Tapeworm anthelmintics		
Tapeworm tablets	Dogs and puppies (6+ weeks)	Bob Martin
Tibs tapeworm tablets	Cats and kittens (6+ months)	Bob Martin
Easy tapewormer tablets	Cats and dogs[a]	Johnson's Veterinary
Flavoured tapeworm tablets	Cats and dogs	Johnson's Veterinary
Dual anthelmintics		
All-in-one wormer	Dogs, small dogs and puppies[a]	Bob Martin
Dual wormer tablets	Dogs	Bob Martin
Cats' dual wormer tablets	Cats and kittens (6+ months)	Bob Martin
Panacur (granules, liquid, paste, tablets)	All	Hoechst Roussel Vet
Telmin KH	Cats and dogs	Jansson-Cilag
Twin wormer tablets	Cats and dogs[a]	Johnson's Vet
Vetzyme combined wormer	All	Seven Seas Vet
Multiwormer	Cats and dogs and large breeds[a]	Sherley's
One dose wormer	Dogs, small dogs and puppies[a]	Sherley's

[a] Separate versions available

Other types of worms

Other possible, but extremely rare, sources of helminth infection in the UK include the hookworm (*Ancyclostoma caninum* and *A. braziliense*), found in the intestine of cats, dogs and various other carnivores. It is responsible for cutaneous larva migrans (ancylostomiasis). Human infection results from direct skin contact with larvae in areas contaminated with animal faeces. The condition is often asymptomatic, although self-limiting pustular skin eruptions may occur.

Dirofilariasis due to infection with the dog heartworm, *Dirofilaris immitis*, is restricted to warmer climates. If the climate warms in the southern UK, it could occur here in the future. The adult worm resides in the pulmonary artery and the right ventricle of its canine host. Mosquitoes are involved in the life-cycle. Pulmonary symptoms are extremely rare; the disease is usually self-limiting.

Fungal infections

Ringworm

The most common fungal infections transmitted from pets to humans are the dermatophytes, *Trichophyton mentagrophytes, T. verrucosum* and *Microsporum canis*. They cause ringworm, which is a skin disease acquired by contact with infectious humans or animals. The disease occurs worldwide. There are other species – involving human or soil reservoirs of infection.

Trichophyton infection in humans is acquired from horses and cattle; Microsporum is acquired from dogs. Transmission is by direct contact with the infected individual, or indirectly via blankets and brushes. The infective agent may remain for months in dry, cool, shaded environments. Animals act as reservoirs of infection, generating spores that contaminate the environment. Dogs, horses and, especially, cats and kittens are the main sources of infection among pets.

In humans, ring-shaped scaly papules appear on the scalp and spread peripherally, with loss of hair within four to 14 days of infection; eventually, a scaly erythematous plaque develops. In animals, similar lesions to humans appear one to four weeks after infection. Cats infected with *M. canis* present a 'moth-eaten' appearance; lesions on dogs are discrete, circular, crusty areas of alopecia.

The condition is often self-limiting if untreated, but may last up to three months. Oral griseofulvin has been used for many years in association with topical antifungal preparations, on both humans and animals. In animals, the skin is usually brushed before application of natamycin or econazole. This is when zoonotic infection typically occurs in humans.

Control is effected by keeping animals well fed and in sunlight. All grooming tools and equipment should be disinfected with formalin. Direct contact with the animal should be avoided as far as possible.

Histoplasmosis

Although *Histoplasma capsulatum* can be isolated from many different animals, including cats and dogs, zoonotic transmission to humans usually occurs in persons involved in breeding birds. The most commonly implicated pet is the pigeon. The fungal spore is usually spread by inhalation of dust from soil rich in animal faeces. Outbreaks have occurred following soil and dust disturbance during building works.

Symptoms in humans include influenza-like symptoms with cough, headache and muscle pain. With heavy infection, breathing difficulties can develop. Clinical disease is treated with amphotericin B. Exposure to dust contaminated by bird droppings should be avoided in endemic areas; masks should be worn and infected soil sprayed with formalin.

Crytococcosis

This is another dust-borne disease associated with pigeons, which is caused by species of the fungus Cryptococcus. It can invade skin, lungs, joints and subcutaneous tissue. Humans are relatively resistant to the organism, unless they are taking corticosteroids or have diabetes mellitus. Treatment and control are as for histoplasmosis (*see above*).

Protozoal infections

Toxoplasmosis

The causative agent is the intracellular protozoan parasite *Toxoplasma gondii*. Toxoplasma infection is common in cats, but rarely causes clinical symptoms. Cats are infected by eating raw meat, birds or mice containing parasite cysts. The cats excrete oocysts for about ten days when first infected. Intermediate hosts are rodents and farm animals, which ingest oocysts from infected soil.

Farm animals, especially sheep, in which *T. gondii* causes enzootic abortion, are involved in the infective life-cycle. A veterinary vaccine (Toxovax) is available.

Humans have been infected by eating vegetables contaminated by cat faeces or by eating undercooked meat containing bradyzoites. Some cases have been associated with drinking raw milk, particularly goats' milk.

Toxoplasmosis does not pose a significant health risk to most healthy humans, although it can be dangerous in immunocompromised patients or those receiving immunosuppressive therapy following transplantation surgery. It also presents a risk to pregnant women who have not previously encountered the parasite and have not developed an immune response. This can result in trans-placental infection, leading to foetal defects.

Ocular toxoplasmosis usually occurs as a posterior uveitis and is usually congenitally acquired.

The most common symptom in adults is generalised or localised lymphadenopathy; fever and sore throat may also be present. As with Toxocara, recent infections may be diagnosed using ELISA.

Steroids and anthelmintics have been used for treatment with varying success. Preventive measures are particularly important for pregnant women. They should be advised:

- not to handle cat litter trays
- to wash vegetables thoroughly before consumption
- to wear gloves whilst gardening to guard against inadvertent contact with buried faeces.

Similarly, contamination of animal feedstuffs with cat faeces should be prevented.

Leishmaniasis

This is a serious protozoal disease in humans and dogs that is common in Mediterranean countries and Asia. It is rarely seen in the UK, usually only being associated with recently imported animals. The disease is usually transmitted by sandflies. The main symptom is a painful ulcer at the site of infection, persisting for several months, with residual scarring. Treatment is with antimony derivatives and amphotericin B.

Rickettsial infections

Cat scratch fever

Cat scratch disease (CSD) is associated with contact with a cat (but not necessarily an actual scratch). It is thought to be caused by infection with a rickettsial organism, *Bartonella henslae*. It also occurs occasionally in dogs and cattle. Symptoms include localised lymph node enlargement near the scratch; sometimes fever and rash are present. Treatment is with neoarsphenamine.

Psittacosis

Serious zoonotic diseases from companion animals are relatively rare, but some can be dangerous, even resulting in death. One zoonose that can kill humans is psittacosis. During one recent ten-year period, there were 2500 cases in Britain, including 11 deaths. Infection is unlikely from birds that have been kept as family pets for years; it is much more likely to derive from newly imported birds. The most commonly identified sources of infection are psittacines (parrots) and other exotic birds, although ducks may also be implicated.

Psittacosis (parrot fever) is a febrile bacterial disease caused by the Gram negative bacterium *Chlamydia psittaci*, found in birds of the parrot family, and in pigeons, budgerigars, ducks and turkeys. In birds, it is mainly a latent infection.

There are two direct mechanisms of transfer of the organism to man; by inhalation of air contaminated with faeces or plumage; or by direct contact with dead birds, usually during post-mortem examination. However, a history of close contact with birds cannot be found in up to 20% of cases, and in other cases may have been very brief. The infective agent may survive in dust for many years, and indirect infection may occur in these instances by inhaling dust-borne organisms.

Outbreaks of the disease are usually confined to aviary and quarantine workers, poultry processing workers and veterinarians, although pet owners may also be infected. Control is exercised through import licences, where appropriate, and quarantine. Well-ventilated poultry processing plants and safe disposal of infected carcasses are also advised.

Chlamydial infection in pregnant women can be life-threatening, causing abortion or neonatal death. As a precaution, contact with birds during pregnancy should be minimised. Symptoms range from a mild influenza-like condition, with joint and muscle pains, atypical pneumonia, diarrhoea and vomiting, to endocarditis, myocarditis and renal problems, with immunocompromised patients at risk of encephalitis and meningitis. In animals, most infections are asymptomatic, except for respiratory disease in parrots.

The condition is treated with antibiotics: tetracycline and erythromycin are effective within seven to ten days. Pet birds may be given oxytetracycline in their feed.

Spirochaete infection

Lyme disease

Lyme disease is a tick-borne disease, endemic in the northern states of the USA, but also present in the UK, particularly in the southern counties of England and parts of Scotland.

Lyme disease is caused by the spirochaete *Borrelia burgdorferi*, of which at least ten genospecies are known. Between 10 and 20% of sheep in the New Forest area of southern England are infected with *B. garinii*. This is the most widely occurring of the four variants found in the UK.

The disease is transmitted to humans through the bite of the infected sheep tick: *Ixodes ricinus* in Europe; *I. scapularis* (formerly called *I. dammini*) in eastern USA; and *I. pacificus* in western USA. The sheep tick feeds on a variety of wild-life, including mice, voles, hedgehogs, hares, blackbirds, deer, rabbits and rodents. Pheasants are thought to be particularly important in the epidemiology of Lyme disease in the UK. In England, approximately 20 million farm-reared pheasants are released into woodlands each year to increase numbers for shooting. In some areas, they may provide a larger reservoir of infection than other species. Dogs can also be infected and act as carriers for ticks.

Icinus ricinus has three development stages: larval, nymph and adult. Apart from the adult male, each life stage feeds once on a host. The two motile stages must attach to a host, feed and fall off before transforming into the next stage. If no blood-providing host is available, the ticks perish; therefore, an important aspect of a successful life-cycle is host availability and diversity. The entire life-cycle may extend over two to three years, depending on the geographic region.

Ticks ingest *Borellia* during their blood meals on an infected animal. The bacterium migrates from the gut to the salivary glands. After moulting to the next development stage, the tick may transmit the bacterium to another animal when they next feed.

The risk of humans developing Lyme disease after being bitten by an infected tick has been estimated at around 20%.

Typically, redness of skin expands from the bite area, often producing a large erythematous ring within three days to several weeks; smaller rings may appear on other parts of the body and last for several days. The disease may be long term, with symptoms ranging from mild to severe and debilitating (including possibly chronic fatigue syndrome). Cardiac, neurological and joint involvement may also develop.

The symptom most frequently presented in the pharmacy is a swelling of the elbow joint. This is often treated with a non-steroidal anti-inflammatory agent, but does not improve. Patients may seek a pharmacist's opinion as to what can be done about this annoying condition when a cortisone injection has been suggested by the physician. The first thing to ascertain is whether the person has been in an environment where they could have been bitten by a tick. Typically, this could be while exercising a dog in long grass in the vicinity of wild deer, perhaps in one of the large parkland areas to be found around the country, where an infected tick could have been picked up. The patient may be unaware that a bite has been inflicted. A positive response would lead one to suspect Lyme disease. Dogs that are affected may show fever and arthritic like symptoms.

Early-stage Lyme disease responds well to oral antibiotics, including doxycycline and amoxycillin, which are generally prescribed for two to three weeks. Later-stage disease may be more difficult to treat, and the choice of drugs and treatment is the subject of considerable discussion. Tetracycline and ampicillin have been used in dogs, with topical organophosphate lotions.

Pet owners should be advised to take care when walking in areas likely to harbour ticks. A vaccine is available to guard against the US strains of *Borrelia*, but due to considerable genetic divergence, no such prophylactic exists in Europe.

Viral infections

Canine viruses are specific to dogs and, therefore, do not usually pose a zoonotic risk. As dogs seem to be susceptible to sub-clinical infections of certain human enteroviruses and coxsackie viruses, they may play a part in the epidemiology of these infective agents.

Canine distemper

Canine distemper is caused by a virus closely related to the virus causing measles in humans. It is rarely seen, except in dog rescue homes, because of an effective immunisation programme. There has been some discussion as to whether canine distemper is implicated in the development of multiple sclerosis or Paget's disease; there is little evidence to support these theories.

Influenza

Aquatic birds throughout the world are reservoirs for all influenza A viruses. The virus spreads by faecal-oral transmission in untreated water. There is evidence that transmission of avian influenza viruses or virus genes to humans may occur through pigs acting as an intermediate host. It is believed that this may then be transmitted to other mammals, including humans and domestic pets, by the airborne route. It is more likely to be a problem in farm environments; such transfers have been reported only rarely.

Orf – contagious pustular dermatitis

Although mainly considered to be an occupational zoonosis associated with sheep farming, there have been occasional instances of working dogs contracting orf. As these animals are often considered to be pets, a brief description is included here.

Orf was a word used in Scotland to describe a disease of sheep characterised by a pustular dermatitis of the mouth and feet. The word is derived from an old Nordic word, 'Hrufa', meaning a scab or boil. The strains of virus that cause orf in sheep, goats, dogs and humans are members of the pox family of viruses that includes pseudo-cowpox, true cowpox and smallpox. The infective agent is known as the orf virus.

Sheep and goats are the main natural reservoirs of the infective agent. Transmission is by direct or indirect contact with the superficial lesions through skin abrasions. Where animals have injured their mouths by eating gorse or other prickly plants, infection occurs swiftly. Young kids and lambs transfer the virus from their lips to maternal teats and udders.

Transfer to humans, mainly sheep farmers and their staff, and to working dogs (far less frequently), is generally by direct contact in the working environment.

In humans, primary lesions are usually on the hands and forearms; the lips may be affected by transference from the hands. Initially, there is a single painful red area at the site of contact, which lasts from three to six weeks; this develops to a pustule, from which fluid exudes. The back may also be involved. In animals, the minor form of the disease is characterised by vesicles, followed by ulcers on the lips, especially at the corner of the mouth. In the severe form, the inside of the mouth is involved. The animal tends to rub its muzzle on its legs to gain some relief from the painful condition, transmitting the virus to the feet. Pustules may be present at other sites on the body which, after ten to 12 days, become thick brownish black scabs that, if lifted, reveal a red, 'angry' lesion.

The condition is self-limiting in humans, but antibiotics are often prescribed to contain any potential secondary infection. If orf affects a flock, the affected animals should be isolated, and their lesions painted with crystal violet and covered with an appropriate dressing. Antibiotics may be given. The animals should be kept apart from the healthy flock for about two weeks after recovery, when they should be dipped. Any lesions on the feet or lower legs may be treated with a footbath.

Anyone treating an infected animal should ensure scrupulous hygiene, scrubbing up with disinfectant, to prevent carrying the virus from one animal to another and to prevent self-infection. A veterinary vaccine is available to reduce the chance of animals becoming infected.

Rabies

Rabies is probably the best known animal-borne viral disease, as it has well-known symptoms.

There are an estimated 15 000 cases of the disease worldwide each year. Untreated, the disease is fatal to humans, cats, dogs, gerbils, guinea pigs, hamsters, rabbits and wild mammals. Because of strict quarantine rules and an extensive animal vaccination programme, rabies has been eradicated in the UK, New Zealand and several other countries for many years. However, pharmacists can provide useful information for those intending to visit, or having recently returned from, countries where the disease is endemic. High-risk areas include most of the countries of Africa, Asia (except Taiwan and Japan) and Latin America.

Rabies is caused by the Rhabdoviridae, a widespread family of highly infectious viruses. There are at least 27 different rhabdoviruses in animals; some can infect man and cause disease. The virus is enveloped and bullet-shaped (70 nm × 170 nm). Rabies is usually transmitted by the bite of an infected animal, with saliva containing the virus.

Until fairly recently, most human cases of rabies arose from a dog bite; this is still the case in developing countries. However, since 1990, 74% of human rabies deaths in the USA have been caused by variants of rabies virus associated with bats. Some USA deaths have occurred when no animal bite is involved. In such cases, rabies is assumed to be the result of contaminated saliva or other body fluids having entered the person's body through an abrasion, a cut on the skin or moist tissues in the lips or eyes. In rare instances, infection may proceed by an airborne route (e.g. following exposure to air in caves densely populated with rabid bats).

Once in the human host, the virus seeks out a nerve and travels along nerves to the brain, where it multiplies and leads to full-blown disease.

The incubation period can be from ten days to seven years (the usual period is up to two months). If immunisation is given within three days of the bite, rabies is usually prevented. During this early incubation stage, the condition is reversible. The incubation period becomes shorter the nearer the bite is to the head. Once symptoms appear, death is almost invariably the outcome.

Symptoms include fever, behavioural changes, headaches, spasmodic contractions of the muscles that facilitate swallowing, convulsions and, ultimately, death. Rabies is sometimes called 'hydrophobia' because in its terminal stages, patients refuse to drink liquids and react violently in attempts to give them fluids orally.

People travelling to countries where the disease is endemic should avoid stroking seemingly docile pets (especially dogs) and any wild animals. In western Canadian parks, racoons appear very tempting to feed and pet, particularly if they are in family groups; but racoons can carry rabies. Travellers should be advised to seek assistance as quickly as possible from local Health Authorities if bitten, to allow tests on the animal to determine the presence of rabies. It is important to gather as much information about the animal as possible. Unfortunately, not all rabies vaccines used abroad meet the levels of safety and efficacy found in UK products. If the risk is considered high, pre-exposure vaccination before departure may be appropriate. The rabies vaccine is an inactivated-virus vaccine and is given as a series of three injections, on days 0, 7 and 21 or 28. There are three different types, each of which is considered safe during pregnancy:

- RVA rabies vaccine contains thimerosal as preservative
- HDCV contains small amounts of neomycin
- PCEC contains no preservative, but it does contain small amounts of neomycin, chlortetracycline and amphotericin B.

These options allow a choice for those people likely to suffer an adverse reaction to one of the vaccines caused by agents used in its formulation.

Other sources of zoonoses

This chapter has considered those zoonoses derived from companion animals and that pharmacists might encounter in community practice. In rural areas, however, clients can present with a variety of other conditions resulting from contact with farm animals and wildlife. A discussion of these conditions is beyond the scope of this chapter. Fortunately, there are few wildlife zoonoses in the UK, compared with many other countries, but some of these are of considerable importance.

For example, the first recorded death from pigeon lung caused by proximity to feral pigeons has raised fears that a sharp increase in the birds' population poses a previously unsuspected threat to health. A newspaper report stated that a 37 year-old mother of five contracted the illness as a result of pigeons nesting outside her home (Dobson, 2000). In Britain, an estimated 2000 people each year are catching infections from wild pigeons that can carry up to 60 diseases. Badgers are considered to be a major reservoir of *Mycobacterium bovis* infection for cattle; magpies are responsible for infecting bottles of milk with *Campylobacter jejuni*; and some birds (e.g. collared doves) are often heavily infected with *Chlamydia*. Chance encounters with injured or dead wild animals may lead to unfortunate consequences if simple rules of hygiene are not observed. Within the currently changing climate, there exists the potential for a number of new zoonoses to develop.

The role of the pharmacist

Just over half of all households in the UK are thought to own at least one pet, with companion species (e.g. cats and dogs) the most favoured. Figures of around 7.5 million and just under 7 million are generally quoted for the numbers of cats and dogs respectively in the UK. Over half a million cat or dog owners alone are thought to visit a pharmacy daily; other animals (e.g. horses, cage birds, ornamental fish and, occasionally, exotic pets) are also popular.

The fact that companion animals and farm animals can affect human health renders the pharmacist's involvement in pet care extremely important. It should be seen as an extension of the counselling and information role normally associated with pharmaceutical care. Health hazards for owners can be minimised when nutrition, care, prophylaxis appropriate to the animal and personal physical hygiene are all observed correctly.

Much of pet care (and some large animal care) is of a prophylactic nature. It is, therefore, possible to satisfy requests for assistance without contravening the Veterinary Surgeons' Act 1966, which effectively restricts diagnosis and treatment of animal diseases to veterinary surgeons or owners. Pharmacists can advise on availability of suitable medicines, provided it is the owner who makes the final choice. However, pharmacists cannot diagnose or suggest cures.

One exception to this is that fish are excluded from the requirements of the Veterinary Surgeons' Act, allowing pharmacists to treat them (Kayne, 1993). However, there are very few licensed medicines available.

Although there are some highly successful large farm suppliers in the UK, most pharmacists tend to restrict their veterinary activities to the pet market. The market for pet-care products (e.g. toys, collars, chews and confectionery) is worth around £150 million per year. Until recently, more than 90% of certain veterinary products (e.g. companion animal anthelmintics, which alone have a market value of £10 million), have been sold from pet shops and supermarkets. Veterinary surgeons, agricultural merchants and pharmacies supply the remainder.

References

Britton J, Lewis S (1997). Pet birds and lung cancer. *BMJ* 313: 1218–1219.

Chakrabarti A (1985). Some epidemiological aspects of animal scabies in human population. *Int J Zoon* 12: 39–52.

Coren S (1997). Allergic patients do not comply with doctors' advice to stop owning pets. Letters. *BMJ* 314: 517.

Dobson R (2000). Mother killed by pigeon disease. *Sunday Times* 21 May.

Hardy G (1981). The seeing-eye dog: an infection risk in hospital? *Can Med Ass J* 124: 698–700.

Hartley E L, Shames C (1959). Man and dog: a psychological analysis. *Gaines Veterinary Symposium* 9: 4–7.

Hugh-Jones M E, Hubbert W T, Hagstad H V (1995). *Zoonoses: Recognition, Control and Prevention.* Ames, Iowa: Iowa State University Press.

Kayne S B (1993). Fish and the pharmacist. *Pharm J* 250: 542–544.

Kayne S B (1995). Fleas. (Letter). *Pharm J* 255: 72.

Talan D A (1999). Report on treatment of pet bites. *N Engl J Med* 340: 138–140.

Further reading

Bell J C, Palmer S R, Payne J M (1988). *The Zoonoses.* London: Edward Arnold.

Cockrum E L (1997). *Rabies, Lyme Disaease, Hanta Virus.* Tucson: Fisher Books.

Gunter B (1999). *Pets and People: The Psychology of Pet Ownership.* London: Whurr Publishers.

Jepson M H, Spencer B J (1992). What the community pharmacist should know about horse wormers. *Pharm J* 233: 601–603.

Kayne S B (1995). The pharmacist's role in pet care. *Pharm J* 254: 515–517.

West G, ed. (1988). *Black's Veterinary Dictionary*, 16th edn. London: A & C Black.

Useful addresses

Children in Hospital and Animal Therapy Association (CHATA)
87 Longland Drive
London N20 8HD
Tel: 020 8445 7883

The Pet Bereavement Support Service
c/o Blue Cross
Shilton Road
Burford
Oxfordshire OX18 4PF
Tel: 0800 0966606

Index